Simple TOC

CHAPTER 1 THE SKELETAL SYSTEM, 1

CHAPTER 2 THE MUSCULAR SYSTEM, 23

CHAPTER 3 OTHER SKELETAL MUSCLES, 395

CHAPTER 4 THE NERVOUS SYSTEM, 405

CHAPTER 5 THE ARTERIAL SYSTEM, 415

CHAPTER 6 TISSUE STRUCTURE AND OTHER SYSTEMS OF THE BODY, 421

MUSCULOSKELETAL ANATOMY COLORING BOOK

JOSEPH E. MUSCOLINO, DC

Owner, The Art and Science of Kinesiology
Stamford, Connecticut
(www.learnmuscles.com)

ELSEVIER

ELSEVIER

3251 Riverport Lane
St. Louis, Missouri 63043

MUSCULOSKELETAL ANATOMY COLORING BOOK,
THIRD EDITION

ISBN: 978-0-323-47731-4

Copyright © 2018, Elsevier Inc. All Rights Reserved.
Previous editions copyrighted 2010, 2004.

All rights reserved. No part of this publication may be reproduced or transmitted in any form or by any means, electronic or mechanical, including photocopying, recording, or any information storage and retrieval system, without permission in writing from the publisher. Details on how to seek permission, further information about the Publisher's permissions policies and our arrangements with organizations such as the Copyright Clearance Center and the Copyright Licensing Agency, can be found at our website: www.elsevier.com/permissions.

This book and the individual contributions contained in it are protected under copyright by the Publisher (other than as may be noted herein).

Notices

Practitioners and researchers must always rely on their own experience and knowledge in evaluating and using any information, methods, compounds or experiments described herein. Because of rapid advances in the medical sciences, in particular, independent verification of diagnoses and drug dosages should be made. To the fullest extent of the law, no responsibility is assumed by Elsevier, authors, editors or contributors for any injury and/or damage to persons or property as a matter of products liability, negligence or otherwise, or from any use or operation of any methods, products, instructions, or ideas contained in the material herein.

International Standard Book Number: 978-0-323-47731-4

Content Strategist: Brandi Graham
Content Development Manager: Luke Held
Content Development Specialist: Kelly Skelton
Publishing Services Manager: Julie Eddy
Project Manager: Mike Sheets
Design Direction: Ashley Miner

Printed in the United States of America

Last digit is the print number: 9 8 7 6 5

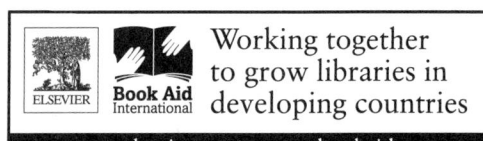

Introduction

Sciences have long been taught in a classroom format in which an instructor lectures to students and the students have textbooks to read at home. Unfortunately, lecture format and textbook reading do not cater to the kinesthetic element of learning that is present in all of us. Toward that end, coloring books of anatomy and physiology are useful tools for approaching and learning class material in a manner that is not possible via lecture and textbook format alone. However, I do not believe that coloring books should replace quality classroom instruction and quality textbooks; rather I believe that coloring books of anatomy and physiology are valuable adjunctive learning tools that should be used in conjunction with classroom learning and textbook reading.

For this reason, I recommend the *Musculoskeletal Anatomy Coloring Book* to aid you as you endeavor to learn the structure and function of the musculoskeletal system, as well as the other major systems of the human body. With regard to an adjunct textbook for learning muscles and how the musculoskeletal system functions, I recommend *The Muscular System Manual: The Skeletal Muscles of the Human Body*, 4th edition (Elsevier, 2017) and *Kinesiology: The Skeletal System and Muscle Function*, 3rd edition (Elsevier, 2017). For learning the kinesthetic skill of muscle and bone palpation, I recommend *The Muscle and Bone Palpation Manual*, 2nd edition (Elsevier, 2016). Also, for quizzing muscle attachments and actions, I recommend the *Musculoskeletal Anatomy Flash Cards* available on the accompanying Evolve site.

Beyond being simply a coloring book, this book is also designed to help the reader learn the information in a number of ways. First, regarding muscles, the two hurdles for the new student are learning the attachments (origins and insertions) and actions of the muscles. In the chapter on muscles (Chapter 2), the text information of the attachments is written next to the locations on the illustration where the actual muscle attachments are located. As you color the muscles from attachment to attachment, I recommend that you integrate this written information by saying the attachments out loud. To help learn the actions of the muscles, arrows that visually demonstrate the line(s) of pull of the muscle have been placed within the muscle. As you color in these arrows, note the actions that are caused by the line of pull demonstrated by the arrows.

Putting the attachment and action information together with the illustration, and kinesthetically coloring at the same time, allow for a fuller integration of the information that you need to learn!

This book is also designed to allow the student to quiz himself/herself. Throughout the book, wherever you find blank lead lines pointing to a structure, use that opportunity to quiz yourself on being able to identify the structure. The answer key starts on page 461. There are also quiz questions on muscle attachments and actions that are located at the end of each section of Chapter 2. Further, on each right-hand page of a 2-page muscle spread in Chapter 2, there are illustrations showing the individual muscle being studied within its larger group of muscles. For another opportunity to quiz yourself, write in the directional terms around these illustrations (e.g., anterior, posterior, lateral, etc.). Check your answers by turning to the illustrations at the beginning of each section in Chapter 2.

Although this book covers every major system of the human body, its emphasis is the musculoskeletal system. More specifically, the major emphasis of this book is the muscular system.

This book is organized into six chapters. The introduction sections in Chapters 2 and 6 contain valuable text information toward understanding the systems that are covered in those chapters. I strongly recommend reading this entire introduction, and the introductory text in Chapters 2 and 6 before you begin coloring. Chapters 1 through 3 cover the musculoskeletal system. Of these chapters, Chapter 2, which covers the major skeletal muscles of the body, is divided into 10 sections. Chapters 4 and 5 cover the nervous system and arterial system, the understanding of which is important toward learning innervation and arterial supply to the skeletal muscles. Chapter 6 covers tissue structure and the other major systems of the human body. The answer key to the self-testing pages that are included throughout the book is located after Chapter 6.

Regarding the use of colors, of course you may use any that you like to color the various structures. However, there are certain colors standardly used for the anatomical structures of the human body, and I recommend the following to you as guidelines:

- Red is classically used for blood vessels that carry "oxygenated" blood (arteries of the systemic circulation and veins of the pulmonic circulation) and blue is used for all blood vessels that carry "deoxygenated" blood (veins of the systemic circulation and arteries of the pulmonic circulation).
- Red is also used for coloring the muscles of the body. Therefore, to make muscles distinct from blood vessels that have been colored red, perhaps a different shade (I recommend a lighter shade) of red can be used for the muscles.
- The attachments of muscles (tendons and aponeuroses) and other fibrous fascia are usually colored white; given that the page is already white, you may simply leave them uncolored. However, since this is a coloring book and the purpose of this book is to learn kinesthetically by coloring, I recommend that you do color them. A light shade of color would be best.
- Yellow is classically used for nerves.
- As for coloring bones, I recommend the following:
    1. When coloring the bones in Chapter 1, color the entire bone lightly with a light shade of color, different from those used above; a light yellow to beige color is most often used. Then use a darker color to color over the landmarks on the bone that you feel are important to you and you want to learn. This will help these landmarks to visually stand out as well as help root them kinesthetically.
    2. When coloring the bones in Chapter 2, I recommend that you use a different color for each of the muscle's two bony attachments (if there are more than two different bony attachments for a particular muscle, you may use more colors). Further, I recommend that you color the attachment of the muscle that is usually fixed (i.e., the origin) with a darker color to convey upon it a feeling of being heavier and more stable. Conversely, I recommend that you use a lighter color for the attachment that usually moves (i.e., the insertion) to convey a feeling of being lighter and therefore more mobile.
- Cartilage is always lightly shaded; pale blue is usually used.
- When coloring the many systems of Chapter 6, beyond the conventionally used colors that are mentioned above, please note the following: the liver is usually a fairly dark brown, the gall bladder is usually green, fat is usually yellow, lymph is usually green, and the brain and spinal cord are usually a light brown.
- The purpose of this book is for you to learn by coloring, and hopefully enjoy yourself along the way. If you prefer to use colors different from those recommended above, and it will add to your enjoyment and learning, please do so. They are only guidelines. Most important is that you enjoy and learn!

Because this is a coloring book and not a textbook, the text in this book has been kept to a minimum. This has been done for two reasons: (1) excessive text tends to clutter the page and obscure visualization of the structures being colored and learned; and (2) the inclusion of text forces the illustrations to be smaller, which also makes visualization and coloring more difficult. Further, I feel that coloring books are best used as adjuncts to textbooks, not as a replacement. Although this coloring book can certainly stand on its own, in many ways it is a companion to *The Muscular System Manual: The Skeletal Muscles of the Human Body, 4th edition* (Elsevier, 2017), which is strongly recommended for students wishing to learn more about the musculoskeletal system.

However, since an understanding of what is being colored is crucial, and the handiness of having some of that information accessible in the same book is helpful, the introductory text in Chapters 2 and 6 are included. Chapter 2's introduction is a very practical approach that gives you a method to understand how muscles work; the more you understand, the less you have to memorize! Chapter 6's introduction is a brief overview of each of the major systems of the body. I strongly recommend reading these two introductory sections before diving into the coloring.

ACKNOWLEDGMENTS

I would like to begin by thanking Barry Antoniow in Canada for first giving me the idea to develop a musculoskeletal anatomy coloring book. It has been long needed and I appreciate Barry's insight. Since so much of the artwork for this coloring book has come from the *Muscular System Manual*, I would like to acknowledge the beautiful, crisp, and clear illustrations drawn by the artists of that book: the principal artist, Jean Luciano; and the additional artists, Rosa Cervoni, Barbara Haeger, and J.C. Muscolino. The quality of these illustrations greatly aids the reader in learning musculoskeletal anatomy. I also must thank the entire crew over at Mosby, Elsevier Science: Kellie White, who made this project become a possibility; Jennifer Watrous, who worked with me each step of the way in developing it; and Linda McKinley, Celeste Clingan, and their team, who spent a tremendous amount of time in actually assembling and creating this book. I would also like to thank Kelly Skelton, Brandi Graham, Mike Sheets, and Ashley Miner of Elsevier for their invaluable assistance in creating and bringing this new edition to you!

I must thank my entire family for their unending support as I spent hour after hour at the computer working on this book. Without their unconditional support, none of this would have been possible.

Lastly, I would like to say that studying by using coloring books has to be one of the more creative and fun ways to learn anatomy. For this reason, I would like to dedicate this book to my children, Randi and J.C., who have consistently taught me to try to keep creativity and fun in my approach to life.

Table of Contents

INTRODUCTION, v

CHAPTER 1 THE SKELETAL SYSTEM, 1

Bones of the Head – Anterior View, 3
Bones of the Head – Lateral & Inferior Views, 4-5
Bones of the Neck – Anterior View, 6
Bones of the Neck – Posterior View, 7
Bones of the Trunk – Anterior View, 8
Bones of the Trunk – Posterior View, 9
Bones of the Pelvis and Thigh – Anterior View, 10
Bones of the Pelvis and Thigh – Posterior View, 11
Bones of the Leg – Anterior View, 12
Bones of the Leg – Posterior View, 13
Bones of the Foot – Dorsal View, 14
Bones of the Foot – Plantar View, 15
Bones of the Scapula and Arm – Anterior View, 16
Bones of the Scapula and Arm – Posterior View, 17
Bones of the Forearm – Anterior View, 18
Bones of the Forearm – Posterior View, 19
Bones of the Hand – Anterior View, 20
Bones of the Hand – Posterior View, 21

CHAPTER 2 THE MUSCULAR SYSTEM, 23

MUSCLES OF THE HEAD, 32

Muscles of the Head – Anterior View, 32
Muscles of the Head – Lateral View, 33
Occipitofrontalis, 34
Temporoparietalis and Auricularis Muscles, 36
Orbicularis Oculi and Levator Palpebrae Superioris, 38
Corrugator Supercilii, Procerus, 40
Nasalis and Depressor Septi Nasi, 42
Levator Labii Superioris Alaeque Nasi & Levator Labii Superioris, 44
Zygomaticus Minor and Zygomaticus Major, 46
Levator Anguli Oris & Risorius, 48
Depressor Anguli Oris and Depressor Labii Inferioris, 50
Mentalis and Buccinator, 52
Orbicularis Oris, 54
Temporalis & Masseter, 56
Lateral Pterygoid and Medial Pterygoid, 58

MUSCLES OF THE NECK, 66

Muscles of the Neck – Anterior View (Superficial), 66
Muscles of the Neck – Anterior View (Intermediate), 67

Muscles of the Neck – Anterior View (Deep), 68

Muscles of the Neck – Lateral View, 69

Muscles of the Neck – Posterior View (Superficial & Intermediate), 70

Muscles of the Neck – Posterior View (Intermediate & Deep), 71

Trapezius, 72

Splenius Capitis and Splenius Cervicis, 74

Levator Scapulae, 76

The Suboccipital Group, 80

Platysma, 82

Sternocleidomastoid, 84

Sternohyoid and Sternothyroid, 86

Thyrohyoid and Omohyoid, 88

Digastric and Stylohyoid, 90

Mylohyoid and Geniohyoid, 92

Anterior, Middle, and Posterior Scalenes, 94-96

Longus Colli and Longus Capitis, 98

Rectus Capitis Anterior and Rectus Capitis Lateralis, 100

MUSCLES OF THE TRUNK, 112

Muscles of the Trunk – Posterior View (Superficial & Intermediate), 112

Muscles of the Trunk – Posterior View (Deep), 113

Muscles of the Trunk – Anterior View (Superficial & Intermediate), 114

Muscles of the Trunk – Anterior View (Intermediate & Deep), 115

Muscles of the Trunk – Lateral View, 116

Muscles of the Trunk – Cross Section Views, 117

Latissimus Dorsi, 118

Rhomboids Major and Minor, 120

Serratus Anterior, 122

Serratus Posterior Superior and Serratus Posterior Inferior, 124

Erector Spinae Group, 126

Iliocostalis, Longissimus, Spinalis, 128-130

Transversospinalis Group, 132

Semispinalis, Multifidus, Rotatores, 134-136

Quadratus Lumborum, 138

Interspinales and Intertransversarii, 140

Levatores Costarum and Subcostales, 142

Pectoralis Major, 144

Pectoralis Minor and Subclavius, 146

External Intercostals and Internal Intercostals, 148-150

Rectus Abdominis, 152

External Abdominal Oblique and Internal Abdominal Oblique, 154

Transversus Abdominis and Transversus Thoracis, 156

Diaphragm, 158

MUSCLES OF THE PELVIS, 170

Muscles of the Pelvis – Anterior View, 170

Muscles of the Pelvis – Lateral View, 171

Muscles of the Pelvis – Posterior View (Superfic), 172

Muscles of the Pelvis – Posterior View (Deep), 173

Psoas Major, 174

Iliacus, 176

Psoas Minor, 178

Gluteus Maximus, 180

Gluteus Medius and Gluteus Minimus, 182-184

Piriformis, 186

Superior Gemellus, Obturator Internus, Inferior Gemellus, 188-190

Obturator Externus, Quadratus Femoris, 192-194

MUSCLES OF THE THIGH, 202

Muscles of the Thigh – Anterior View (Superficial), 202

Muscles of the Thigh – Anterior View (Deep), 203

Muscles of the Thigh – Posterior View (Superficial), 204

Muscles of the Thigh – Posterior View (Deep), 205

Muscles of the Thigh – Lateral View, 206

Muscles of the Thigh – Medial View, 207

Tensor Fasciae Latae, 208

Sartorius, 210

Rectus Femoris, 212

Vastus Lateralis and Vastus Medialis, 214

Vastus Intermedius and Articularis Genus, 216

Pectineus and Gracilis, 218

Adductor Longus, 220

Adductor Brevis, 222

Adductor Magnus, 224

Biceps Femoris, 226

Semitendinosus and Semimembranosus, 228

MUSCLES OF THE LEG, 238

Muscles of the Leg – Anterior View, 238

Muscles of the Leg – Posterior View (Superficial), 239

Muscles of the Leg – Posterior View (Intermediate), 240

Muscles of the Leg – Posterior View (Deep), 241

Muscles of the Leg – Posterior View, 242

Muscles of the Leg – Medial View, 243

Tibialis Anterior, 244

Extensor Hallucis Longus, 246

Extensor Digitorum Longus and Fibularis Tertius, 248

Fibularis Longus and Fibularis Brevis, 250

Gastrocnemius and Soleus, 252

Plantaris and Popliteus, 254

Tibialis Posterior, 256

Flexor Digitorum Longus, 258

Flexor Hallucis Longus, 260

INTRINSIC MUSCLES OF THE FOOT, 270

Intrinsic Muscles of the Foot – Dorsal View, 270

Intrinsic Muscles of the Foot – Plantar View, 271

Intrinsic Muscles of the Foot – Plantar View, 272

Intrinsic Muscles of the Foot – Plantar View, 273

Extensor Digitorum Brevis & Extensor Hallucis Brevis, 274

Abductor Hallucis & Abductor Digiti Minimi Pedis, 276

Flexor Digitorum Brevis, 278

Quadratus Plantae & Lumbricals Pedis, 280

Flexor Hallucis Brevis & Flexor Digiti Minimi Pedis, 282

Adductor Hallucis, 284

Plantar Interossei & Dorsal Interossei Pedis, 286

MUSCLES OF THE SCAPULA/ARM, 294

Muscles of the Shoulder – Anterior View, 294

Muscles of the Shoulders – Posterior View, 295

Anterior View of Arm (Superficial), 296

Anterior View of Arm (Deep), 297

Medial View of Arm, 298

Lateral View of Arm, 299

Posterior View of Arm, 300

Views of the Glenohumeral Joint (Anterior and Posterior), 301

Supraspinatus and Infraspinatus, 302

Teres Minor and Subscapularis, 304

Teres Major, 306

Deltoid, 308

Coracobrachialis, 310
Biceps Brachii and Brachialis, 312
Triceps Brachii, 314

MUSCLES OF THE FOREARM, 326

Muscles of the Forearm – Anterior View (Superficial), 326
Muscles of the Forearm – Anterior View (Intermediate), 327
Muscles of the Forearm – Anterior View (Deep), 328
Pronators and Supinator, 329
Muscles of the Forearm – Posterior View (Superficial), 330
Muscles of the Forearm – Posterior View (Deep), 331
Muscles of the Forearm/Hand – Posterior View, 332
Muscles of the Forearm/Hand – Posterior View, 333
Pronator Teres & Pronator Quadratus, 334
Flexor Carpi Radialis, Palmaris Longus, Flexor Carpi Ulnaris, 336-338
Brachioradialis, 340
Flexor Digitorum Superficialis & Flexor Digitorum Profundus, 342
Flexor Pollicis Longus, 344
Anconeus, 346
Extensor Carpi Radialis Longus, Extensor Carpi Radialis Brevis, Extensor Carpi Ulnaris, 348-350
Extensor Digitorum & Extensor Digiti Minimi, 352
Supinator, 354
Abductor Pollicis Longus & Extensor Pollicis Brevis, 356
Extensor Pollicis Longus & Extensor Indicis, 358

INTRINSIC MUSCLES OF THE HAND, 372

Palmar View of the Hand (Superficial), 372
Palmar View of the Hand (Superficial Muscular), 373
Palmar View of the Hand (Deep Muscular), 374
Dorsal View of the Hand, 375
Abductor Pollicis Brevis & Flexor Pollicis Brevis, 376
Opponens Pollicis & Opponens Digiti Minimi, 378
Abductor Digiti Minimi Manus & Flexor Digiti Minimi Manus, 380
Palmaris Brevis, 382
Adductor Pollicis & Lumbricals Manus, 384
Palmar Interossei & Dorsal Interossei Manus, 386

CHAPTER 3 OTHER SKELETAL MUSCLES, 395

Abdomen, 396
Perineum, 397
Tongue, 398
Palate, 399
Pharynx, 400
Larynx, 401
Eye, 402
Ear, 403

CHAPTER 4 THE NERVOUS SYSTEM, 405

Cranial Nerves, 406
Spinal Nerve Cross Section, 407
Cervical and Brachial Plexuses, 408-409
Lumbar, Sacral, and Coccygeal Plexuses, 410-411
Lower Extremity Innervation, 412
Upper Extremity Innervation, 413

CHAPTER 5 THE ARTERIAL SYSTEM, 415

Lateral View of Arterial Supply to the Head and Neck, 416
Anterior View of Arterial Supply to the Trunk, 417
Arterial Supply to the Lower Extremity, 418
Arterial Supply to the Upper Extremity, 419

CHAPTER 6 TISSUE STRUCTURE AND OTHER SYSTEMS OF THE BODY, 421

The Cell, 426
Typical Synovial Joint, 436
Integumentary System, 438
Cardiac System, 440
Venous System, 442
Lymphatic System, 444
Respiratory System, 446
Urinary System, 448
Gastrointestinal System, 450
Immune System, 452
Endocrine System, 454
Sensory System, 456
Reproductive System, 459

ANSWER KEY, 461
ILLUSTRATION CREDITS, 476

The Skeletal System 1

GET READY TO EXPLORE:

Bones of the Head
Anterior View of the Bones and Bony
  Landmarks of the Head, 3
Lateral View of the Bones and Bony
  Landmarks of the Head, 4
Inferior View of the Bones and Bony
  Landmarks of the Head, 5

Bones of the Neck
Anterior View of the Bones and Bony
  Landmarks of the Neck, 6
Posterior View of the Bones and Bony
  Landmarks of the Neck, 7

Bones of the Trunk
Anterior View of the Bones and Bony
  Landmarks of the Trunk, 8
Posterior View of the Bones and Bony
  Landmarks of the Trunk, 9

Bones of the Pelvis and Thigh
Anterior View of the Bones and Bony
  Landmarks of the Right Pelvis and Thigh, 10
Posterior View of the Bones and Bony
  Landmarks of the Right Pelvis and Thigh, 11

Bones of the Leg
Anterior View of the Bones and Bony
  Landmarks of the Right Leg, 12
Posterior View of the Bones and Bony
  Landmarks of the Right Leg, 13

Bones of the Foot
Dorsal View of the Bones and Bony
  Landmarks of the Right Foot, 14
Plantar View of the Bones and Bony
  Landmarks of the Right Foot, 15

Bones of the Scapula/Arm
Anterior View of the Bones and Bony
  Landmarks of the Right Scapula/Arm, 16
Posterior View of the Bones and Bony
  Landmarks of the Right Scapula/Arm, 17

Bones of the Forearm
Anterior View of the Bones and Bony
  Landmarks of the Right Forearm, 18
Posterior View of the Bones and Bony
  Landmarks of the Right Forearm, 19

Bones of the Hand
Palmar View of the Bones and Bony
  Landmarks of the Right Hand, 20
Dorsal View of the Bones and Bony
  Landmarks of the Right Hand, 21

An asterisk (*) following a number indicates that the structure is a bony landmark rather than a bone. Answers to labeling exercises are on p. 461.

More review activities on Evolve at http://evolve.elsevier.com/Muscolino/muscular/

THE SKELETAL SYSTEM 3

ANTERIOR VIEW OF THE BONES AND BONY LANDMARKS OF THE HEAD

4 THE SKELETAL SYSTEM

LATERAL VIEW OF THE BONES AND BONY LANDMARKS OF THE HEAD

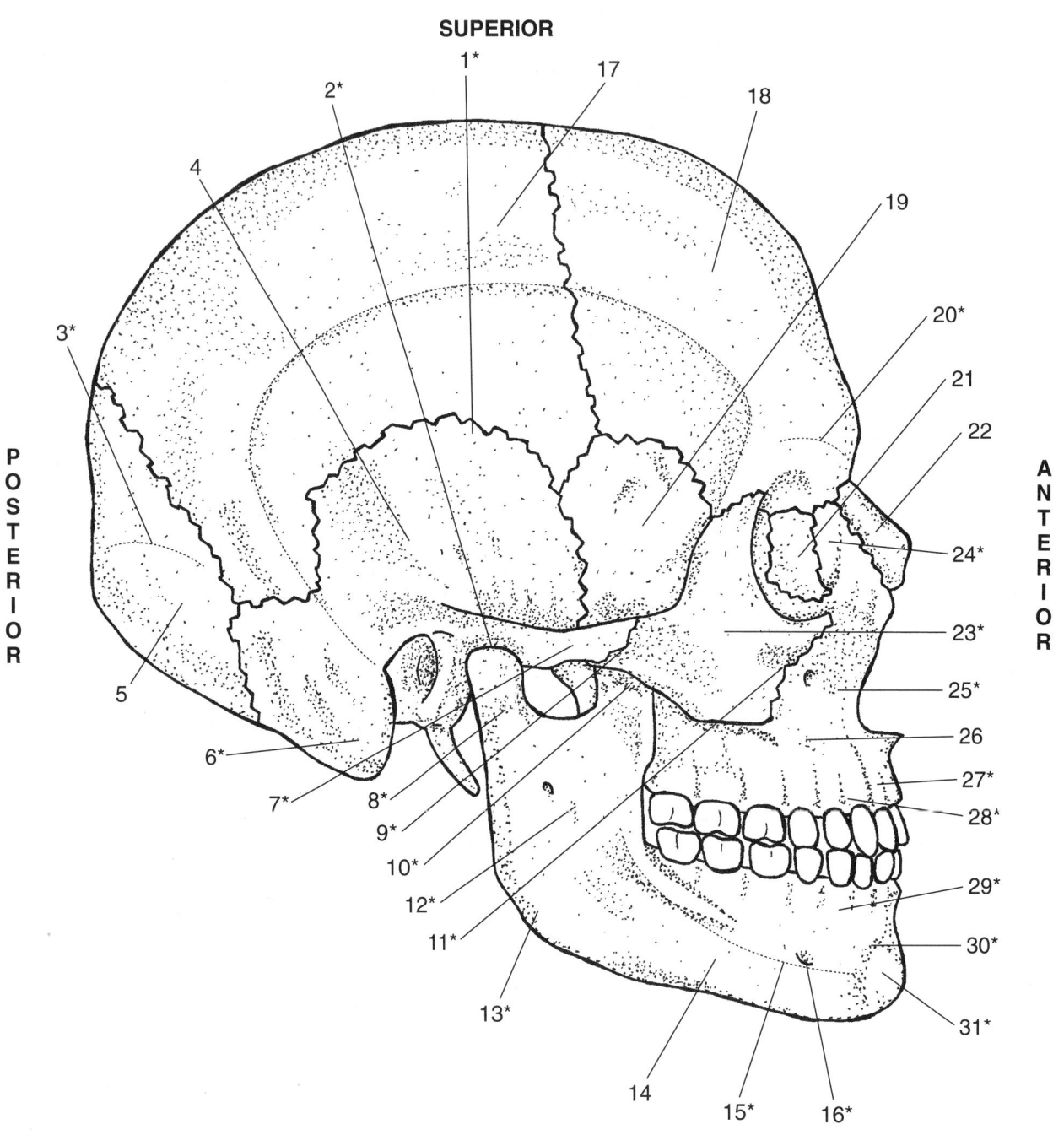

THE SKELETAL SYSTEM 5

INFERIOR VIEW OF THE BONES AND BONY LANDMARKS OF THE HEAD

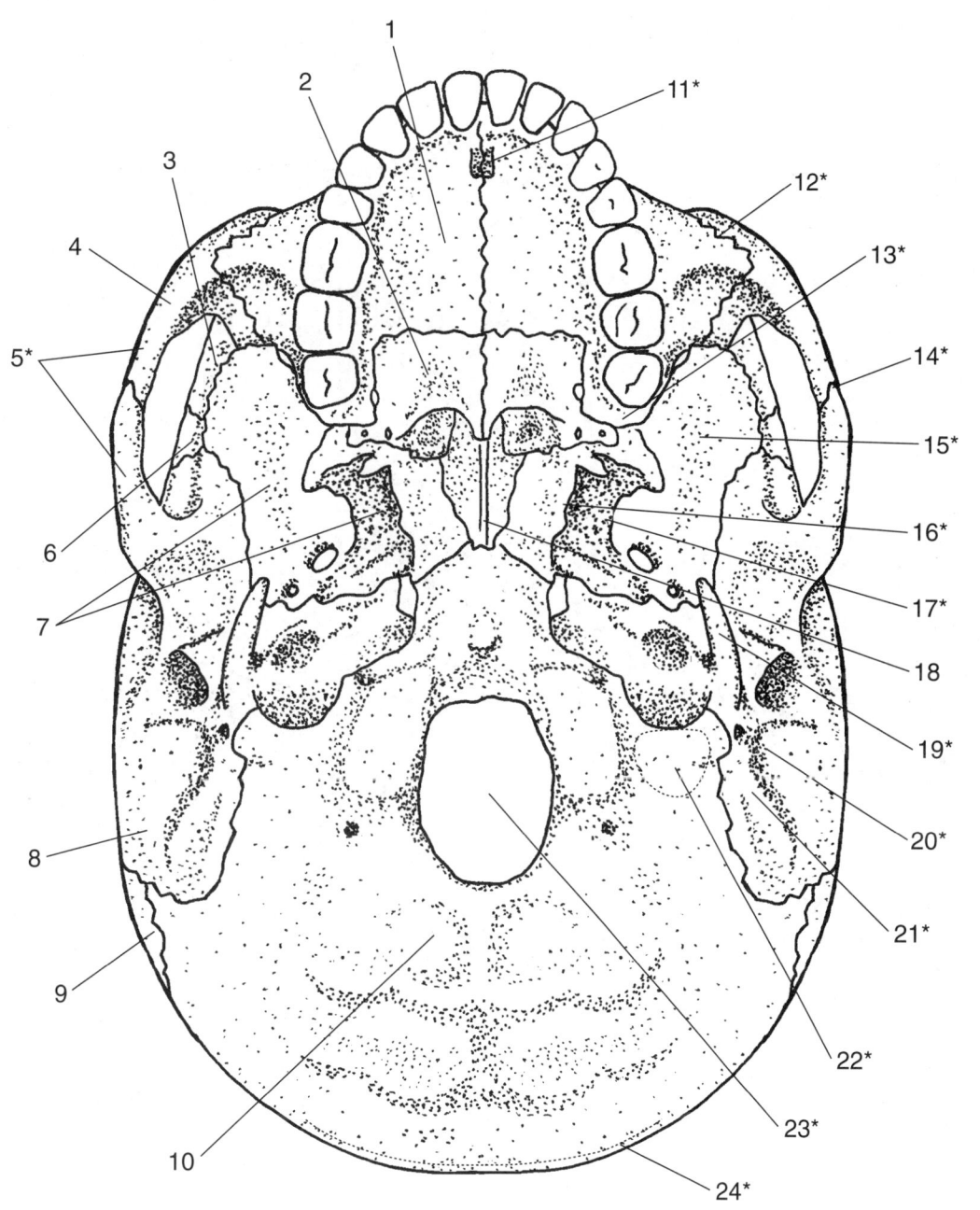

THE SKELETAL SYSTEM

ANTERIOR VIEW OF THE BONES AND BONY LANDMARKS OF THE NECK

THE SKELETAL SYSTEM

POSTERIOR VIEW OF THE BONES AND BONY LANDMARKS OF THE NECK

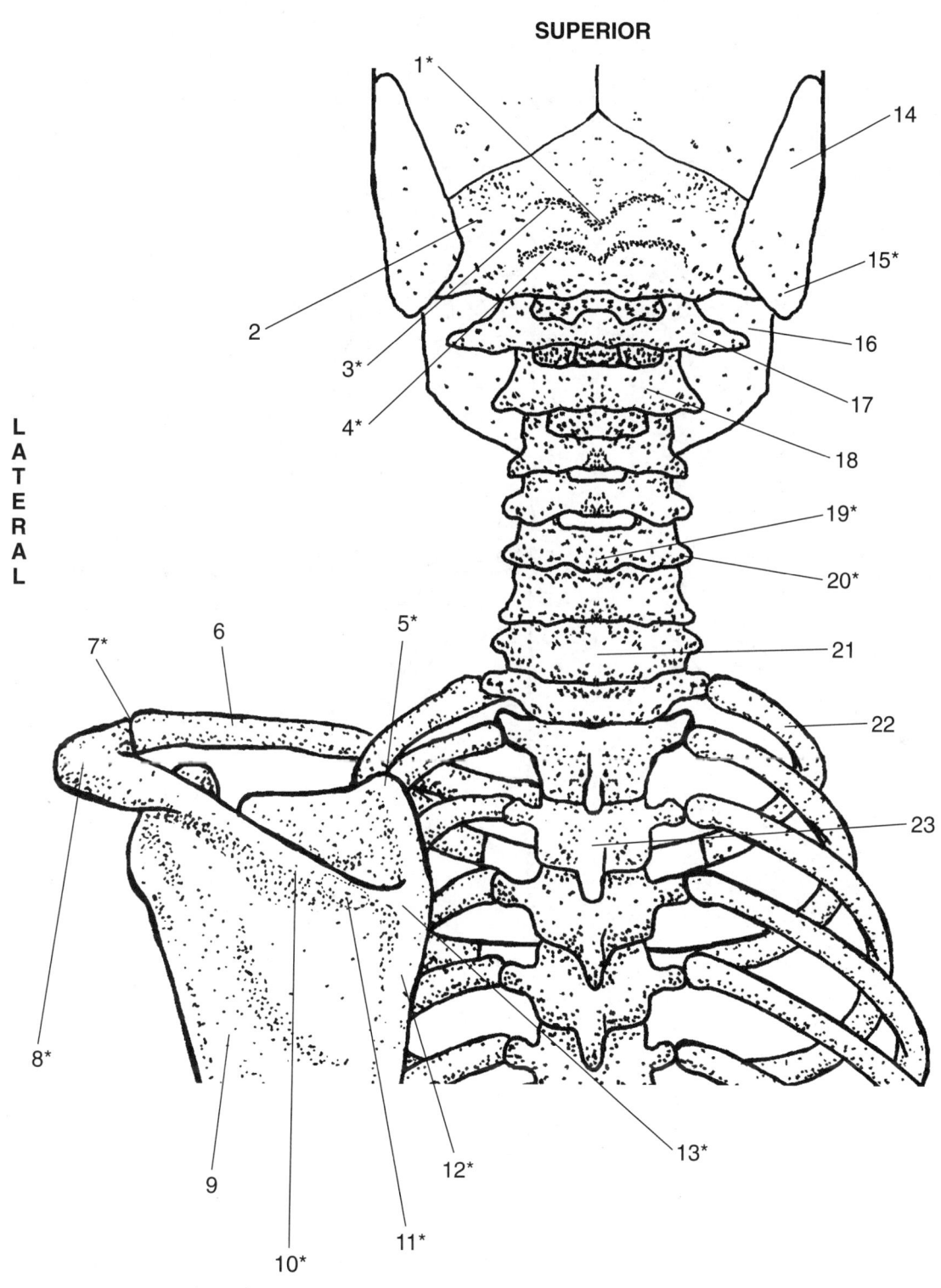

THE SKELETAL SYSTEM

ANTERIOR VIEW OF THE BONES AND BONY LANDMARKS OF THE TRUNK

THE SKELETAL SYSTEM

POSTERIOR VIEW OF THE BONES AND BONY LANDMARKS OF THE TRUNK

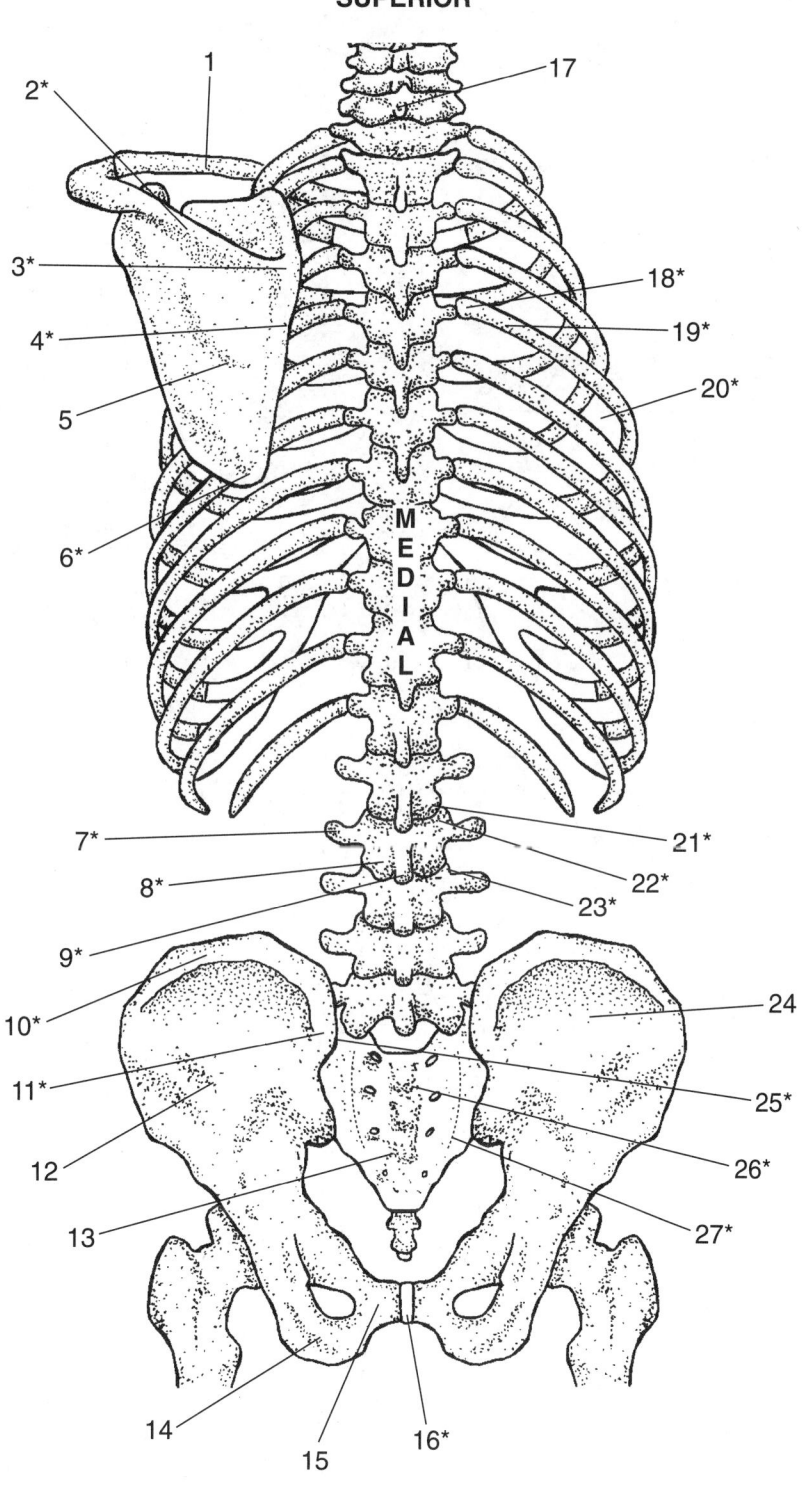

10 THE SKELETAL SYSTEM

ANTERIOR VIEW OF THE BONES AND BONY LANDMARKS OF THE RIGHT PELVIS AND THIGH

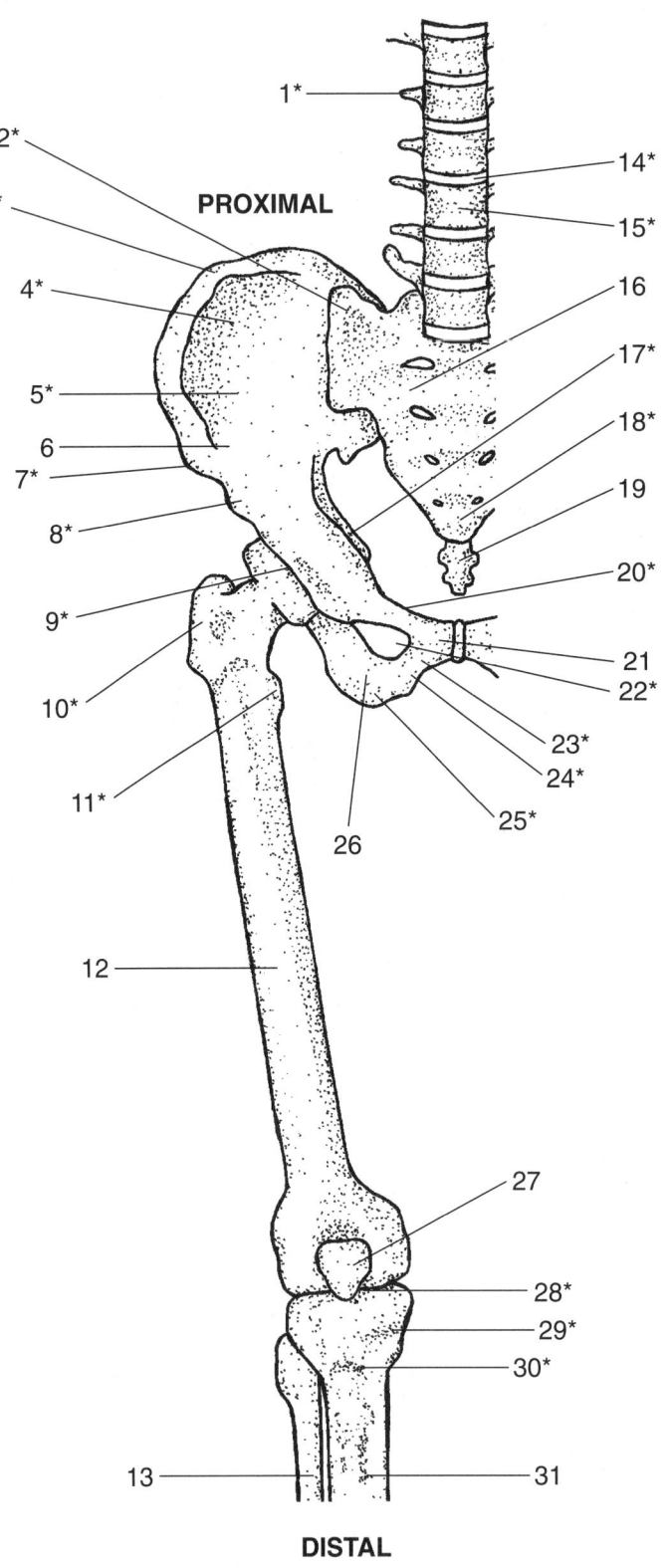

THE SKELETAL SYSTEM

POSTERIOR VIEW OF THE BONES AND BONY LANDMARKS OF THE RIGHT PELVIS AND THIGH

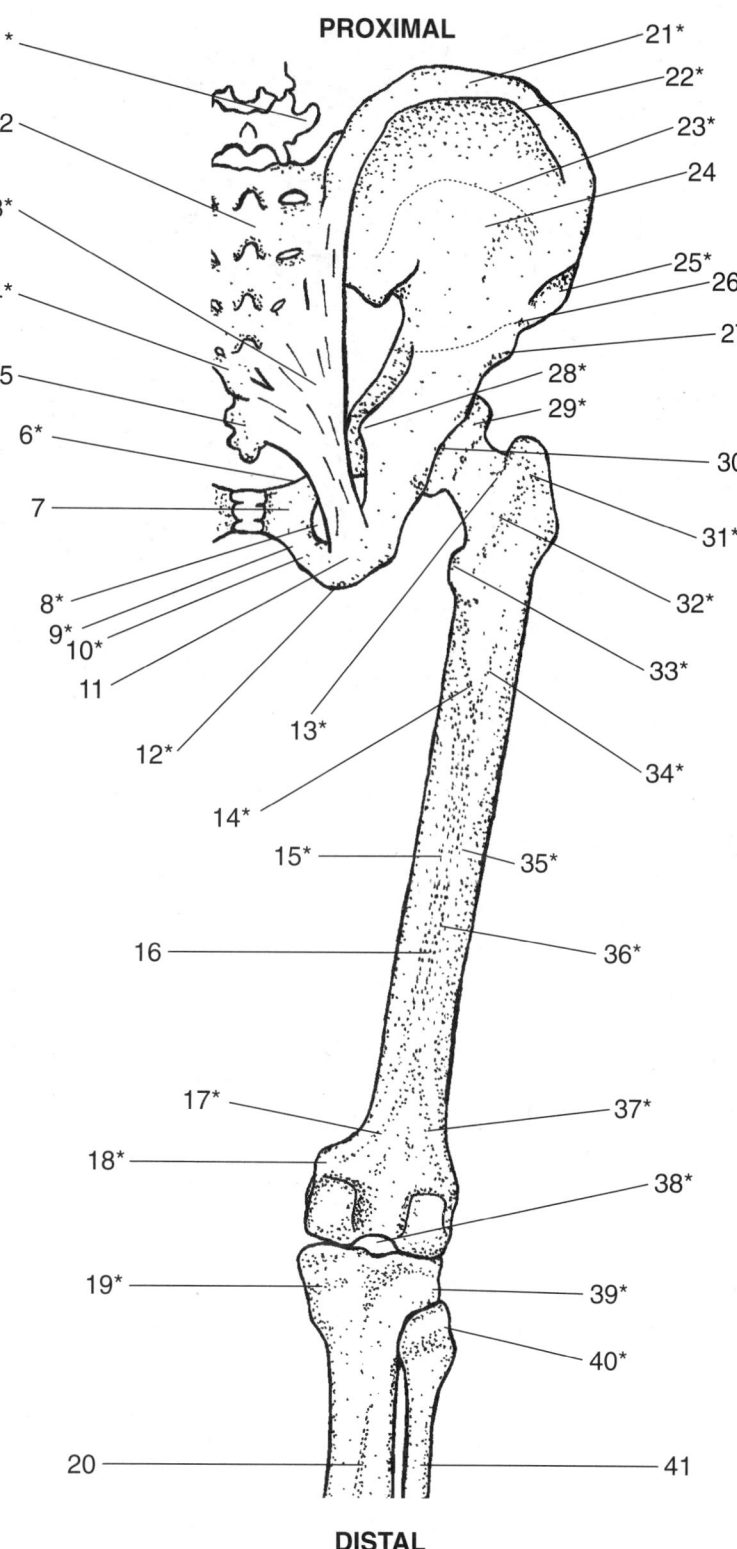

12 THE SKELETAL SYSTEM

ANTERIOR VIEW OF THE BONES AND BONY LANDMARKS OF THE RIGHT LEG

THE SKELETAL SYSTEM

POSTERIOR VIEW OF THE BONES AND BONY LANDMARKS OF THE RIGHT LEG

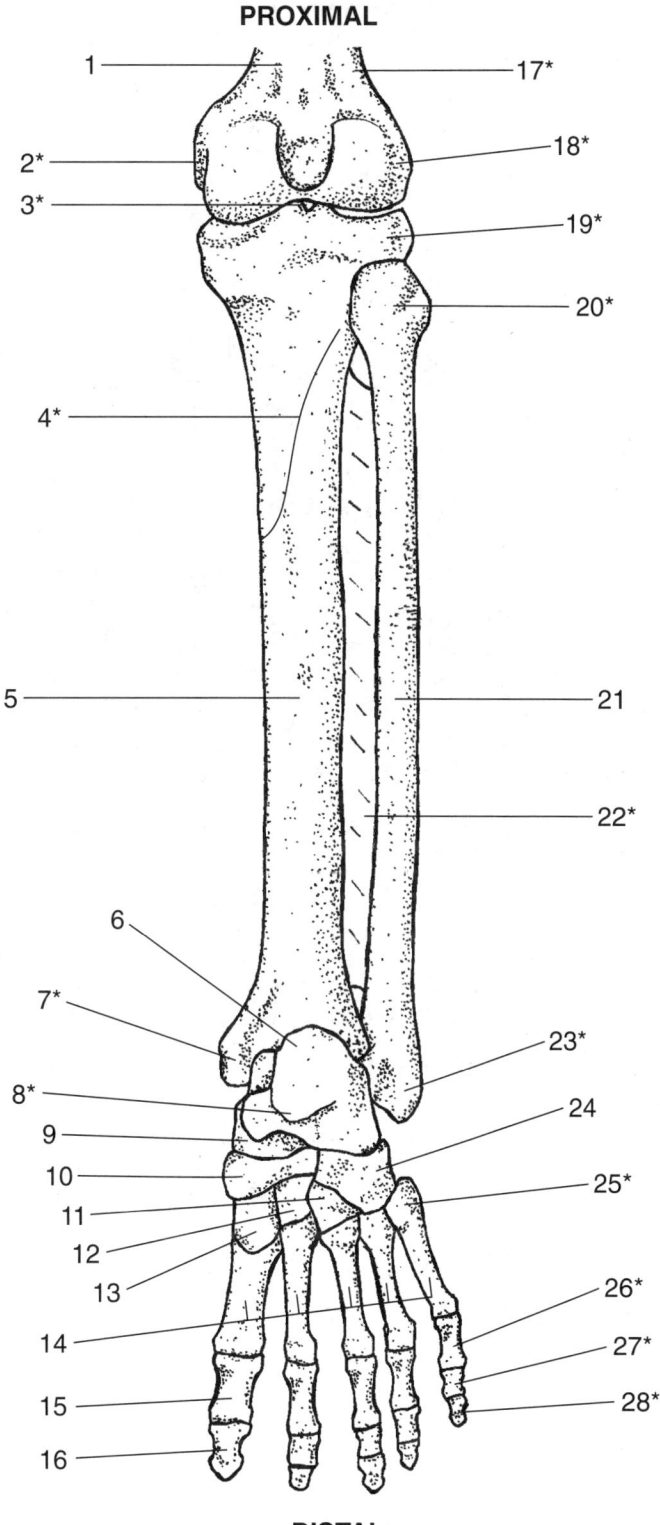

14 THE SKELETAL SYSTEM

DORSAL VIEW OF THE BONES AND BONY LANDMARKS OF THE RIGHT FOOT

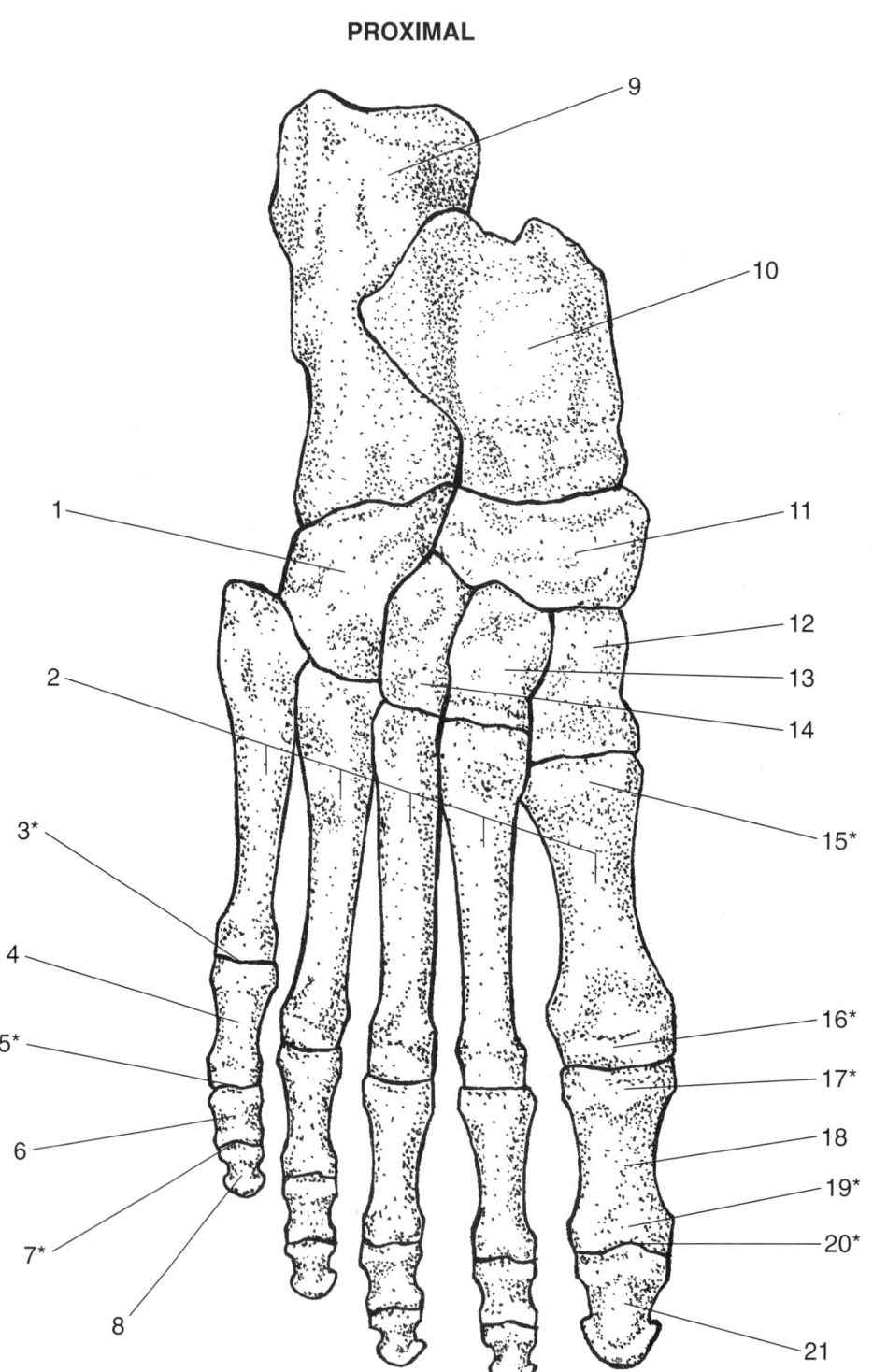

THE SKELETAL SYSTEM

PLANTAR VIEW OF THE BONES AND BONY LANDMARKS OF THE RIGHT FOOT

16 THE SKELETAL SYSTEM

ANTERIOR VIEW OF THE BONES AND BONY LANDMARKS OF THE RIGHT SCAPULA/ARM

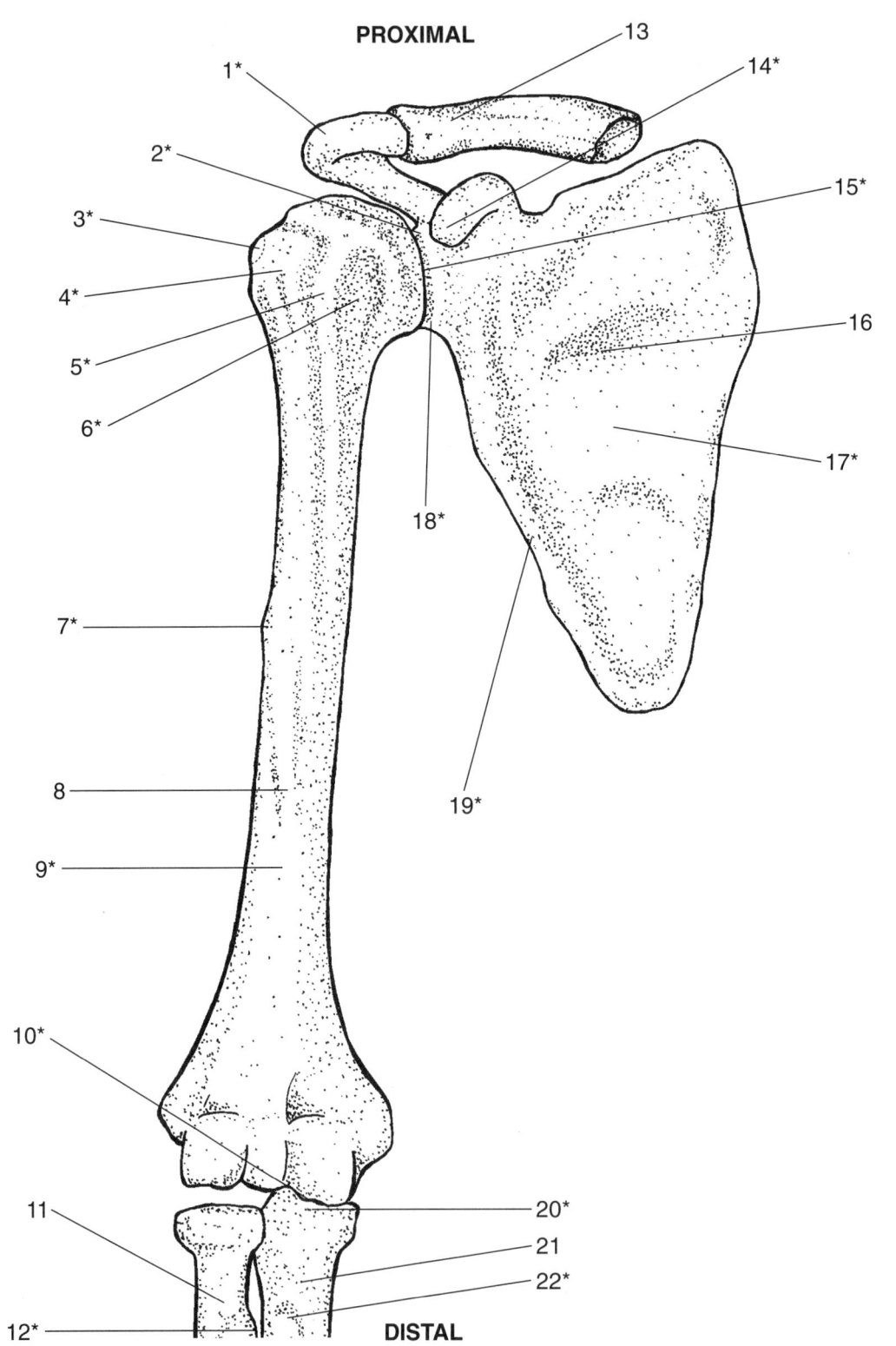

THE SKELETAL SYSTEM

POSTERIOR VIEW OF THE BONES AND BONY LANDMARKS OF THE RIGHT SCAPULA/ARM

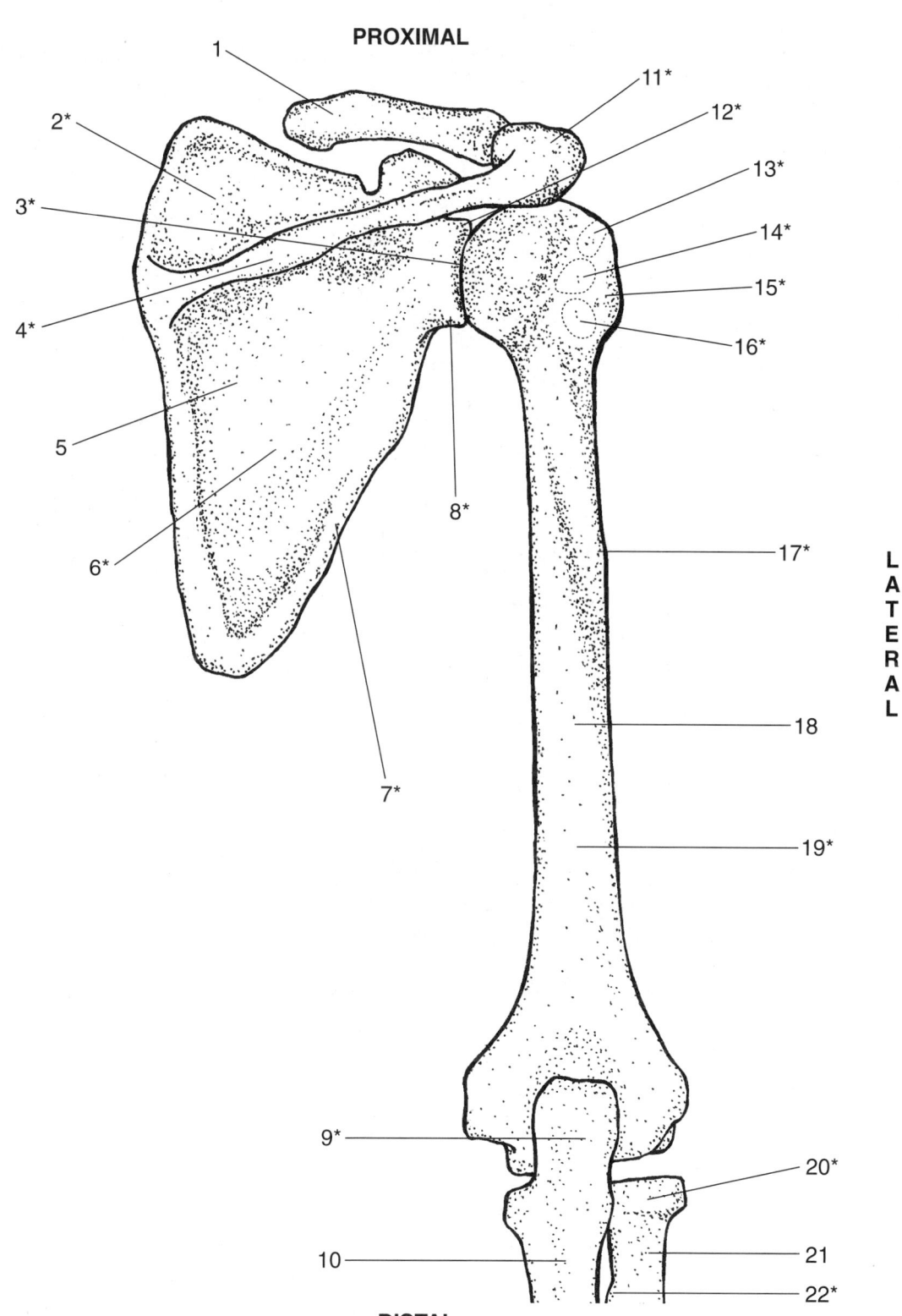

THE SKELETAL SYSTEM

ANTERIOR VIEW OF THE BONES AND BONY LANDMARKS OF THE RIGHT FOREARM

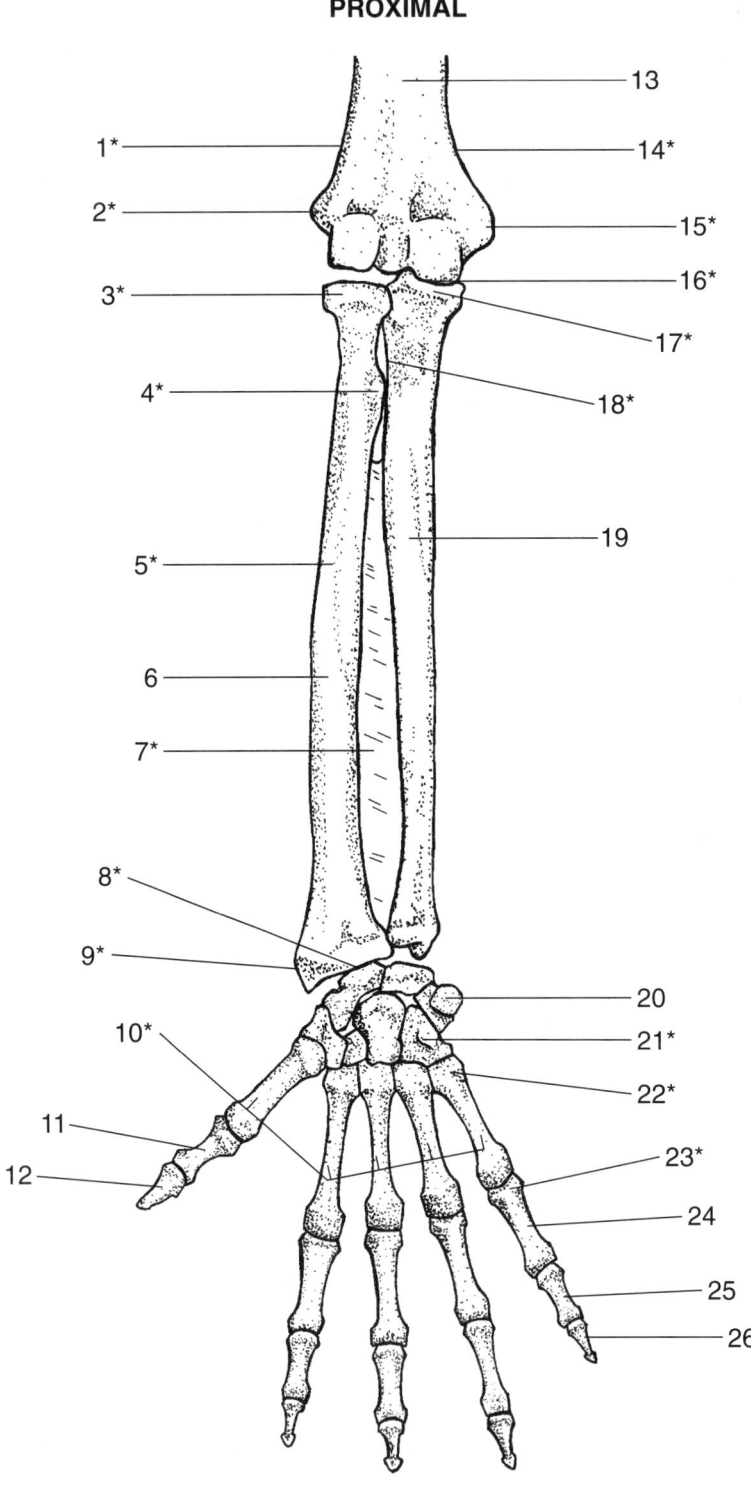

THE SKELETAL SYSTEM

POSTERIOR VIEW OF THE BONES AND BONY LANDMARKS OF THE RIGHT FOREARM

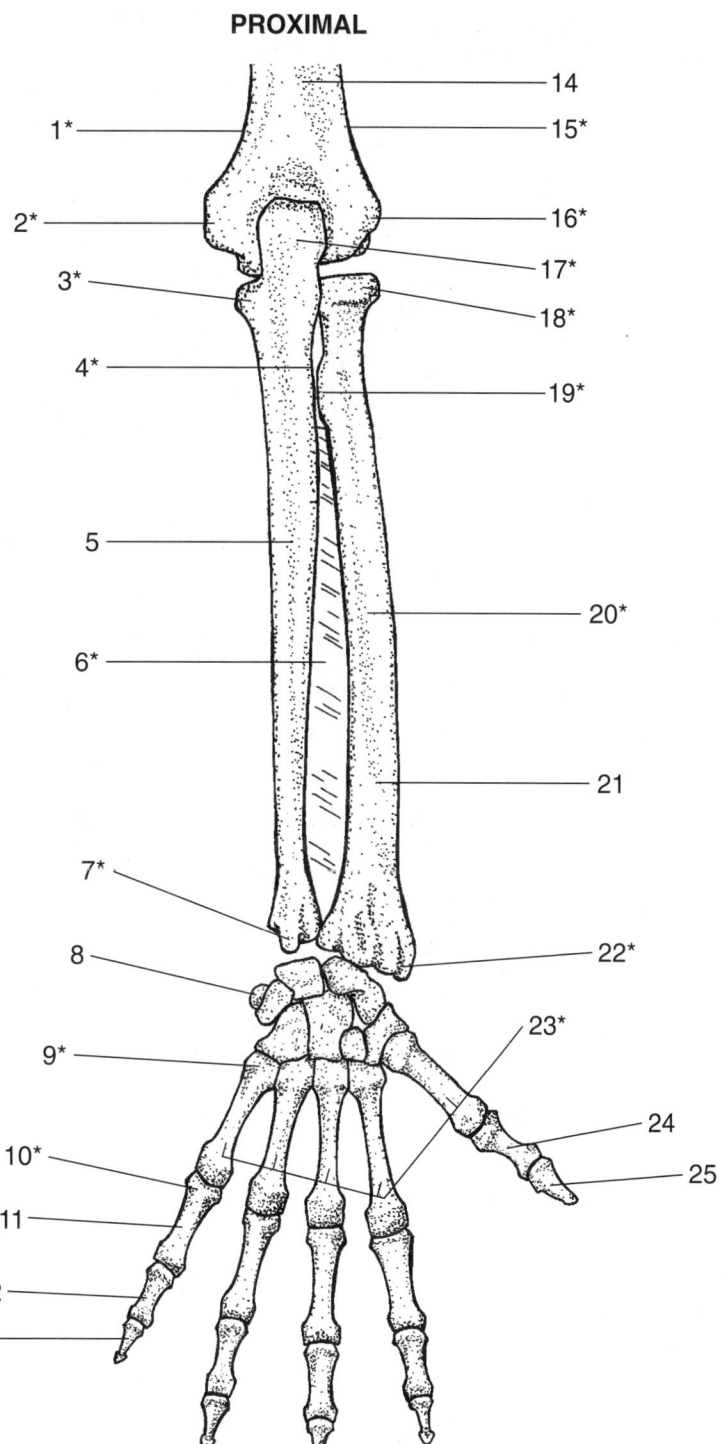

THE SKELETAL SYSTEM

PALMAR VIEW OF THE BONES AND BONY LANDMARKS OF THE RIGHT HAND

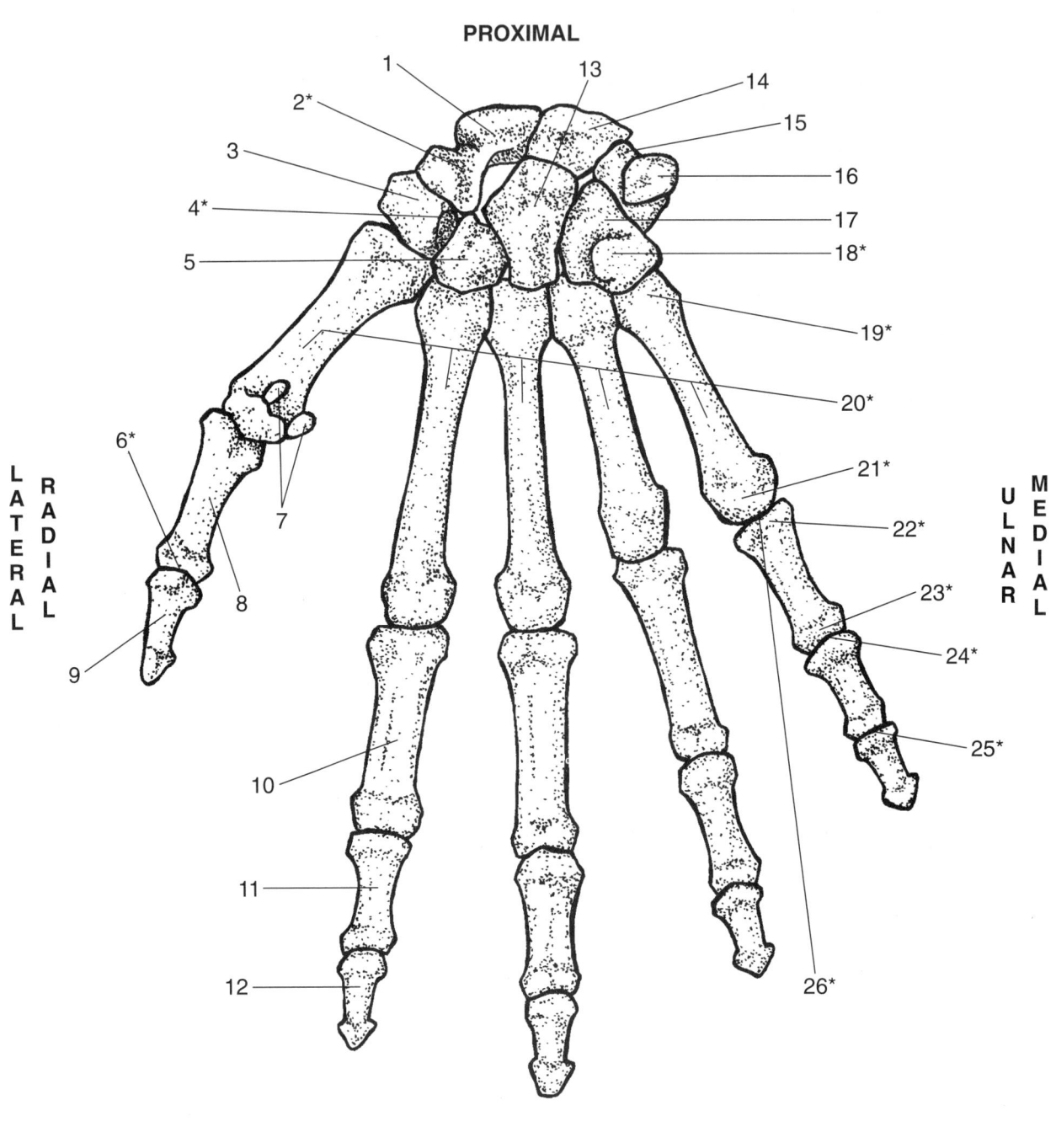

THE SKELETAL SYSTEM

DORSAL VIEW OF THE BONES AND BONY LANDMARKS OF THE RIGHT HAND

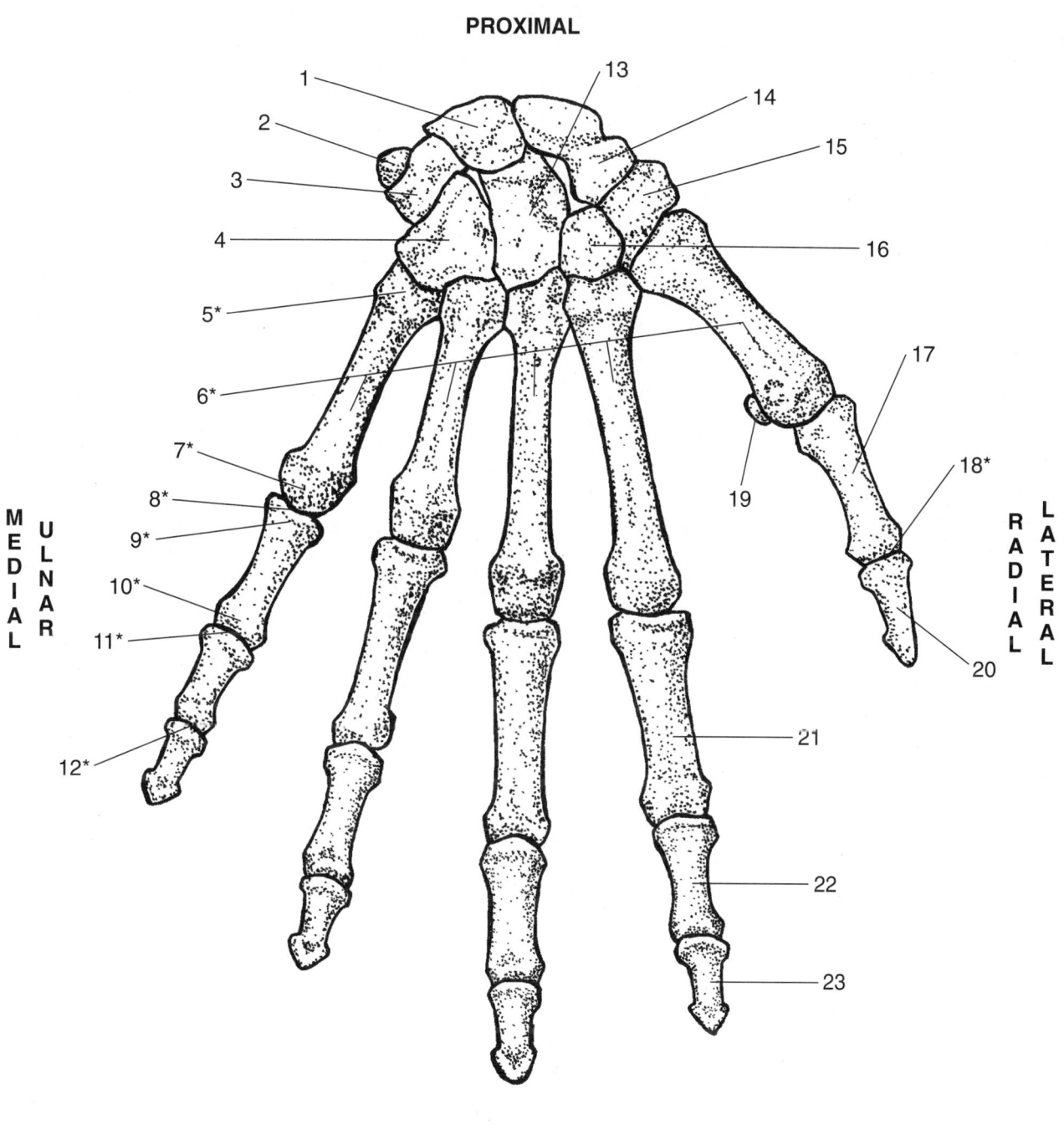

The Muscular System 2

Get Ready to Explore:

Muscles of the Head
Occipitofrontalis, 34
Temporoparietalis, 36
Auricularis Anterior, Superior, and Posterior, 36
Orbicularis Oculi, 38
Levator Palpebrae Superioris, 38
Corrugator Supercilii, 40
Procerus, 40
Nasalis, 42
Depressor Septi Nasi, 42
Levator Labii Superioris Alaeque Nasi, 44
Levator Labii Superioris, 44
Zygomaticus Minor, 46
Zygomaticus Major, 46
Levator Anguli Oris, 48
Risorius, 48
Depressor Anguli Oris, 50
Depressor Labii Inferioris, 50
Mentalis, 52
Buccinator, 52
Orbicularis Oris, 54
Temporalis, 56
Masseter, 56
Lateral Pterygoid, 58
Medial Pterygoid, 58

Muscles of the Neck
Trapezius ("Trap"), 72
Splenius Capitis, 74
Splenius Cervicis, 74
Levator Scapulae, 76
Rectus Capitis Posterior Major, 78
Rectus Capitis Posterior Minor, 78
Obliquus Capitis Inferior, 80
Obliquus Capitis Superior, 80
Platysma, 82
Sternocleidomastoid ("SCM"), 84
Sternohyoid, 86
Sternothyroid, 86
Thyrohyoid, 88
Omohyoid, 88

Digastric, 90
Stylohyoid, 90
Mylohyoid, 92
Geniohyoid, 92
Anterior Scalene, 94
Middle Scalene, 94
Posterior Scalene, 96
Longus Colli, 98
Longus Capitis, 98
Rectus Capitis Anterior, 100
Rectus Capitis Lateralis, 100

Muscles of the Trunk
Latissimus Dorsi ("Lat"), 118
Rhomboids Major and Minor, 120
Serratus Anterior, 122
Serratus Posterior Superior, 124
Serratus Posterior Inferior, 124
The Erector Spinae Group, 126
Iliocostalis, 128
Longissimus, 128
Spinalis, 130
The Transversospinalis Group, 132
Semispinalis, 134
Multifidus, 134
Rotatores, 136
Quadratus Lumborum ("QL"), 138
Interspinales, 140
Intertransversarii, 140
Levatores Costarum, 142
Subcostales, 142
Pectoralis Major, 144
Pectoralis Minor, 146
Subclavius, 146
External Intercostals, 148
Internal Intercostals, 150
Rectus Abdominis, 152
External Abdominal Oblique, 154
Internal Abdominal Oblique, 154
Transversus Abdominis, 156
Transversus Thoracis, 156
Diaphragm, 158

More review activities on Evolve at http://evolve.elsevier.com/Muscolino/muscular/

THE MUSCULAR SYSTEM

Muscles of the Pelvis
Psoas Major, 174
Iliacus, 176
Psoas Minor, 178
Gluteus Maximus, 180
Gluteus Medius, 182
Gluteus Minimus, 184
Piriformis, 186
Superior Gemellus, 188
Obturator Internus, 188
Inferior Gemellus, 190
Obturator Externus, 192
Quadratus Femoris, 194

Muscles of the Thigh
Tensor Fasciae Latae ("TFL"), 208
Sartorius, 210
Rectus Femoris, 212
Vastus Lateralis, 214
Vastus Medialis, 214
Vastus Intermedius, 216
Articularis Genus, 216
Pectineus, 218
Gracilis, 218
Adductor Longus, 220
Adductor Brevis, 222
Adductor Magnus, 224
Biceps Femoris, 226
Semitendinosus, 228
Semimembranosus, 228

Muscles of the Leg
Tibialis Anterior, 244
Extensor Hallucis Longus, 246
Extensor Digitorum Longus, 248
Fibularis Tertius, 248
Fibularis Longus, 250
Fibularis Brevis, 250
Gastrocnemius ("Gastroc"), 252
Soleus, 252
Plantaris, 254
Popliteus, 254
Tibialis Posterior, 256
Flexor Digitorum Longus, 258
Flexor Hallucis Longus, 260

Intrinsic Muscles of the Foot
Extensor Digitorum Brevis, 274
Extensor Hallucis Brevis, 274
Abductor Hallucis, 276
Abductor Digiti Minimi Pedis, 276
Flexor Digitorum Brevis, 278
Quadratus Plantae, 280
Lumbricals Pedis, 280
Flexor Hallucis Brevis, 282
Flexor Digiti Minimi Pedis, 282
Adductor Hallucis, 284
Plantar Interossei, 286
Dorsal Interossei Pedis, 286

Muscles of the Scapula/Arm
Supraspinatus, 302
Infraspinatus, 302
Teres Minor, 304
Subscapularis, 304
Teres Major, 306
Deltoid, 308
Coracobrachialis, 310
Biceps Brachii, 312
Brachialis, 312
Triceps Brachii, 314

Muscles of the Forearm
Pronator Teres, 334
Pronator Quadratus, 334
Flexor Carpi Radialis, 336
Palmaris Longus, 336
Flexor Carpi Ulnaris, 338
Brachioradialis, 340
Flexor Digitorum Superficialis, 342
Flexor Digitorum Profundus, 342
Flexor Pollicis Longus, 344
Anconeus, 346
Extensor Carpi Radialis Longus, 348
Extensor Carpi Radialis Brevis, 348
Extensor Carpi Ulnaris, 350
Extensor Digitorum, 352
Extensor Digiti Minimi, 352
Supinator, 354
Abductor Pollicis Longus, 356
Extensor Pollicis Brevis, 356
Extensor Pollicis Longus, 358
Extensor Indicis, 358

Muscles of the Hand
Abductor Pollicis Brevis, 376
Flexor Pollicis Brevis, 376
Opponens Pollicis, 378
Opponens Digiti Minimi, 378
Abductor Digiti Minimi Manus, 380
Flexor Digiti Minimi Manus, 380
Palmaris Brevis, 382
Adductor Pollicis, 384
Lumbricals Manus, 384
Palmar Interossei, 386
Dorsal Interossei Manus, 386

Note: Throughout this chapter, muscle attachments are indicated by italics.

THE MUSCULOSKELETAL SYSTEM

For all movement of the body, the musculoskeletal system is involved. The musculoskeletal system is comprised of the bones of the skeleton, the joints located between the bones, and the muscles that move the bones at the joints of the body.

Skeletal System

The skeletal system is composed of bones that create a skeletal structure for support of the body. On a tissue level, bones are made up of spongy bone (that as its name implies, has spaces like a sponge) and compact bone (that as its name implies, is tightly compacted tissue). Of primary importance to the musculoskeletal system is: bones provide rigid levers to which muscles can attach and these bones are located within body parts. When a muscle contracts, the muscle pulls on a bone, and the body part that the bone is located within may move. Bones also function to protect internal organs, provide a reservoir of calcium, and house bone marrow that makes blood cells. Bones are usually divided into four major categories based upon their shape. These categories are: long and short bones, flat bones, round bones, and irregular bones.

Joints

Structurally, a joint is where two or more bones are joined together by soft (connective) tissue; functionally, a joint allows movement. Structurally, there are three types of joints in the body: fibrous, cartilaginous, and synovial. Fibrous joints are united by tough fibrous tissue, and cartilaginous joints are united by cartilaginous tissue. However, the most movement is allowed by synovial joints, which is the only type of joint that has a joint cavity. A typical synovial joint is a joint in which the two bones are connected by a double-layered capsule of soft tissue. This joint capsule has an outer fibrous layer that is lined with an inner synovial membrane. The joint capsule encloses a joint cavity that has synovial fluid within it; the synovial fluid is created by the synovial membrane. The joint (articular) surfaces of the bones are covered with cartilage for cushioning. Synovial joints are often classified based on the number of axes about which they permit motion. There are uniaxial, biaxial, triaxial, and nonaxial synovial joints. Outside of the joint (defined as being outside of the joint capsule) are ligaments that connect the two bones to each other. These ligaments function to hold the bones in proper alignment by limiting movement and preventing dislocation. There are also muscles located outside of the joint. These muscles attach to the bones via their tendons, crossing the joint that is located between the bones. When a muscle contracts, it can create movement.

Muscle Cell Structure and Function

A muscle is an organ made up of many muscle cells that are longitudinal in shape (long and thin). For this reason, a muscle cell is also known as a *muscle fiber*. These muscle fibers are arranged into groups known as *fascicles*. Fibrous fascia connective tissue encases each individual muscle fiber (endomysium), each fascicle (perimysium), and the entire muscle (epimysium). The continuation of this fibrous fascia creates the tendon (called an aponeurosis if its shape is broad and flat) that attaches a muscle to a bone. Each muscle fiber is composed of myofibrils that run longitudinally within the fiber. These myofibrils are divided into sarcomeres that are arranged end to end. Each sarcomere is in turn composed of longitudinally oriented protein filaments known as *actin* and *myosin*; actin filaments are thin, and myosin filaments are thick. The actin filaments are attached to the boundaries of the sarcomere, known as *Z lines*; the myosin filaments are located in the center of the sarcomere. When a stimulus comes from the nervous system, this stimulus travels into the interior of the muscle fiber via the transverse ("T") tubules. This message to contract causes stored calcium ions in the sarcoplasmic reticulum (endoplasmic reticulum) of the muscle fiber to be released into the sarcoplasm (cytoplasm). The calcium ions bond to the actin, exposing active sites on the actin to which the myosin heads attach, forming cross-bridges. These myosin cross-bridges then bend, thereby pulling the actin filaments in toward the center (NOTE: this sliding of the filaments along each other gives the name to this process, the *sliding filament theory*); this causes the sarcomere to shorten. When the sarcomeres shorten, the myofibril shortens. When the myofibrils shorten, the muscle fiber shortens. When enough muscle fibers shorten, the muscle shortens, creating a pulling force on its attachments. If this pulling force is sufficient, motion of the body parts to which the muscle is attached will occur.

The Basics of Muscle Structure and Function

A muscle attaches via its tendons from one bone to another bone. In so doing, a muscle crosses the joint that is located between the two bones (Fig. 2.1).

When a muscle contracts, it attempts to shorten toward its center. If the muscle is successful in shortening toward its center, then the two bones to which it is attached will have a force exerted on them that will pull them toward each other (Fig. 2.2).

Since the bony attachments of the muscle are within body parts, if the muscle moves a bone, then the body part that the bone is within moves. In this way, muscles can cause movement of parts of the body. When a muscle contracts and shortens as described here, this type of contraction is called a *concentric contraction* and the muscle that is concentrically contracting is called a "mover."

26 THE MUSCULAR SYSTEM

Figure 2.1. The location of a muscle is shown; it attaches from one bone to another bone and crosses the joint that is located between the two bones.

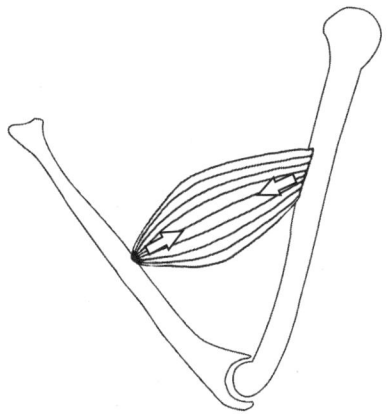

Figure 2.2. A muscle is shown contracting and shortening (a concentric contraction).

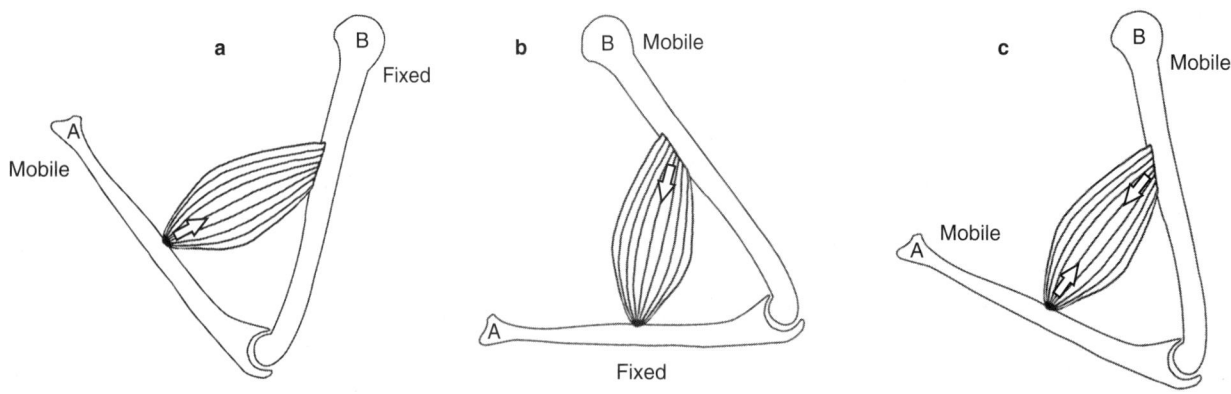

Figure 2.3. The three scenarios of a muscle concentrically contracting are shown.
In Figure 2.3a, Bone A moves toward Bone B.
In Figure 2.3b, Bone B moves toward Bone A.
In Figure 2.3c, Bone A and Bone B both move toward each other.

Figure 2.4. The right brachialis muscle at rest (medial view).

It is worth noting that whether a muscle is successful in shortening toward its center is determined by the strength of the pulling force of the muscle compared with the resistance force (the force necessary to actually move one or both body parts that the muscle is attached to). The force necessary to move a body part is usually the force necessary to move the weight of the body part. However, other forces may be involved.

If the force of a muscle's contraction is less than the resistance force, the muscle lengthens as it contracts. This type of contraction is called an eccentric contraction and the muscle that is eccentrically contracting is called an "antagonist." If the force of muscle's contraction is equal to the resistance force, the muscle stays the same length as it contracts. This type of contraction is called an isometric contraction and the muscle that is isometrically contracting is called a "fixator" or "stabilizer."

What Happens When a Muscle Concentrically Contracts?

Assuming that a muscle contracts with sufficient strength to shorten toward its center, let's look at the possible scenarios that can occur. If we call one of the attachments of the muscle "Bone A" and the other attachment of the muscle "Bone B," then we see that there are three possible scenarios (Fig. 2.3):
1. Bone A will be pulled toward Bone B.
2. Bone B will be pulled toward Bone A.
3. Both Bone A and Bone B will be pulled toward each other.

In this manner, a muscle creates a joint action. To fully describe this joint action, we must state which body part has moved and we also must state at which joint the movement has occurred. As an example to illustrate these concepts, let's look at the brachialis muscle. One attachment of the brachialis is onto the humerus of the arm and the other attachment of the brachialis is onto the ulna of the forearm. In attaching to the arm and the forearm, the brachialis crosses the elbow joint that is located between these two body parts (Fig. 2.4).

When the brachialis contracts, it attempts to shorten toward its center and exerts a pulling force on the forearm and the arm.

Scenario 1: The usual result of the brachialis contracting is that the forearm will be pulled toward the arm. This is because the forearm is lighter than the arm and therefore would be likely to move before the arm would. (Additionally, if the arm were to move, the trunk would have to move as well, which makes it even less likely that the arm will be the attachment that will move.) To fully describe this action, we call it *flexion of the forearm at the elbow joint* (Fig. 2.5a). In this scenario, the arm is the attachment that is fixed and the forearm is the attachment that is mobile.

Scenario 2: However, it is possible for the arm to move toward the forearm. If the forearm were to be fixed in place, perhaps because the hand is holding onto an immovable object, then the arm would have to move instead. This action is called *flexion of the arm at the elbow joint* (Fig. 2.5b). In this scenario, the forearm is the attachment

THE MUSCULAR SYSTEM

Figure 2.5. The three scenarios that can result from a concentric contraction of the brachialis muscle.

Figure 2.5a Flexion of the forearm at the elbow joint. The arm is fixed and the forearm is mobile, moving toward the arm.

Figure 2.5b Flexion of the arm at the elbow joint. The forearm is fixed (in our illustration, the hand is holding onto an immovable bar) and the arm is mobile, moving toward the forearm.

Figure 2.5c Flexion of the forearm and the arm at the elbow joint. Neither attachment is fixed so both are mobile, moving toward each other.

that is fixed and the arm is the attachment that is mobile. This scenario can be called a "reverse action" because the attachment that is usually fixed, the arm, is now mobile, and the attachment that is usually mobile, the forearm, is now fixed.

Scenario 3: Since the contraction of the brachialis exerts a pulling force on the forearm and the arm, it is possible for both of these bones to move. When this occurs, there are two actions: flexion of the forearm at the elbow joint and flexion of the arm at the elbow joint (Fig. 2.5c). In this case, both bones are mobile and neither one is fixed.

It is important to realize that the brachialis does not intend nor choose which attachment will move, or if both attachments will move. When a muscle contracts, it merely exerts a pulling force toward its center. Which attachment moves is determined by other factors. The relative weight of the body parts is the most common factor. However, another common determinant is when the central nervous system directs another muscle in the body to contract.

The contraction of this second muscle "fixes" (stops from moving) one of the attachments of our mover muscle. (If this occurs, this second muscle that contracts to fix a body part would be called a "fixator" or "stabilizer" muscle.) It follows that if one attachment is fixed, then the other attachment would be mobile.

Beginning the Process of Learning Muscles

Essentially, when learning about muscles, there are two major aspects that must be learned: the attachments and actions of the muscle. Generally speaking, attachments of a muscle must be memorized. However, there are times when clues are given about the attachments of a muscle by the muscle's name. For example, the name *coracobrachialis* tells us that the muscle has one attachment on the coracoid process of the scapula and that its other attachment is on the brachium (i.e., the humerus). Similarly, the name *zygomaticus major* tells us that this muscle attaches onto the zygomatic bone (and that there must be another muscle called the *zygomaticus minor*).

Unlike muscle attachments, muscle actions do not have to be memorized. Instead, by understanding the simple concept that a muscle pulls at its attachments to move a body part, the action or actions of a muscle can be reasoned out.

5-Step Approach to Learning Muscles

When first confronted with having to study and learn about a muscle, I recommend the following approach:
1. Look at the name of the muscle to see if it gives you any "free information" that saves you from having to memorize attachments or actions of the muscle.
2. Learn the general location of the muscle well enough to be able to visualize the muscle on your body. At this point, you need only know it well enough to know: (1) which joint it crosses, (2) where it crosses the joint, and (3) how it crosses the joint, i.e., what direction its fibers are running.
3. Use this general knowledge of the muscle's location to figure out the actions of the muscle.
4. Go back and learn (memorize, if necessary) the specific attachments of the muscle.
5. Now look at the relationship of this muscle to other muscles (and other soft tissue structures) of the body. Look at the following: Is this muscle superficial or deep? And, what other muscles (and other soft tissue structures) are located near this muscle?

Figuring Out a Muscle's Actions (Step 3)

Once you have a general familiarity with a muscle's location on your body, then it is time to begin the process of reasoning out the actions of the muscle. The most important thing that you must look at is: *the direction of the muscle fibers relative to the joint that it crosses.*

By doing this, you can see: the line of pull of the muscle relative to the joint.

This line of pull will determine the actions of the muscle, i.e., how the contraction of the muscle will cause the body parts to move at that joint.

The approach that I like to have my students follow is to ask the following three questions of themselves:
1. *What joint does the muscle cross?*
2. *Where does the muscle cross the joint?*
3. *How does the muscle cross the joint?*

Question 1—What Joint Does the Muscle Cross?

I always recommend to my students that the first question to ask and answer in figuring out the actions of a muscle is to simply know what joint it crosses. The following rule applies: If a muscle crosses a joint, then it will have an action at that joint. For example, if we look at the coracobrachialis, knowing that it crosses the shoulder joint tells us that it must have an action at the shoulder joint.

We may not know what the exact action of the coracobrachialis is yet, but at least we now know at what joint it has its actions. To figure out exactly what these actions are, we need to look at the next two questions. (It is worth pointing out that the converse of this rule is also generally true, that is: if a muscle does not cross a joint, then it will not have an action at that joint.)

Questions 2 and 3:—Where Does the Muscle Cross the Joint? and How Does the Muscle Cross the Joint?

These two questions must be looked at together. The "where" of a muscle crossing a joint is whether it crosses the joint anteriorly, posteriorly, medially, or laterally. It is helpful to place a muscle into one of these broad groups because the following general rules apply: muscles that cross a joint anteriorly will usually flex a body part at that joint, and muscles that cross a joint posteriorly will usually extend a body part at that joint*; muscles that cross a joint laterally will usually abduct or laterally flex a body part at that joint, and muscles that cross a joint medially will usually adduct a body part at that joint. The "how" of a muscle crossing a joint is whether it crosses the joint with its fibers running vertically or horizontally. This is also very important.

To illustrate this idea, lets look at the pectoralis major muscle. The pectoralis major has two parts, a clavicular head and a sternocostal head. The "where" of these two heads of the pectoralis major crossing the shoulder joint is the same, that is, they both cross the shoulder joint anteriorly. But the "how" of these two heads crossing the shoulder joint is very different. The clavicular head crosses the shoulder joint with its fibers running vertically, therefore it flexes the arm at the shoulder joint (because it pulls the arm upward in the sagittal plane, which is flexion). However, the sternocostal head crosses the shoulder joint with its fibers running horizontally, therefore it adducts the arm at the shoulder joint (because it pulls the arm from lateral to medial in the frontal plane, which is adduction).

With a muscle that has a horizontal direction to its fibers, there is another factor that must be considered when looking at "how" this muscle crosses the joint. That is whether the muscle attaches to the first place on the bone that it reaches, or whether the muscle wraps around the bone before attaching to it. Muscles that run horizontally (in the transverse plane) and wrap around the bone before attaching to it create a rotation action when they contract and pull on the attachment. For example, the sternocostal head of the pectoralis major does not attach to the first point on the humerus that it reaches. Instead, it continues to wrap around the shaft of the humerus to attach onto the lateral lip of the bicipital groove of the humerus. When the sternocostal head pulls, it medially rotates the arm at the shoulder joint (in addition to adducting it).

In essence, by asking the three questions: What joint does a muscle cross?, Where does the muscle cross the joint?, and How does the muscle cross the joint?, we are trying to determine the direction of the muscle fibers relative to the joint. Determining this will give us the line of pull of the muscle relative to the joint and that will give us the actions of the muscle, saving us the trouble of having to memorize this information!

Functional Groups Approach

The best method for approaching and learning each and every action of a new muscle that you first encounter to learn is to use the reasoning of step 3 of the 5-step approach. You have learned that for each aspect of the direction of fibers for a muscle, you apply the questions of where and how the muscle crosses the joint. This reasoning is solid and will lead you to reason out all actions of the muscle that is being studied. However, it can be very repetitive and time consuming as you apply this method to muscle after muscle after muscle that all cross the same joint in the same manner.

Therefore, once you are very comfortable with applying the questions of step 3 for learning the actions of each muscle individually, I recommend that you begin to use your understanding of how muscles function and apply it on a larger scale. Instead of looking at each muscle individually and going through all of the questions of step 3 for that muscle, take a step back and look at the broad functional groups of muscles at each joint. For example, instead of individually using the questions of step 3 to learn that the brachialis flexes the forearm at the elbow joint, and then that the biceps brachii flexes the forearm at the elbow joint, and then that the pronator teres flexes the forearm at the elbow joint, and also the flexor carpi radialis, palmaris longus, etc., etc., it is a simpler and more elegant approach to look at the functional groups of muscles that cross this joint. In other words, the bigger picture is to see that ALL muscles that cross the elbow joint anteriorly flex the forearm at the elbow joint. Looking at the body this way, when you encounter yet another muscle that crosses the elbow joint anteriorly, you can automatically place it into the group of forearm flexors at the elbow joint.

For each joint of the human body, look for the functional groups. In the case of the elbow joint, since it is a pure hinge, uniaxial joint, it is very simple; there are only two functional groups, anterior muscles that flex and posterior muscles that extend.

Triaxial joints such as the shoulder or hip joint will have more functional groups (flexors, extensors, abductors, adductors, medial rotators, and lateral rotators) but the concepts will always be the same. Once you clearly see this concept, the learning of the actions of muscles of the body can be greatly simplified and streamlined.

Reminder About Reverse Actions

Please remember that the reverse actions of a muscle are always possible, even if they have not been specifically listed in this book. For some examples of reverse actions,

---

*Flexion is nearly always an anterior movement of a body part and extension is nearly always a posterior movement of a body part. However, from the knee joint and further distal, flexion is a posterior movement and extension is an anterior movement of the body part.

please see Chapter 3 in *The Muscular System Manual, third edition* (Elsevier, 2010).

A Visual and Kinesthetic Exercise for Learning a Muscle's Actions
The Rubber Band Exercise

An excellent method for learning the actions of a muscle is to place a large colorful rubber band (or large colorful shoelace or string) on your body or the body of a partner, in the same location that the muscle you are studying is located. Hold one end of the rubber band at one of the attachment sites of the muscle and hold the other end of the rubber band at the other attachment site of the muscle. Make sure that you have the rubber band running/oriented in the same direction as the direction of the fibers of the muscle. If it is not uncomfortable, you may even loop or tie the rubber band (or shoelace) around the body parts that are the attachments of the muscle.

Once you have the rubber band in place, pull one of the ends of the rubber band toward the center of the rubber band to see the action that the rubber band/muscle has upon that body part's attachment; return the attachment of the rubber band to where it began and then pull the other end of the rubber band toward the center of the rubber band to see the action that the rubber band/muscle has upon the other body part's attachment.

By placing the rubber band on your body or your partner's body, you are simulating the direction of the muscle's fibers relative to the joint that it crosses. By pulling either end of the rubber band toward the center, you are simulating the line of pull of the muscle relative to the joint that it crosses. The resultant movements that occur are the actions that the muscle would have. This is an excellent exercise to both visually see the actions of a muscle and to kinesthetically experience the actions of a muscle.

This exercise can be used to learn all muscle actions, and can be especially helpful for determining actions that may be a little more difficult to visualize, such as rotation actions.

NOTE: I recommend the use of a large colorful rubber band more than a shoelace or string because when you stretch out a rubber band and place it in the location that a muscle would be, the natural elasticity of a rubber band creates a pull on the attachment sites that nicely simulates the pull of a muscle on its attachments when it contracts. If you can, I recommend that you work with a partner to do this exercise. Have your partner hold one of the "attachments" of the rubber band while you hold the other "attachment." This leaves one of your hands free to pull the rubber band attachment sites toward the center.

A FURTHER NOTE OF CAUTION: If you are using a rubber band, be careful that you do not accidentally let go and have the rubber band hit you or your partner. For this reason, it would be preferable to use a shoelace instead of a rubber band when working near the face.

THE MUSCULAR SYSTEM — Muscles of the Head

ANTERIOR VIEW OF THE HEAD

Anterior view of the face (superficial)

Anterior view of the face (intermediate)

THE MUSCULAR SYSTEM Muscles of the Head

LATERAL VIEW OF THE HEAD

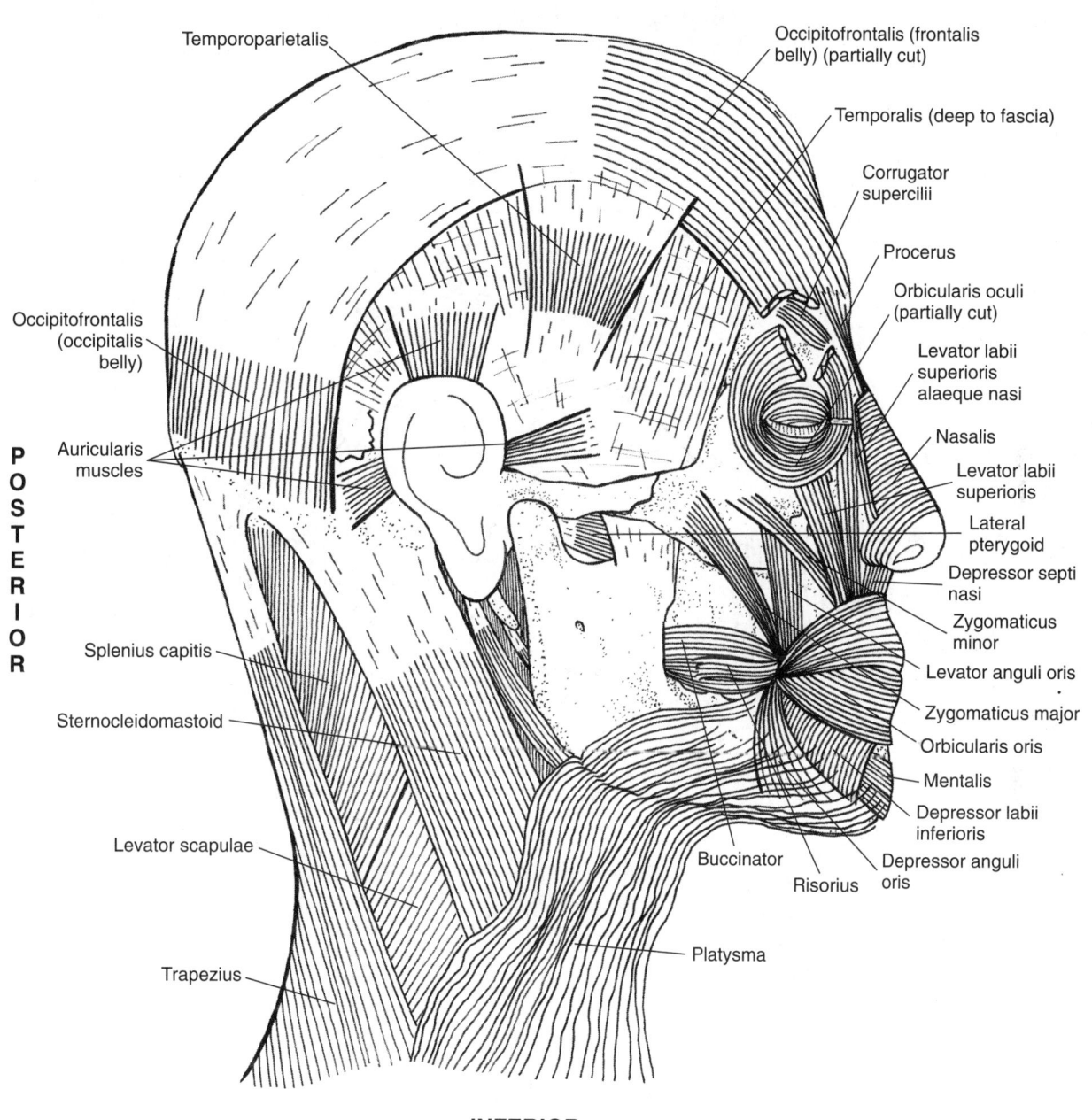

THE MUSCULAR SYSTEM — Muscles of the Head

OCCIPITOFRONTALIS
(PART OF THE EPICRANIUS)
ok-**sip**-i-to-fron-**ta**-lis

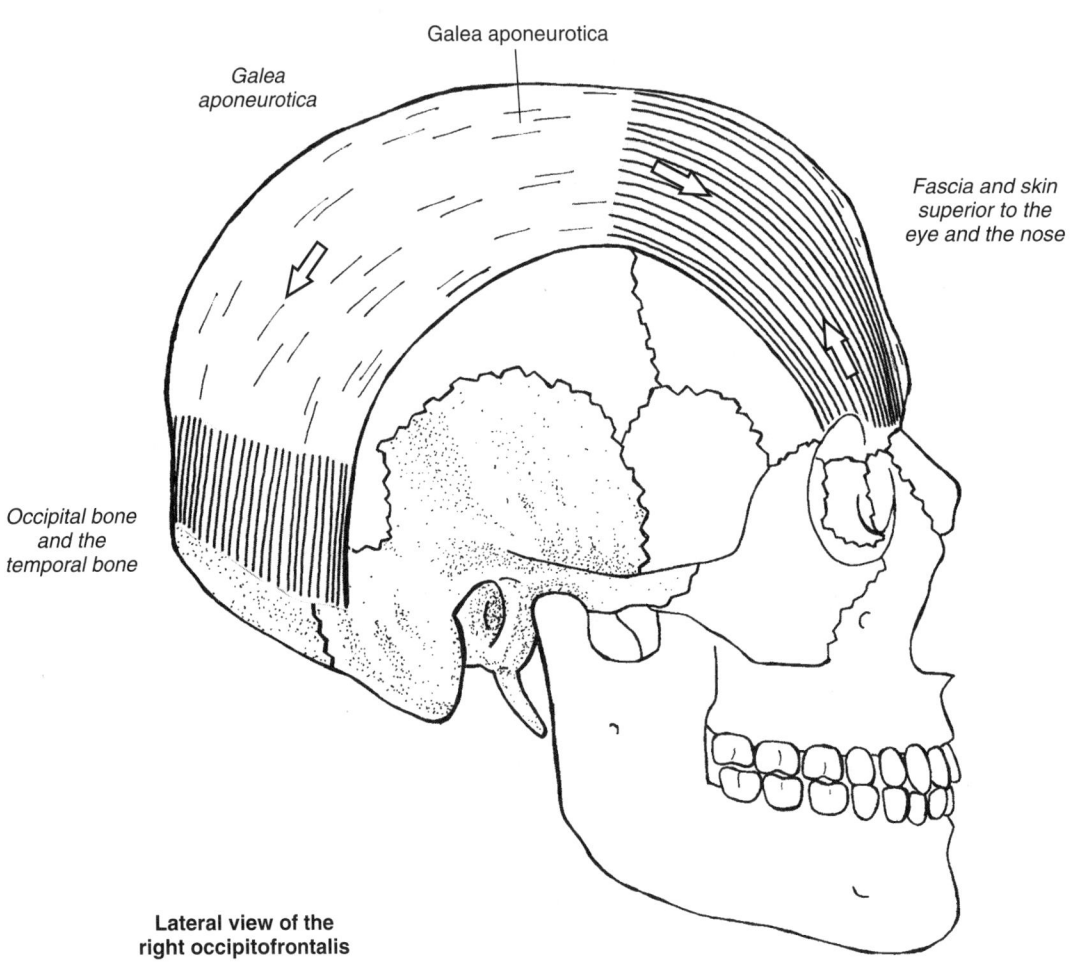

Lateral view of the right occipitofrontalis

Actions
Draws the scalp posteriorly (occipitalis)
Draws the scalp anteriorly (frontalis)
Elevates the eyebrows (frontalis)

Innervation
The facial nerve (CN VII)

Arterial Supply
Occipitalis: the occipital and posterior auricular arteries
Frontalis: supraorbital and supratrochlear branches of the ophthalmic artery

THE MUSCULAR SYSTEM Muscles of the Head

Did You Know?

The occipitofrontalis is often involved in tension headaches.

TEMPOROPARIETALIS
(PART OF THE EPICRANIUS)
tem-po-ro-pa-ri-i-tal-is

Actions
Elevates the ear
Tightens the scalp

Innervation
The facial nerve (CN VII)

Arterial Supply
The superficial temporal and posterior auricular arteries

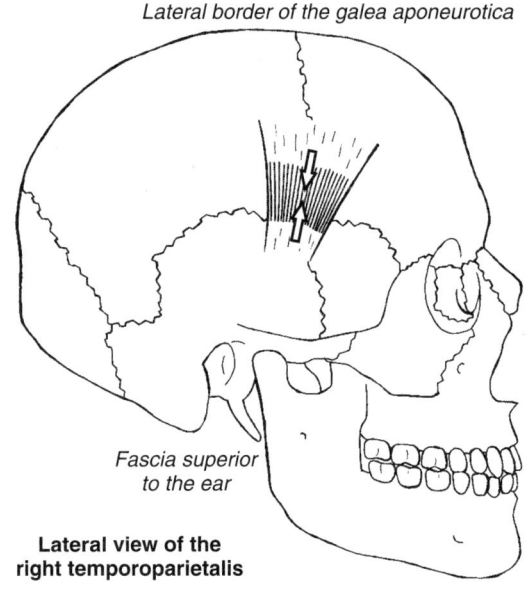

Lateral view of the right temporoparietalis

AURICULARIS ANTERIOR, SUPERIOR, AND POSTERIOR
aw-rik-u-la-ris an-tee-ri-or, sue-pee-ri-or, pos-tee-ri-or

Actions
Draws the ear anteriorly (auricularis anterior)
Elevates the ear (auricularis superior)
Draws the ear posteriorly (auricularis posterior)
Tightens and moves the scalp (auricularis anterior and superior)

Innervation
The facial nerve (CN VII)

Arterial Supply
The superficial temporal and posterior auricular arteries

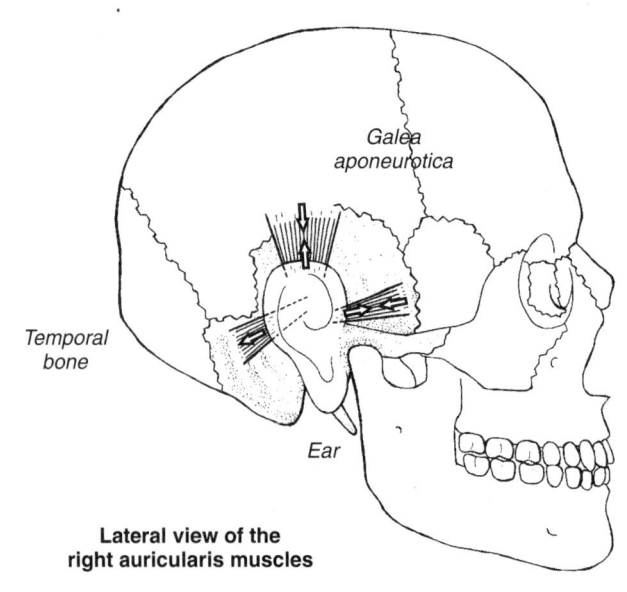

Lateral view of the right auricularis muscles

THE MUSCULAR SYSTEM Muscles of the Head

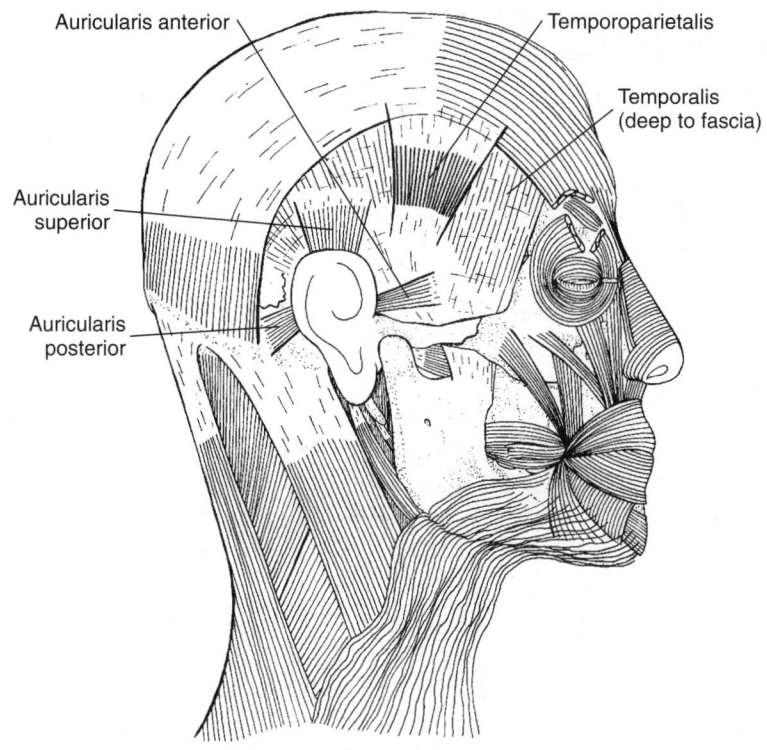

- Auricularis anterior
- Temporoparietalis
- Temporalis (deep to fascia)
- Auricularis superior
- Auricularis posterior

The temporoparietalis is located superficial to the temporalis.

- Temporoparietalis

The actions of moving the ear that are created by the auricularis muscles are largely vestigial and are nonfunctional in many people.

37

ORBICULARIS OCULI
or-**bik**-you-la-ris **ok**-you-lie

Actions
Closes and squints the eye (orbital part)
Depresses the upper eyelid (palpebral part)
Elevates the lower eyelid (palpebral part)
Assists tear transport and drainage (lacrimal part)

Innervation
The facial nerve (CN VII)

Arterial Supply
The branches of the facial artery and superficial temporal artery

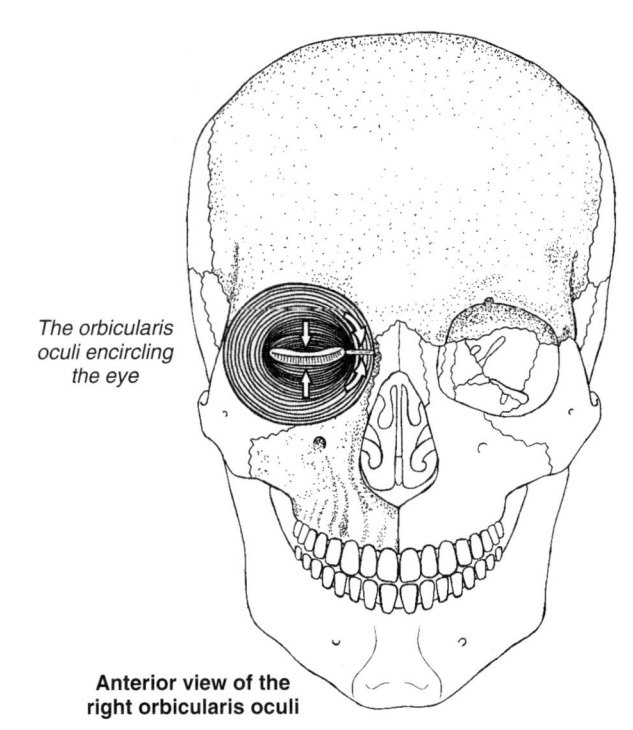

The orbicularis oculi encircling the eye

Anterior view of the right orbicularis oculi

LEVATOR PALPEBRAE SUPERIORIS
le-vay-tor pal-**pee**-bree su-**pee**-ri-**or**-is

Action
Elevates the upper eyelid

Innervation
The oculomotor nerve (CN III)

Arterial Supply
The ophthalmic artery

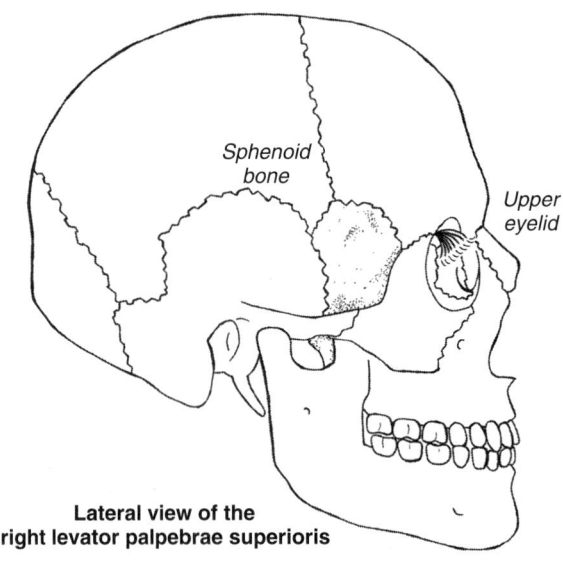

Sphenoid bone

Upper eyelid

Lateral view of the right levator palpebrae superioris

THE MUSCULAR SYSTEM Muscles of the Head

DID YOU KNOW

The portion of the orbicularis oculi located in the eyelids is under both conscious control to blink the eye voluntarily and unconscious control to blink the eye involuntarily (as part of a reflex to protect the eye from possible damage).

DID YOU KNOW

The levator palpebrae superioris is located within the socket of the eye and the upper eyelid.

CORRUGATOR SUPERCILII
kor-u-gay-tor su-per-**sil**-i-eye

Action
Draws eyebrow inferiorly and medially

Innervation
The facial nerve (CN VII)

Arterial Supply
The supratrochlear and supraorbital arteries

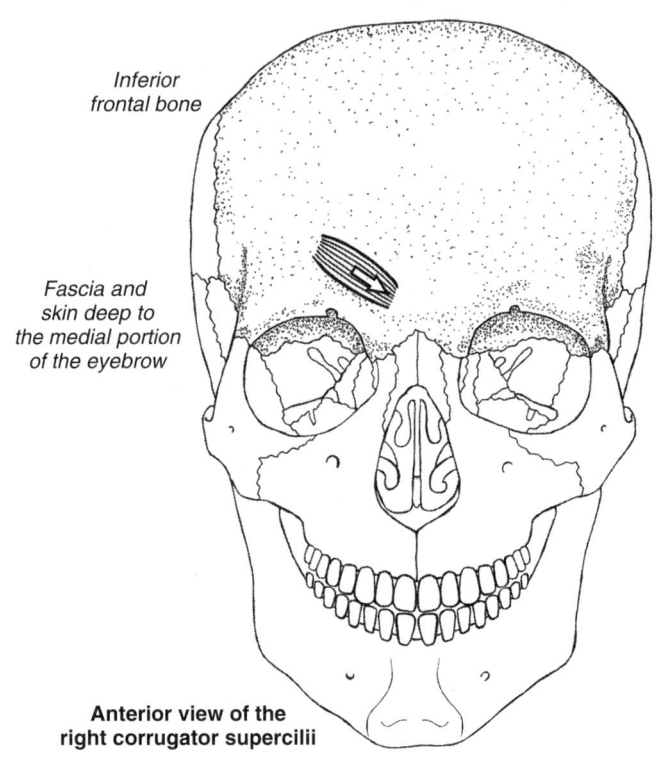

Anterior view of the right corrugator supercilii

PROCERUS
pro-**se**-rus

Actions
Draws down the medial eyebrow
Wrinkles the skin of the nose

Innervation
The facial nerve (CN VII)

Arterial Supply
The facial artery

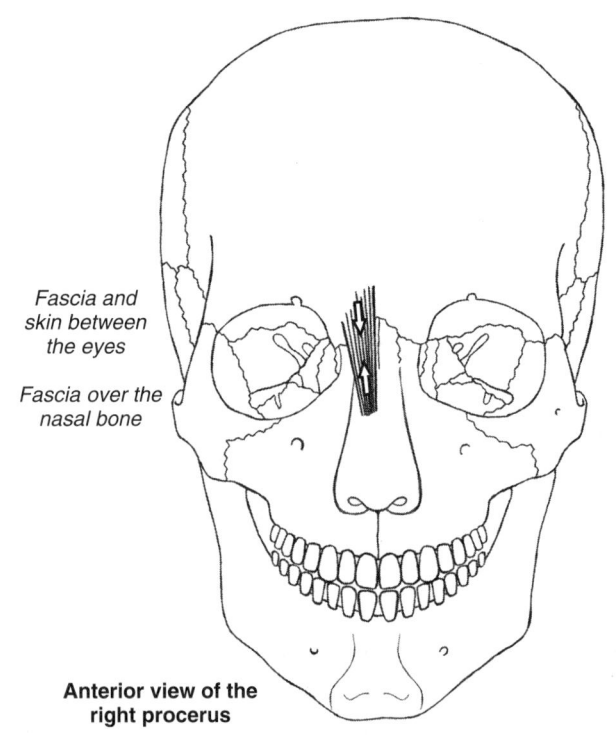

Anterior view of the right procerus

THE MUSCULAR SYSTEM Muscles of the Head

Contraction of the corrugator supercilii contributes to frowning and also assists in shielding the eyes from bright sunlight.

Procerus in Latin means "chief noble" or "prince"; hence the action of the procerus creates an expression that conveys a look of superiority.

NASALIS
nay-**sa**-lis

Action
Flares the nostril (alar part)
Constricts the nostril (transverse part)

Innervation
The facial nerve (CN VII)

Arterial Supply
The facial artery

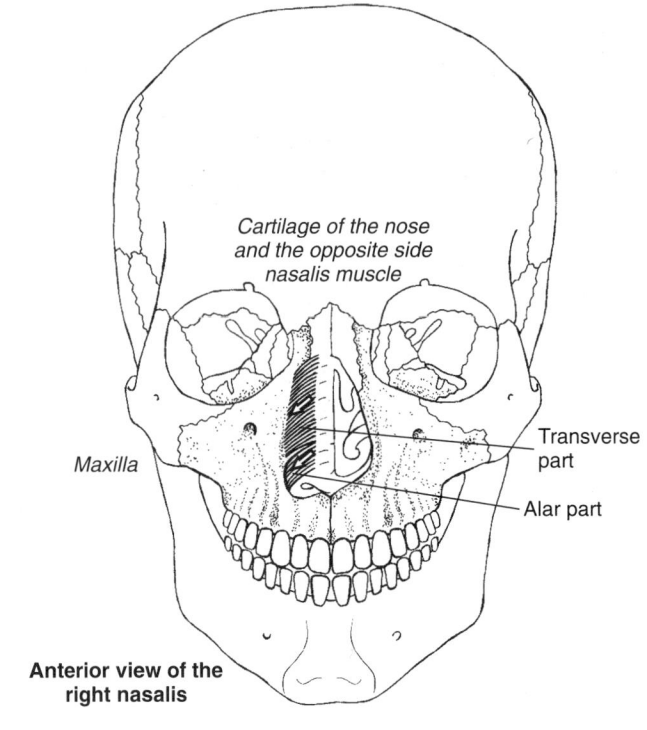

Anterior view of the right nasalis

DEPRESSOR SEPTI NASI
dee-**pres**-or **sep**-ti **nay**-zi

Action
Constricts the nostril

Innervation
The facial nerve (CN VII)

Arterial Supply
The facial artery

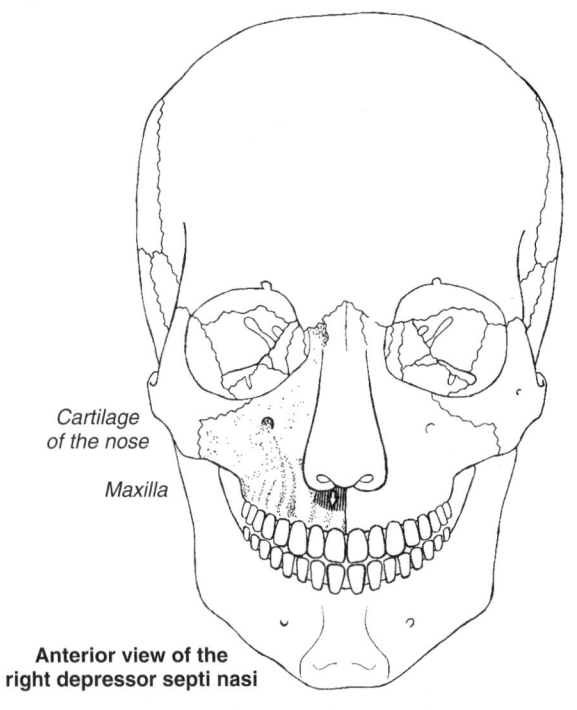

Anterior view of the right depressor septi nasi

THE MUSCULAR SYSTEM Muscles of the Head

The action of flaring the nostril by the nasalis opens the aperture for breathing and can be important for conveying emotional states.

The action of constricting the nostril by the depressor septi nasi closes the aperture for breathing and can also be involved in facial expressions.

LEVATOR LABII SUPERIORIS ALAEQUE NASI

le-**vay**-tor **lay**-be-eye
soo-**pee**-ri-o-ris
a-**lee**-kwe **nay**-si

Actions
Elevates the upper lip
Flares the nostril
Everts the upper lip

Innervation
The facial nerve (CN VII)

Arterial Supply
The infraorbital artery

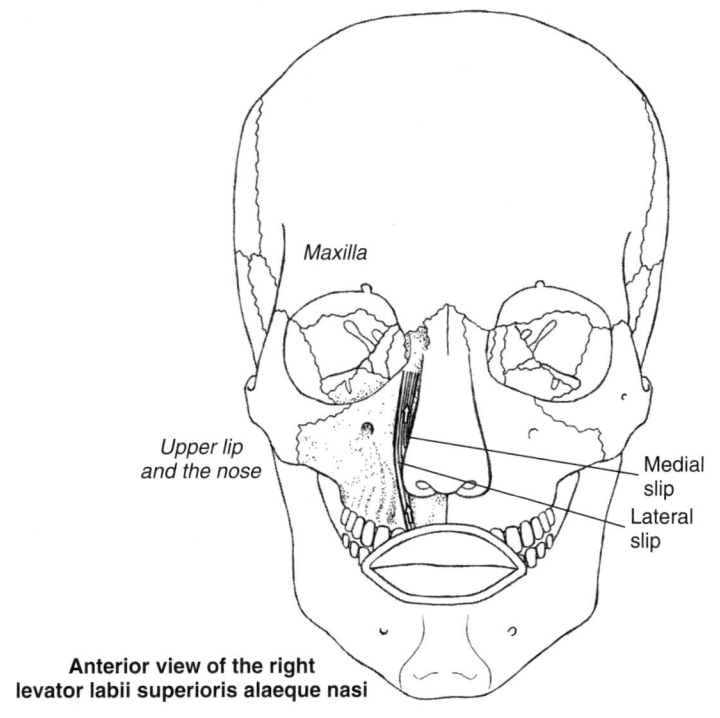

**Anterior view of the right
levator labii superioris alaeque nasi**

LEVATOR LABII SUPERIORIS

le-**vay**-tor **lay**-be-eye
soo-**pee**-ri-o-ris

Actions
Elevates the upper lip
Everts the upper lip

Innervation
The facial nerve (CN VII)

Arterial Supply
The facial artery

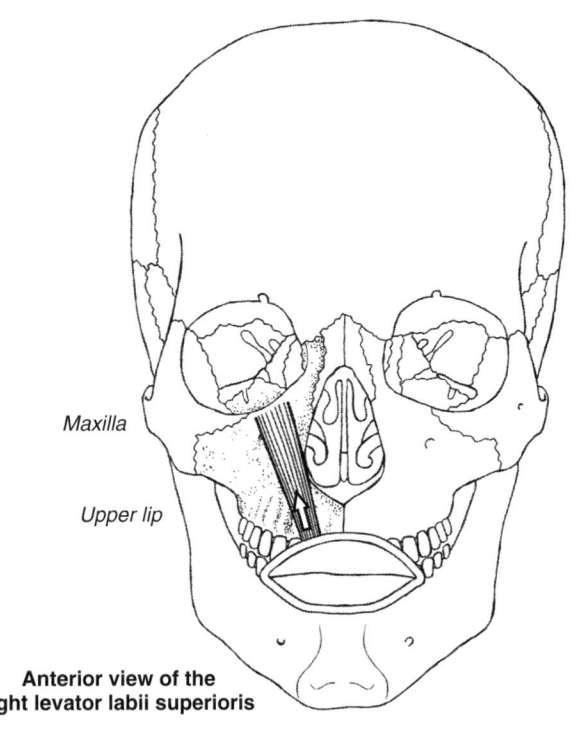

**Anterior view of the
right levator labii superioris**

THE MUSCULAR SYSTEM Muscles of the Head

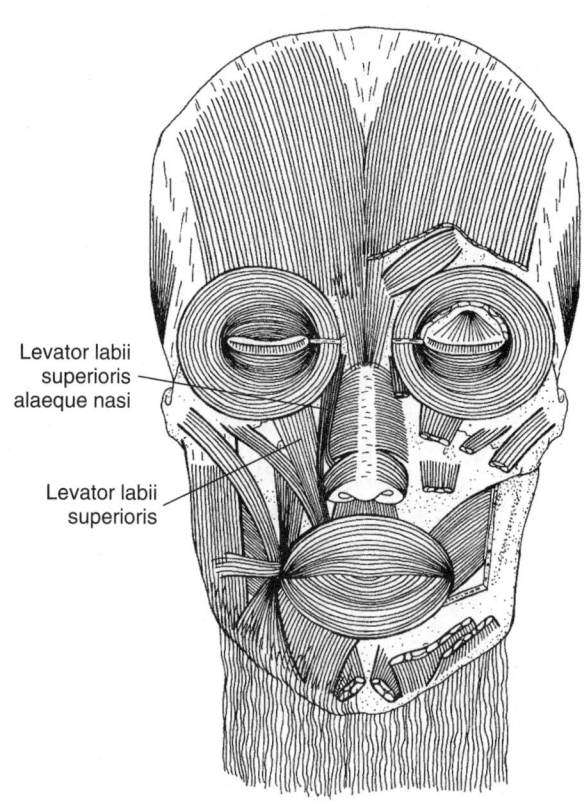

- Levator labii superioris alaeque nasi
- Levator labii superioris

DID YOU KNOW

The levator labii superioris alaeque nasi is a muscle of facial expression that, as its name describes, can move both the mouth and the nose.

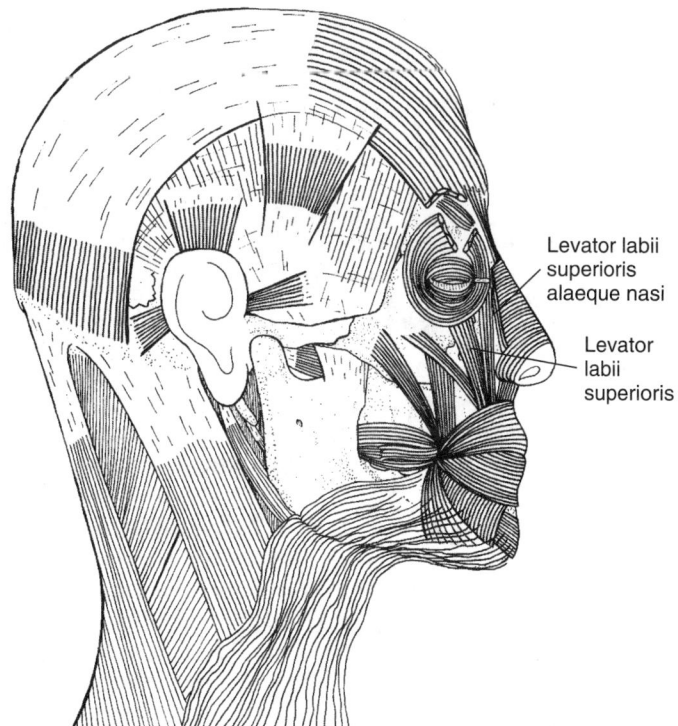

- Levator labii superioris alaeque nasi
- Levator labii superioris

DID YOU KNOW

Contraction of the levator labii superioris muscles lifts the upper lip, which exposes the upper teeth. This action can contribute to a number of facial expressions.

ZYGOMATICUS MINOR
zi-go-**mat**-ik-us **my**-nor

Actions
Elevates the upper lip
Everts the upper lip

Innervation
The facial nerve (CN VII)

Arterial Supply
The facial artery

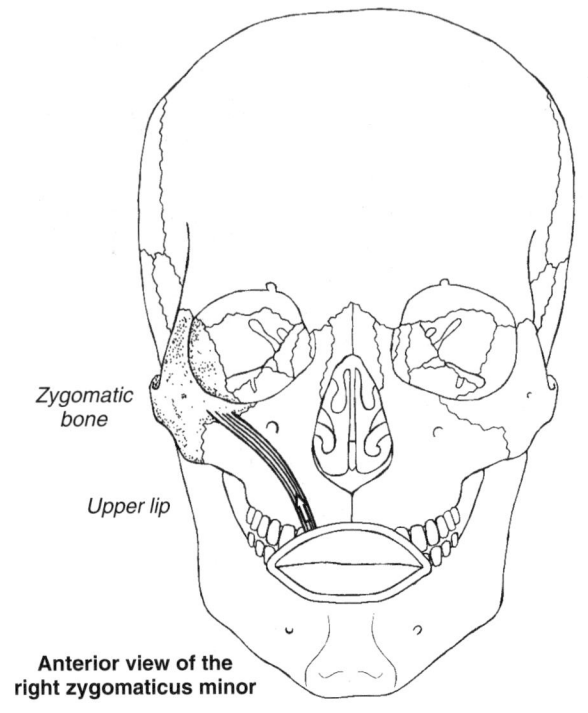

Anterior view of the right zygomaticus minor

ZYGOMATICUS MAJOR
zi-go-**mat**-ik-us **may**-jor

Actions
Elevates the angle of the mouth
Draws laterally the angle of the mouth

Innervation
The facial nerve (CN VII)

Arterial Supply
The facial artery

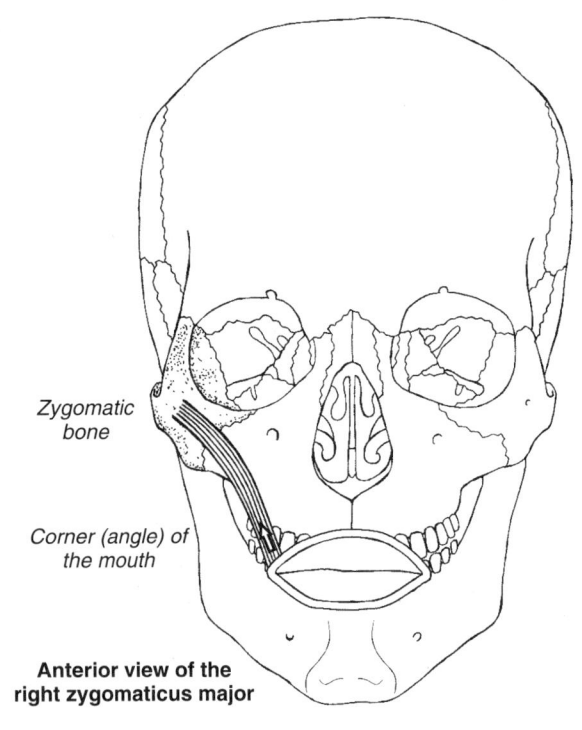

Anterior view of the right zygomaticus major

THE MUSCULAR SYSTEM Muscles of the Head 47

Zygomaticus major
Zygomaticus minor

Zygomaticus minor
Zygomaticus major

DID YOU KNOW?

As the name zygomaticus implies, both zygomaticus muscles attach onto the zygomatic bone.

LEVATOR ANGULI ORIS
le-**vay**-tor **ang**-you-lie **o**-ris

Action
Elevates the angle of the mouth

Innervation
The facial nerve (CN VII)

Arterial Supply
The facial artery

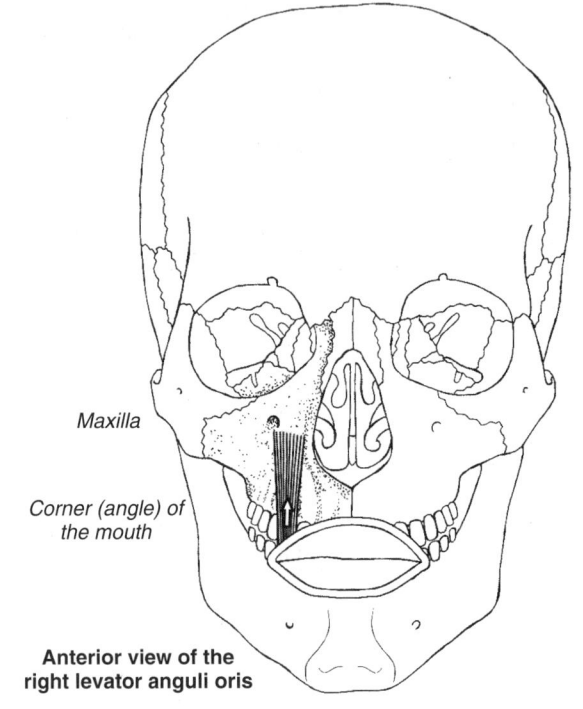

Anterior view of the right levator anguli oris

RISORIUS
ri-**so**-ri-us

Action
Draws laterally the angle of the mouth

Innervation
The facial nerve (CN VII)

Arterial Supply
The facial artery

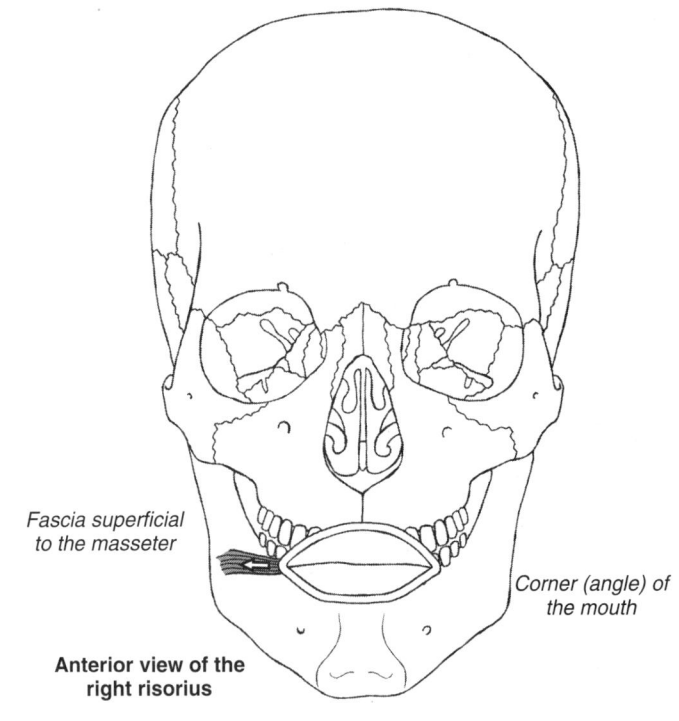

Anterior view of the right risorius

THE MUSCULAR SYSTEM   Muscles of the Head   49

The levator anguli oris is also known as the caninus because contraction of this muscle results in the typical "Dracula" expression wherein the canine teeth are exposed.

The name risorius means "laughing" in Latin; the risorius draws the angle of the mouth laterally, which occurs during laughter.

DEPRESSOR ANGULI ORIS

dee-**pres**-or **ang**-you-lie **o**-ris

Actions
Depresses the angle of the mouth
Draws laterally the angle of the mouth

Innervation
The facial nerve (CN VII)

Arterial Supply
The facial artery

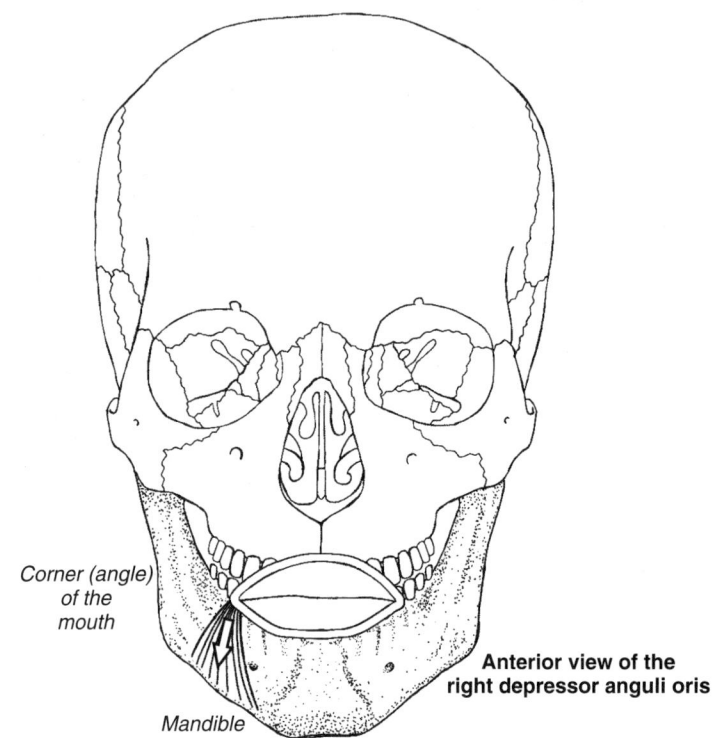

Anterior view of the right depressor anguli oris

DEPRESSOR LABII INFERIORIS

dee-**pres**-or **lay**-be-eye in-**fee**-ri-**o**-ris

Actions
Depresses the lower lip
Draws laterally the lower lip
Everts the lower lip

Innervation
The facial nerve (CN VII)

Arterial Supply
The facial artery

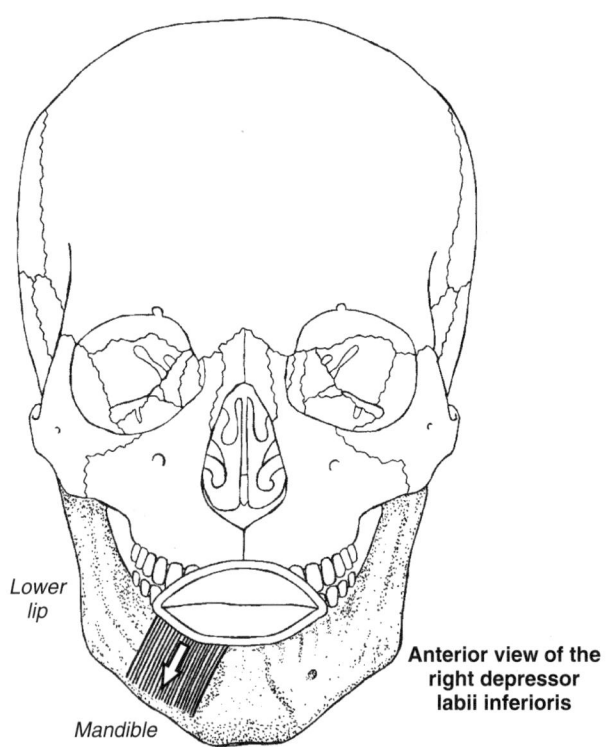

Anterior view of the right depressor labii inferioris

THE MUSCULAR SYSTEM Muscles of the Head   51

Depressor anguli oris
Depressor labii inferioris

Contraction of the depressor anguli oris and depressor labii inferioris muscles contributes to facial expressions of sadness, doubt, and uncertainty.

Depressor labii inferioris
Depressor anguli oris

MENTALIS
men-**ta**-lis

Actions
Elevates the lower lip
Everts and protracts the lower lip
Wrinkles the skin of the chin

Innervation
The facial nerve (CN VII)

Arterial Supply
The facial artery

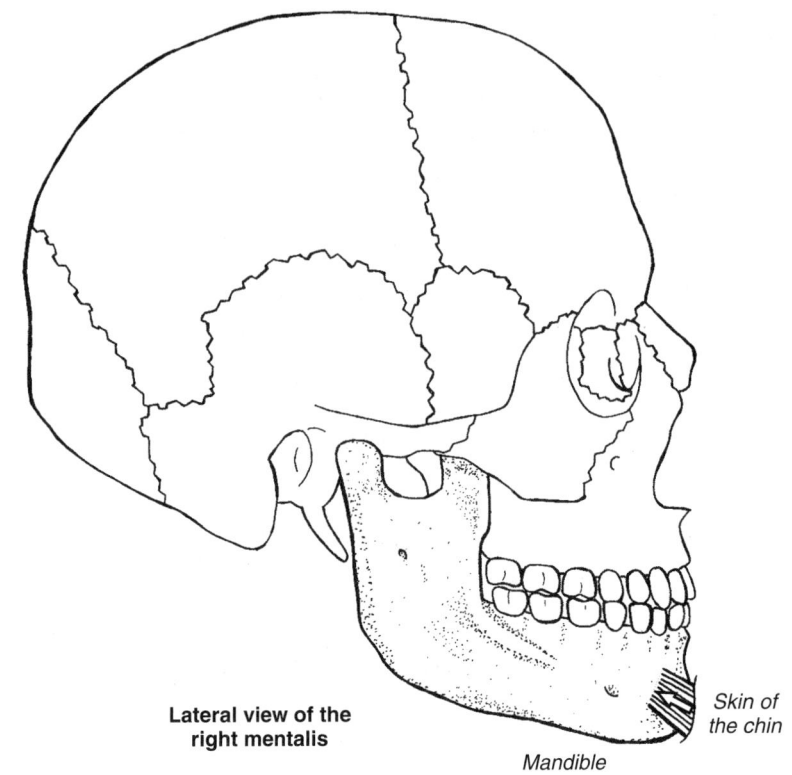

Lateral view of the right mentalis

BUCCINATOR
buk-sin-a-tor

Action
Compresses the cheeks (against the teeth)

Innervation
The facial nerve (CN VII)

Arterial Supply
The maxillary and facial arteries

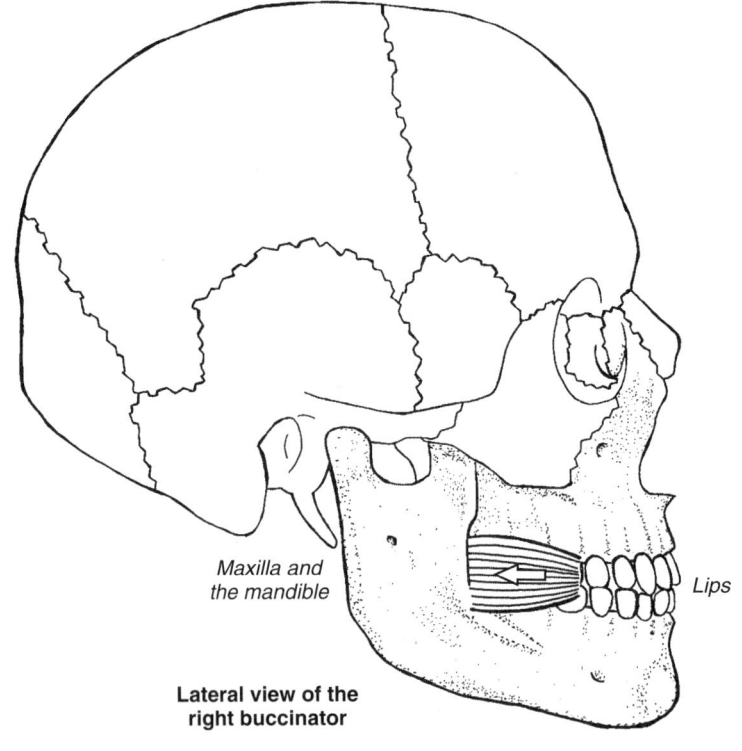

Lateral view of the right buccinator

THE MUSCULAR SYSTEM Muscles of the Head

Strong contraction of the mentalis muscles can make the lower lip stick out, creating the facial expression of pouting.

Contraction of the buccinator muscles is necessary for whistling, blowing up a balloon, and blowing into a brass or woodwind instrument.

ORBICULARIS ORIS
or-**bik**-you-**la**-ris **o**-ris

The orbicularis oris encircling the mouth

Anterior view of the orbicularis oris

Actions	**Innervation**	**Arterial Supply**
Closes the mouth Protracts the lips	The facial nerve (CN VII)	The facial artery

THE MUSCULAR SYSTEM — Muscles of the Head

THE MUSCULAR SYSTEM Muscles of the Head

Contraction of the orbicularis oris causes the lips to close and protrude as in puckering the lips or whistling.

TEMPORALIS
tem-po-**ra**-lis

Actions
Elevates the mandible at the temporomandibular joints

Retracts the mandible at the temporomandibular joints

Innervation
The trigeminal nerve (CN V)

Arterial Supply
The maxillary and superficial temporal arteries

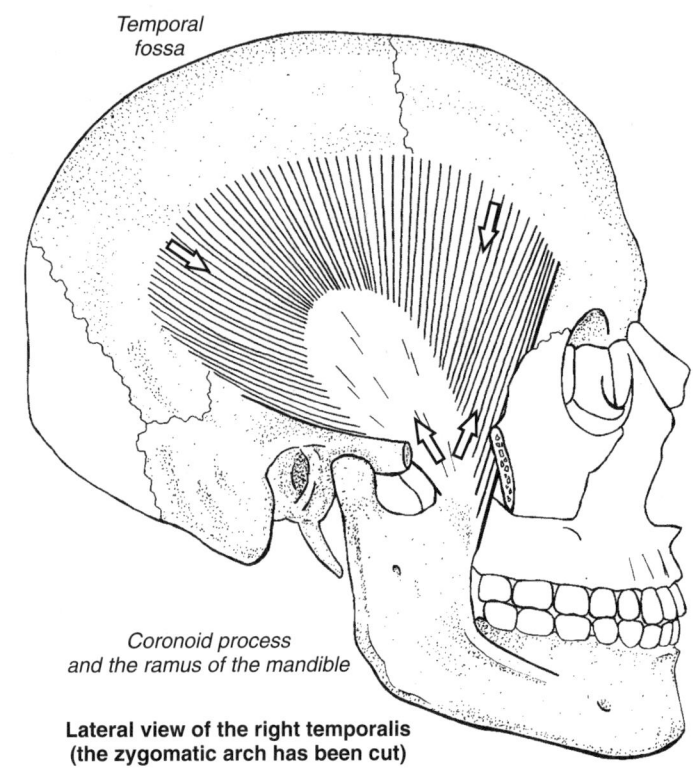

Lateral view of the right temporalis (the zygomatic arch has been cut)

MASSETER
ma-sa-ter

Actions
Elevates the mandible at the temporomandibular joints

Protracts the mandible at the temporomandibular joints

Retracts the mandible at the temporomandibular joints

Innervation
The trigeminal nerve (CN V)

Arterial Supply
The maxillary artery

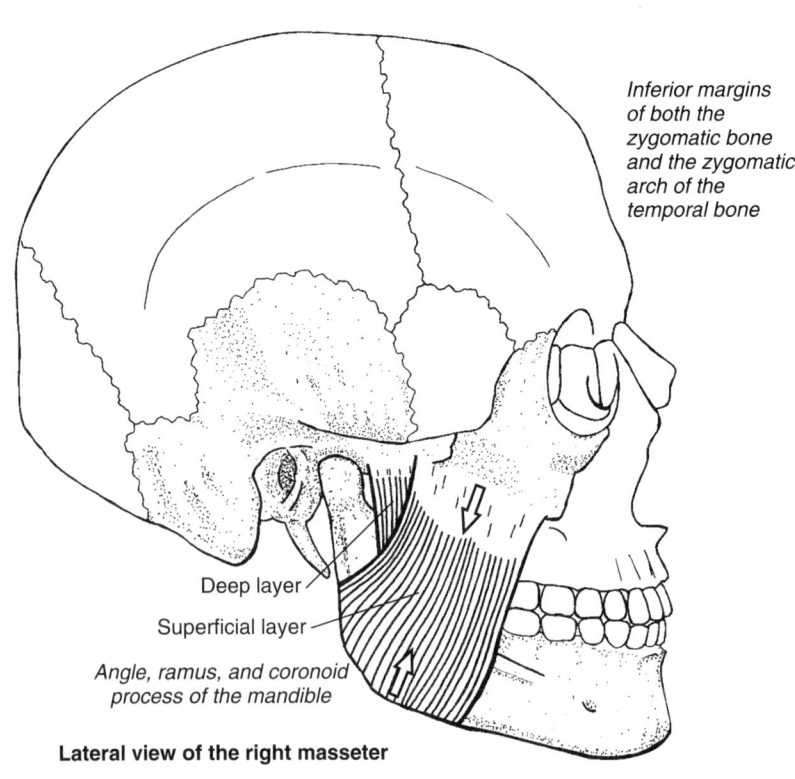

Lateral view of the right masseter

THE MUSCULAR SYSTEM Muscles of the Head

DID YOU KNOW

The temporalis is often involved in tension headaches and temporomandibular joint (TMJ) dysfunction.

Masseter

(Masseter not shown in this view)

DID YOU KNOW

Proportional to its size, the masseter is considered to be the strongest muscle in the human body.

LATERAL PTERYGOID
lat-er-al ter-i-goyd

Actions
Protracts the mandible at the temporomandibular joints
Contralaterally deviates the mandible at the temporomandibular joints

Innervation
The trigeminal nerve (CN V)

Arterial Supply
The maxillary artery

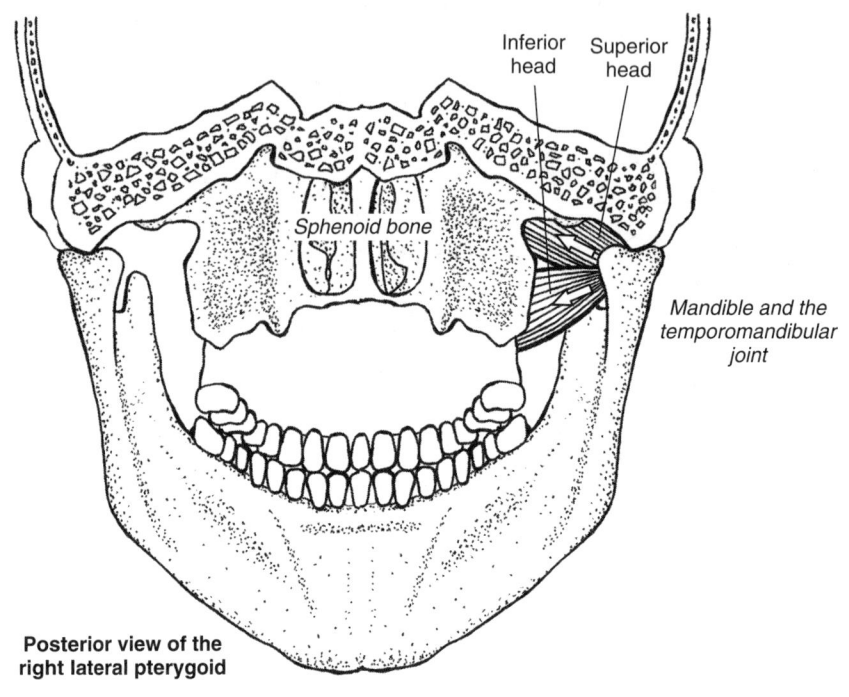

Posterior view of the right lateral pterygoid

MEDIAL PTERYGOID
mee-dee-al ter-i-goyd

Actions
Elevates the mandible at the temporomandibular joints
Protracts the mandible at the temporomandibular joints
Contralaterally deviates the mandible at the temporomandibular joints

Innervation
The trigeminal nerve (CN V)

Arterial Supply
The maxillary artery

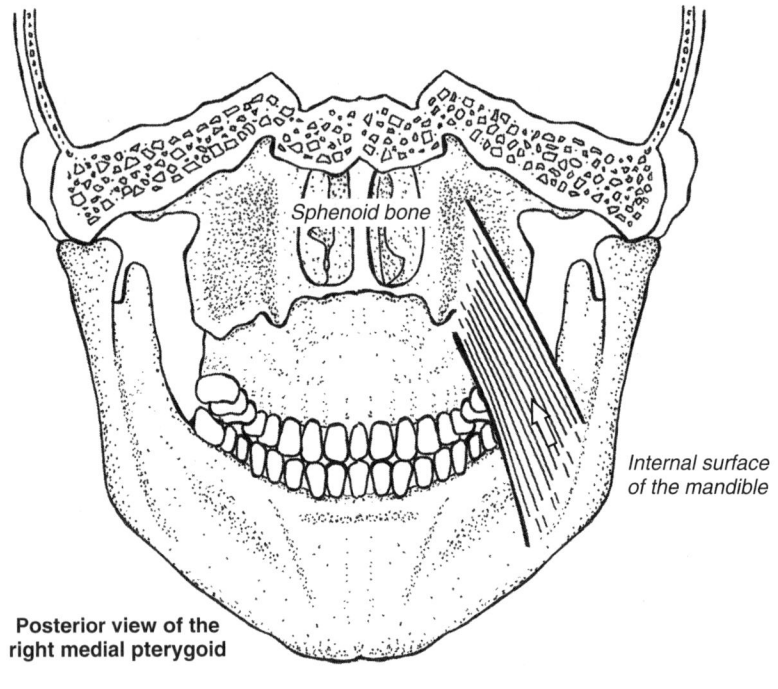

Posterior view of the right medial pterygoid

THE MUSCULAR SYSTEM: Muscles of the Head

 DID YOU KNOW?

The lateral pterygoid has an attachment directly into the capsule and articular disc of the TMJ, making this muscle likely to be involved in TMJ dysfunction.

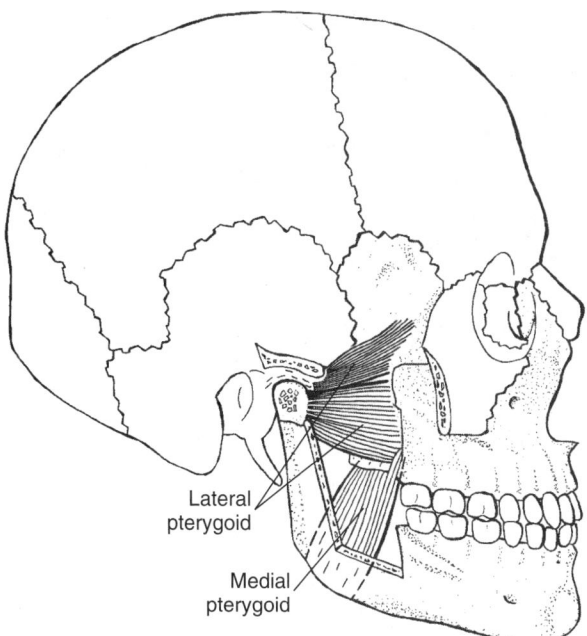

(The mandible has been partially cut away.)

 DID YOU KNOW?

The direction of fibers of the medial pterygoid is essentially identical to the masseter, except that the medial pterygoid is deep to the mandible and the masseter is superficial to the mandible.

60 THE MUSCULAR SYSTEM Muscles of the Head

ANTERIOR VIEW OF THE HEAD

Answers to labeling exercises are on p. 463.

THE MUSCULAR SYSTEM Muscles of the Head 61

LATERAL VIEW OF THE HEAD

Review Questions

Muscles of the Head
Answers to these questions are found on page 463.

1. What muscle of mastication has attachments directly into the capsule and articular disc of the temporomandibular joint?

2. Where is the temporalis relative to the zygomatic arch of the temporal bone?

3. What muscle of facial expression is primarily responsible for making the expression of pouting?

4. What muscles comprise the epicranius?

5. How many muscles of facial expression elevate the angle of the mouth?

6. Where they overlap, which muscle is deeper, the depressor anguli oris or the depressor labii inferioris?

7. What muscle lies medial to the levator labii superioris?

8. How are the depressor labii inferioris and mentalis antagonistic to each other?

9. What muscle of the mouth and nose lies medial and inferior to the orbicularis oculi?

10. What two muscles evert the lower lip?

11. How many muscles of facial expression elevate the upper lip?

12. Which scalp muscle is likely most involved with tension headaches?

13. What happens to the length of the right lateral pterygoid if the mandible laterally deviates to the right?

14. What muscle is located immediately inferior to the orbicularis oris?

15. What three muscles elevate the mandible at the temporomandibular joint?

16. How is the levator anguli oris synergistic with the zygomaticus major?

17. What muscle is synergistic with the nasalis?

18. Where they overlap, which muscle is superficial, the temporalis or the masseter?

19. What muscle helps to close the mouth by bringing the lips together without moving the mandible?

20. What are the two bellies of the occipitofrontalis?

21. How are the lateral and medial pterygoids synergistic with each other?

22. What muscle is immediately inferior to the occipitalis toward the midline of the head?

23. How are the digastric and temporalis antagonistic to each other?

24. What muscle is antagonistic to the nasalis?

25. Into what muscle of the nose does the frontalis blend?

26. How is the risorius synergistic with the zygomaticus major?

More review activities on Evolve at http://evolve.elsevier.com/Muscolino/muscular/

THE MUSCULAR SYSTEM Muscles of the Head

27. What two muscles are synergistic with both actions of the levator labii superioris?

28. The procerus lies superior to what muscle?

29. What is the name of the sheet of fascia that connects the frontalis with the occipitalis?

30. What muscle is antagonistic to the auricularis anterior?

31. What two muscles are immediately superior to the orbicularis oculi?

32. What muscle is antagonistic to the corrugator supercilii?

33. What muscle lies lateral to the levator labii superioris?

34. What muscle's superior attachment is located deep to the zygomaticus minor?

35. What muscle of facial expression creates the typical "Dracula" expression?

36. What muscle is immediately deep to the lateral attachment of the risorius?

37. What muscle attaches to the angle of the mouth and is located inferiorly to the risorius?

38. How are the depressor labii inferioris and mentalis synergistic with each other?

39. What two muscles are located immediately lateral to the orbicularis oris?

40. The depressor anguli oris and depressor labii inferioris both attach into what bone?

41. What muscle is synergistic with the corrugator supercilii?

42. What muscle is a muscle of facial expression of the mouth and nose?

43. What three muscles elevate the upper lip?

44. Which muscle is deeper, the temporoparietalis or the temporalis?

45. What muscle closes and squints the eye?

46. Where they overlap, which muscle is deeper, the depressor labii inferioris or the mentalis?

47. Which muscle is more medial, the zygomaticus major or minor?

48. What muscle of facial expression is primarily used when whistling?

49. What happens to the length of the orbicularis oris when the lips are puckered?

50. What are the two parts of the nasalis?

51. What two muscles lie superficial to the buccinator?

52. What muscle lies superior to the levator labii superioris?

53. What two muscles elevate the ear?

54. What muscle is located immediately medial to the zygomaticus minor?

55. What are the four major muscles of mastication?

56. What is similar and different about the orientation of the masseter and medial pterygoid?

57. What muscle lies immediately lateral to the nasalis?

58. The majority of the corrugator supercilii lies deep to what muscle?

59. What muscle of the nose attaches into only skin and fascia?

60. Name the auricularis muscles.

61. What muscle is superficial to the mentalis?

62. What muscle is located immediately superior to the orbicularis oris at the midline?

63. What muscle of the face is a sphincter muscle?

64. What muscle of facial expression is primarily used when blowing up a balloon?

65. What muscle is immediately inferior to the depressor septi nasi?

66. Which auricularis muscle attaches into the Galea aponeurotica?

67. What muscle of facial expression lies primarily within the eye socket?

68. What muscle of mastication attaches to the internal surface of the angle of the mandible?

69. What does the name *risorius* mean in Latin?

70. What muscle is antagonistic to the levator palpebrae superioris?

71. What action does the occipitofrontalis have upon the eyebrow?

72. Where they overlap, what is the relationship of the auricularis muscles to the temporalis?

73. What five muscles of facial expression attach into the mandible?

74. What happens to the length of the depressor anguli oris if the angle of the mouth is elevated?

75. The name of what facial muscle is derived from the Latin word for prince?

76. What happens to the length of the temporalis when the mandible depresses at the temporomandibular joints?

77. What muscle attaches between the two parts of the nasalis?

78. How many muscles of facial expression draw laterally the angle of the mouth?

THE MUSCULAR SYSTEM — Muscles of the Neck

ANTERIOR VIEW OF THE NECK (SUPERFICIAL)

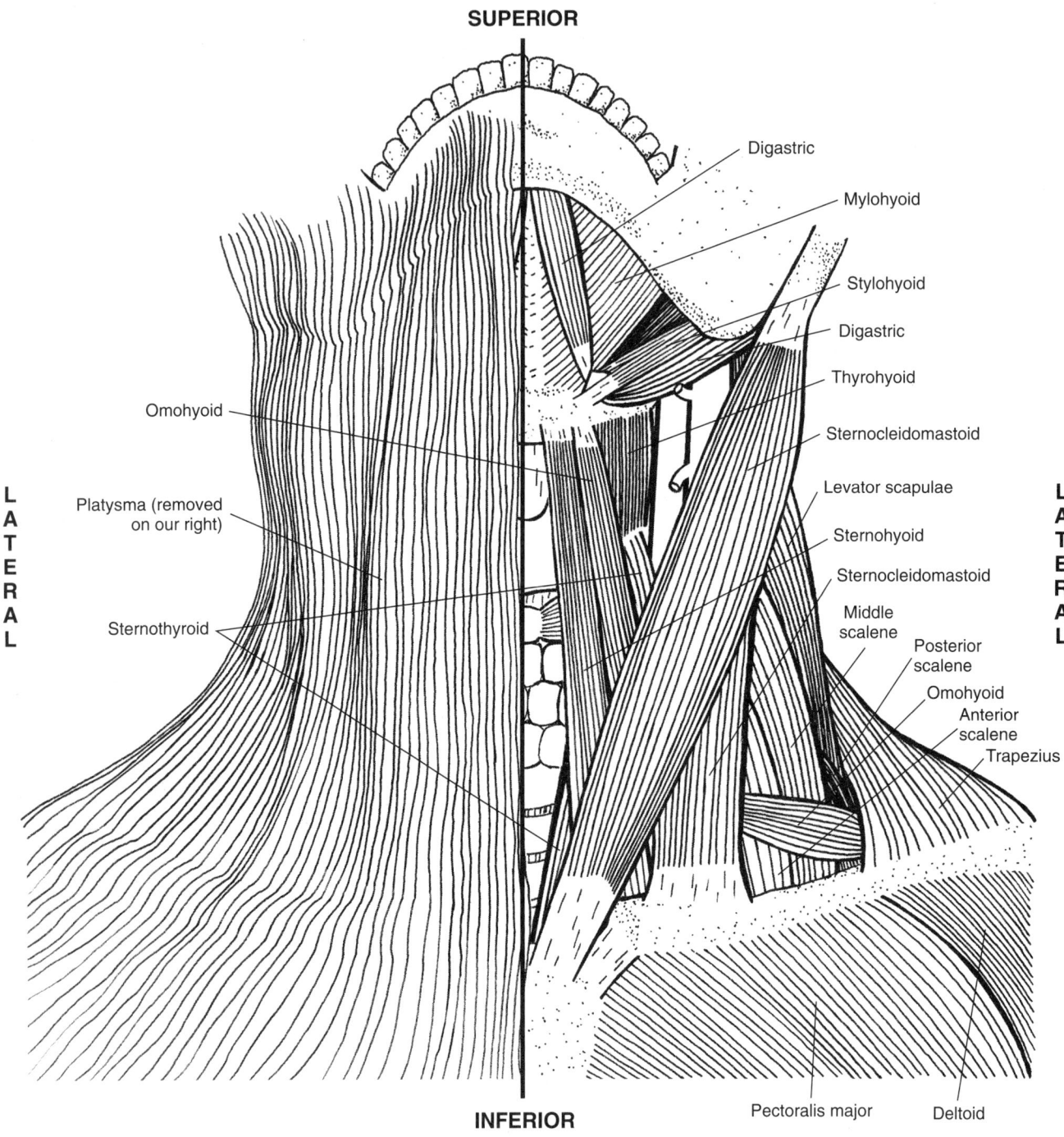

THE MUSCULAR SYSTEM Muscles of the Neck

ANTERIOR VIEW OF THE NECK (INTERMEDIATE)

ANTERIOR VIEW OF THE NECK (DEEP)

THE MUSCULAR SYSTEM Muscles of the Neck

LATERAL VIEW OF THE NECK

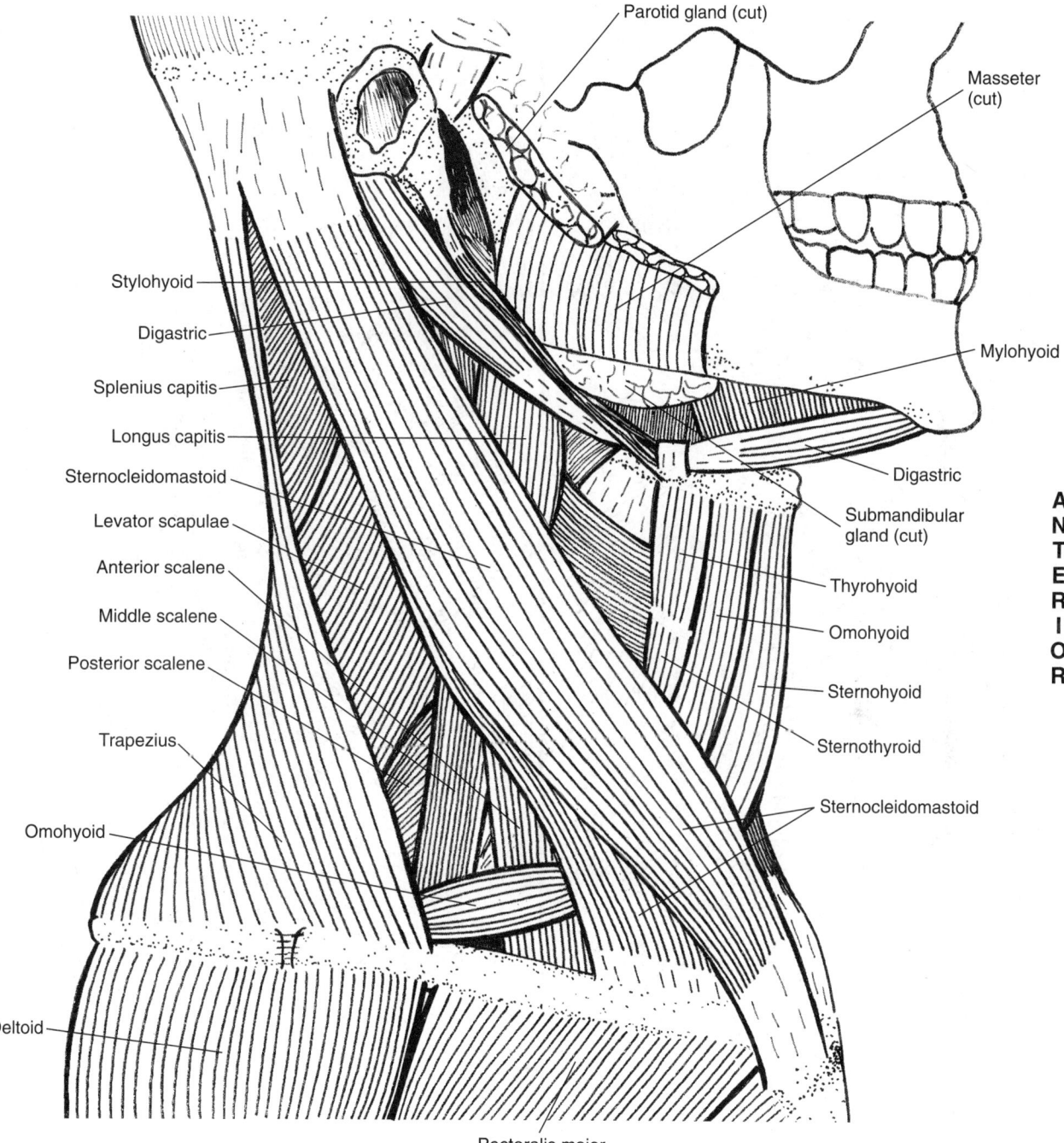

THE MUSCULAR SYSTEM — Muscles of the Neck

POSTERIOR VIEW OF THE NECK (SUPERFICIAL AND INTERMEDIATE)

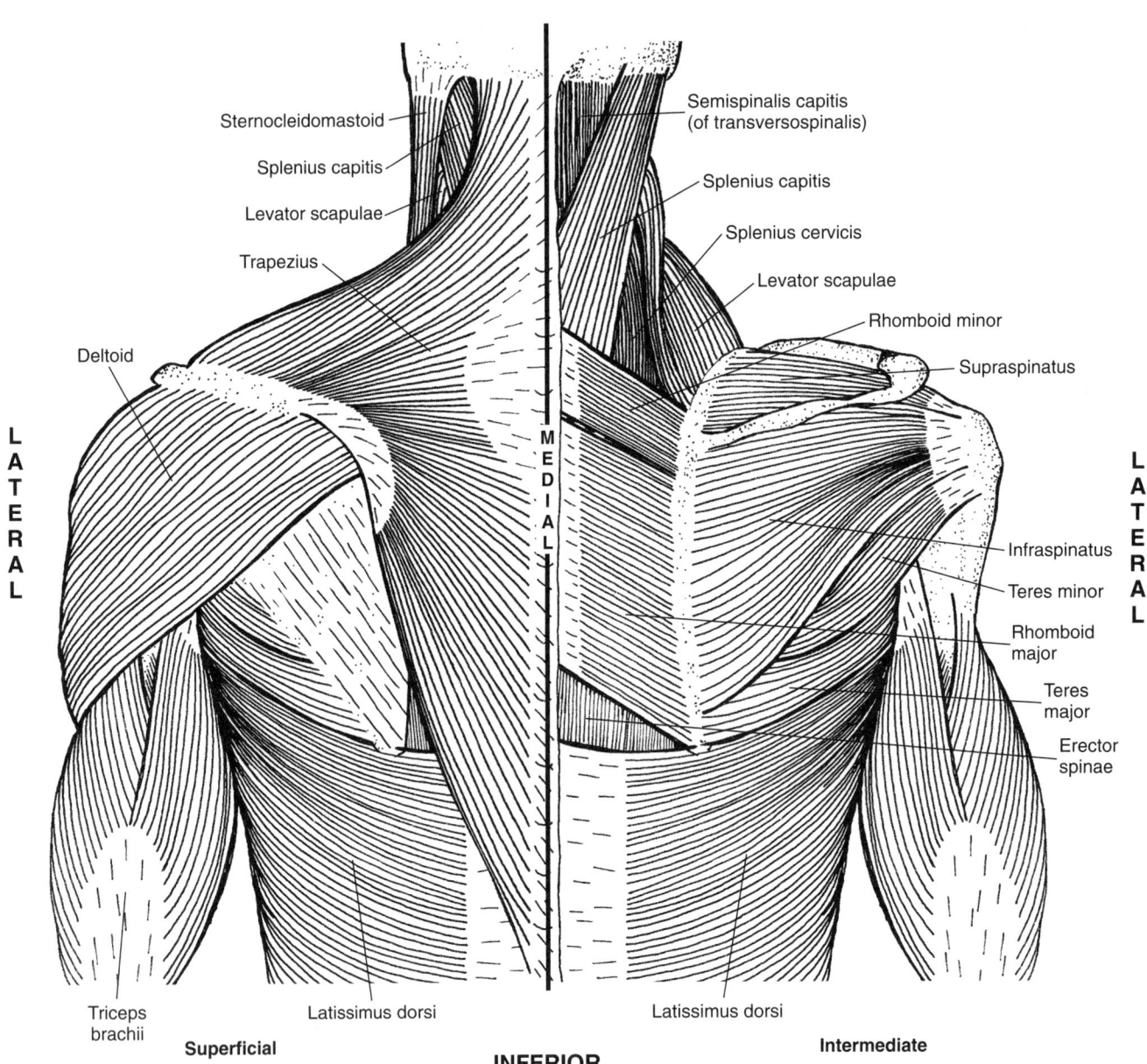

THE MUSCULAR SYSTEM Muscles of the Neck

POSTERIOR VIEW OF THE NECK (INTERMEDIATE AND DEEP)

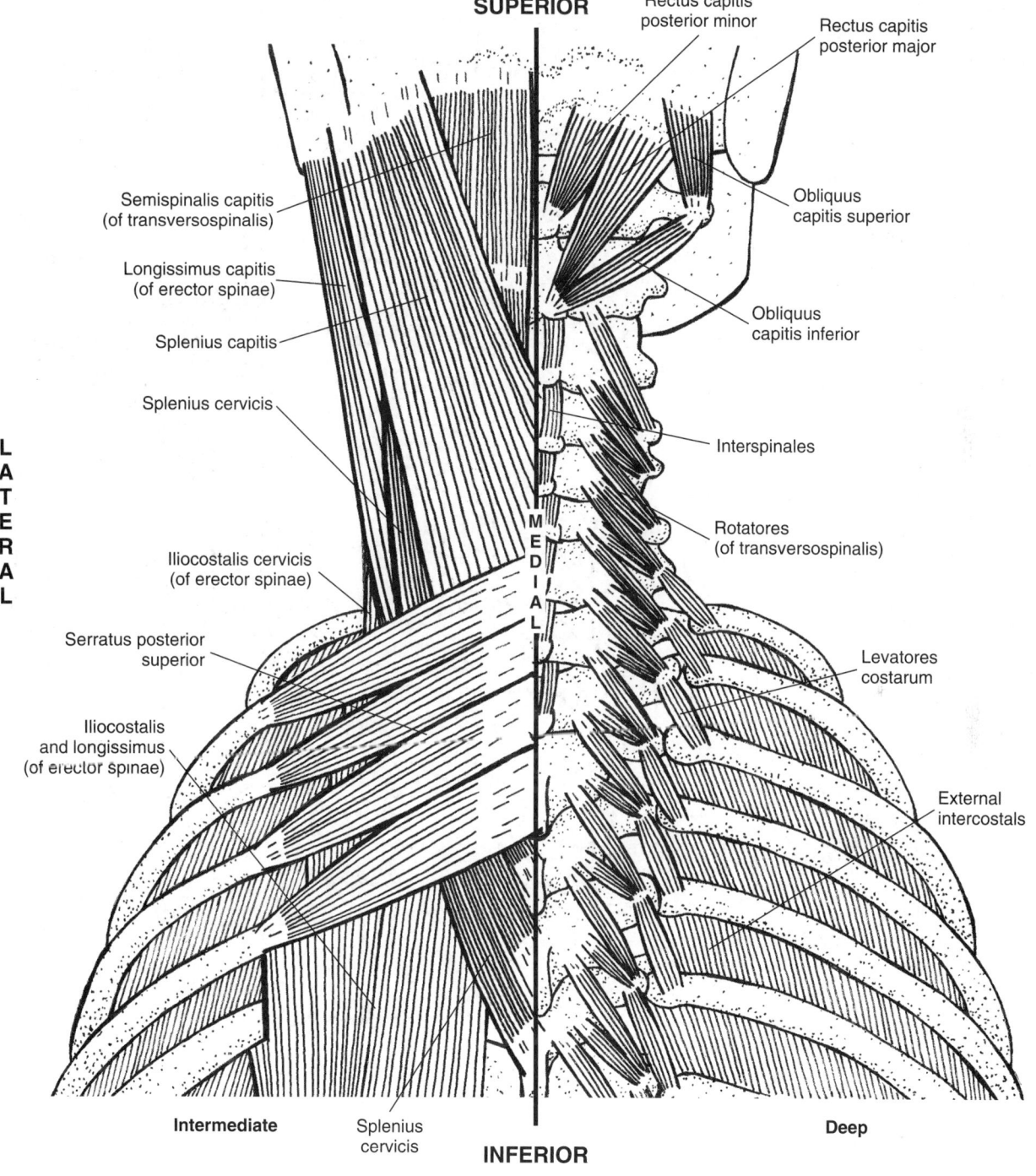

TRAPEZIUS ("TRAP")
tra-**pee**-zee-us

Actions
Lateral flexion of the neck and the head at the spinal joints (upper)
Extension of the neck and the head at the spinal joints (upper)
Contralateral rotation of the neck and the head at the spinal joints (upper)
Elevation of the scapula at the scapulocostal joint (upper)
Retraction (adduction) of the scapula at the scapulocostal joint (entire muscle)
Depression of the scapula at the scapulocostal joint (lower)
Upward rotation of the scapula at the scapulocostal joint (upper and lower)
Extension of the trunk at the spinal joints (middle and lower)

Innervation
Spinal accessory nerve (CN XI)

Arterial Supply
The transverse cervical artery and the dorsal scapular artery

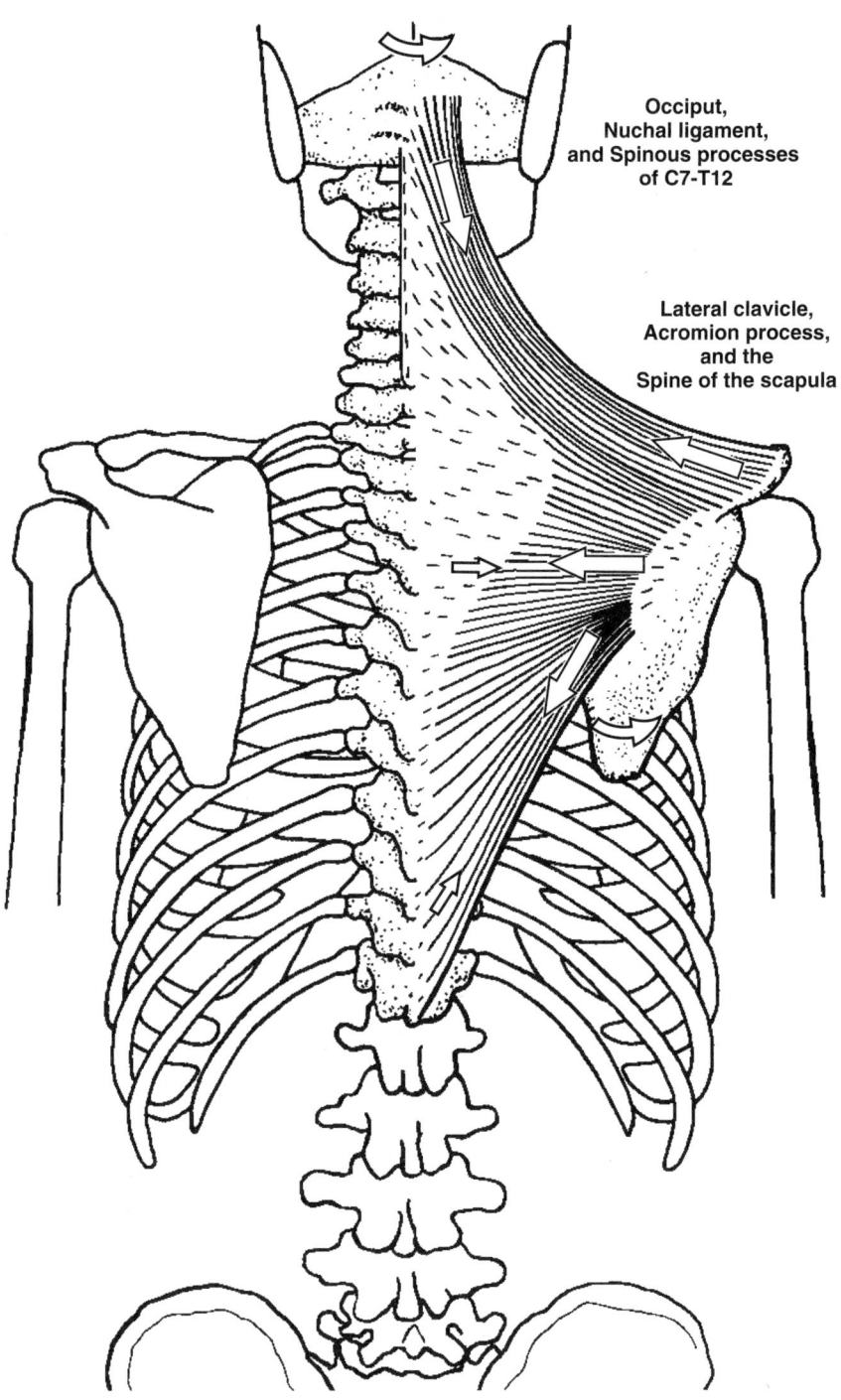

Occiput, Nuchal ligament, and Spinous processes of C7-T12

Lateral clavicle, Acromion process, and the Spine of the scapula

Posterior view of the right trapezius

THE MUSCULAR SYSTEM Muscles of the Neck

The trapezius is considered to have three functional parts: upper, middle, and lower. This muscle is extremely important as it is involved in both postural stabilization and active movement of the head, neck, trunk, and shoulder girdle.

SPLENIUS CAPITIS
splee-nee-us **kap**-i-tis

Actions
Extension of the head and the neck at the spinal joints
Lateral flexion of the head and the neck at the spinal joints
Ipsilateral rotation of the head and the neck at the spinal joints

Innervation
Cervical spinal nerves

Arterial Supply
The occipital artery

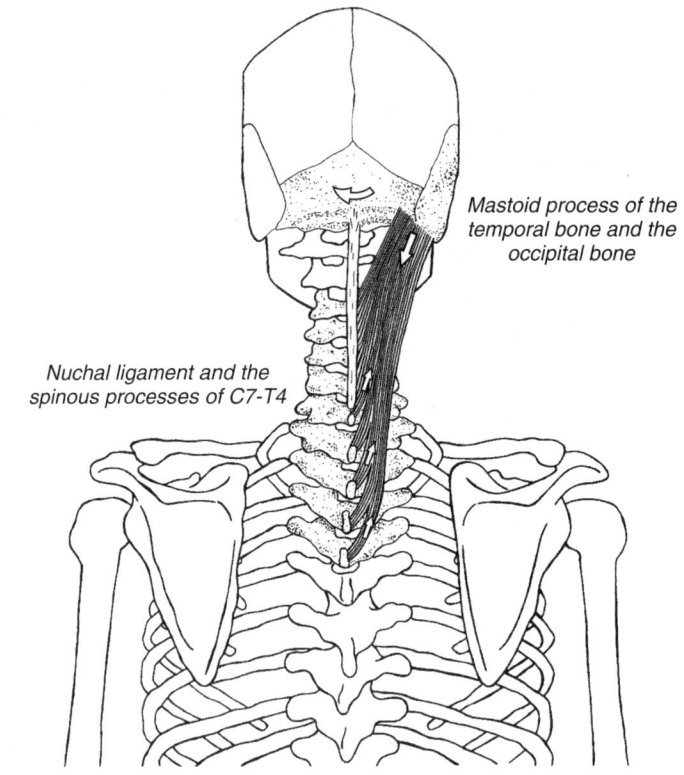

Mastoid process of the temporal bone and the occipital bone

Nuchal ligament and the spinous processes of C7-T4

Posterior view of the right splenius capitis

SPLENIUS CERVICIS
splee-nee-us **ser**-vi-sis

Actions
Extension of the neck at the spinal joints
Lateral flexion of the neck at the spinal joints
Ipsilateral rotation of the neck at the spinal joints

Innervation
Cervical spinal nerves

Arterial Supply
The occipital artery and the dorsal branches of the upper posterior intercostal arteries

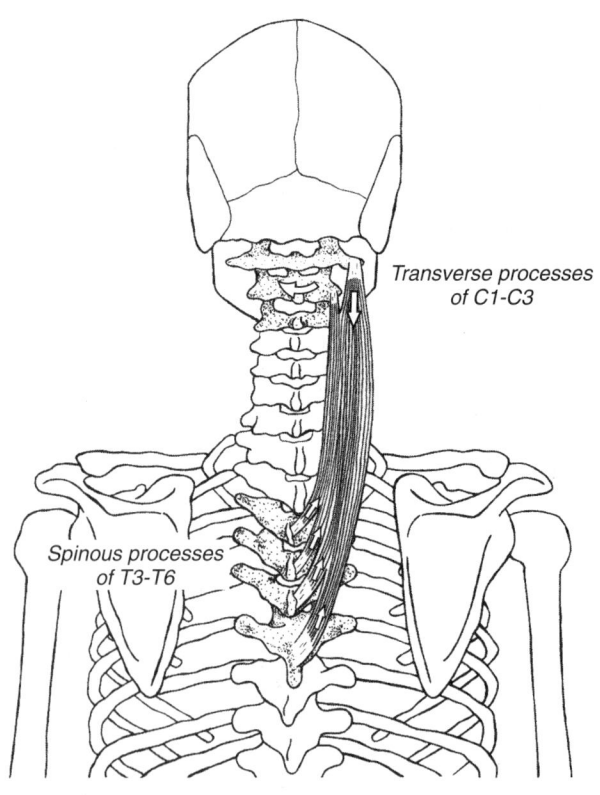

Transverse processes of C1-C3

Spinous processes of T3-T6

Posterior view of the right splenius cervicis

THE MUSCULAR SYSTEM Muscles of the Neck

Because of their "V" shape, the left and right splenius capitis muscles are sometimes called the "golf tee" muscles.

The left and right splenius cervicis muscles also form a "V" shape.

LEVATOR SCAPULAE
le-**vay**-tor **skap**-you-lee

Actions
Elevation of the scapula at the scapulocostal joint
Extension of the neck at the spinal joints
Lateral flexion of the neck at the spinal joints
Ipsilateral rotation of the neck at the spinal joints
Downward rotation of the scapula at the scapulocostal joint
Retraction (adduction) of the scapula at the scapulocostal joint

Innervation
Dorsal scapular nerve

Arterial Supply
The dorsal scapular artery

Transverse processes of C1-C4

Medial border of the scapula, from the superior angle to the root of the spine of the scapula

Posterior view of the right levator scapulae

THE MUSCULAR SYSTEM Muscles of the Neck

The levator scapulae has a twist in its fibers so that the most superior fibers on the scapula attach the most inferiorly on the spine, and vice versa.

RECTUS CAPITIS POSTERIOR MAJOR
(OF THE SUBOCCIPITAL GROUP)

rek-tus kap-i-tis pos-tee-ri-or may-jor

Actions
Extension of the head at the atlanto-occipital joint
Lateral flexion of the head at the atlanto-occipital joint
Ipsilateral rotation of the head at the atlanto-occipital joint
Extension and ipsilateral rotation of the atlas at the atlantoaxial joint

Innervation
The suboccipital nerve

Arterial Supply
The occipital artery and the deep cervical artery

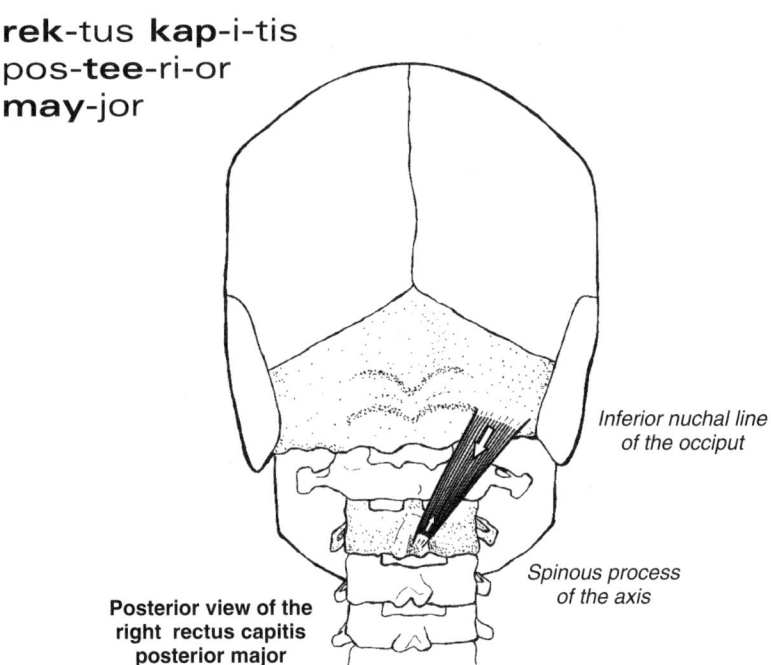

Posterior view of the right rectus capitis posterior major

- Inferior nuchal line of the occiput
- Spinous process of the axis

RECTUS CAPITIS POSTERIOR MINOR
(OF THE SUBOCCIPITAL GROUP)

rek-tus kap-i-tis pos-tee-ri-or my-nor

Action
Protraction of the head at the atlanto-occipital joint
Extension of the head at the atlanto-occipital joint

Innervation
The suboccipital nerve

Arterial Supply
The occipital artery and muscular branches of the vertebral artery

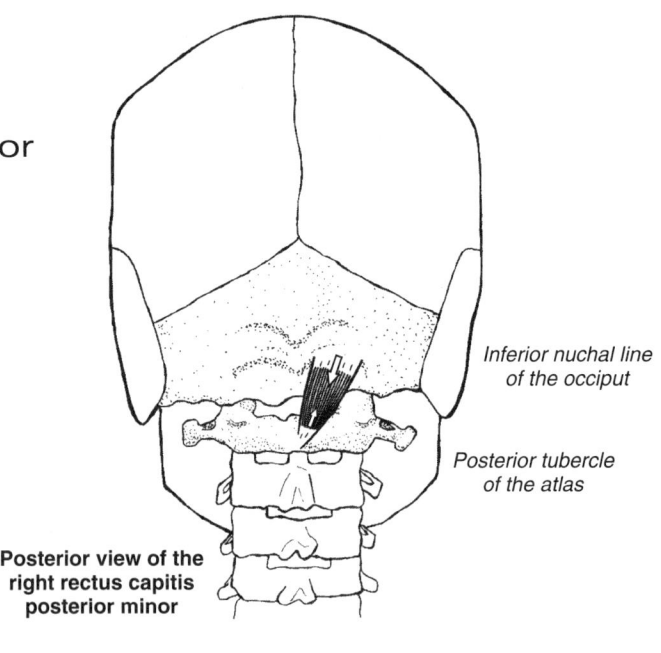

Posterior view of the right rectus capitis posterior minor

- Inferior nuchal line of the occiput
- Posterior tubercle of the atlas

THE MUSCULAR SYSTEM Muscles of the Neck

DID YOU KNOW

The rectus capitis posterior major is the largest of the suboccipital group. The suboccipital group is primarily important as the postural stabilizer of the head.

DID YOU KNOW

The rectus capitis posterior minor has an additional attachment that asserts its pull into the dura mater, making this muscle extremely likely to cause headaches when it is tight.

OBLIQUUS CAPITIS INFERIOR
(OF THE SUBOCCIPITAL GROUP)
ob-**lee**-kwus **kap**-i-tis in-**fee**-ri-or

Action
Ipsilateral rotation of the atlas at the atlantoaxial joint

Innervation
The suboccipital nerve

Arterial Supply
The deep cervical artery and the descending branch of the occipital artery

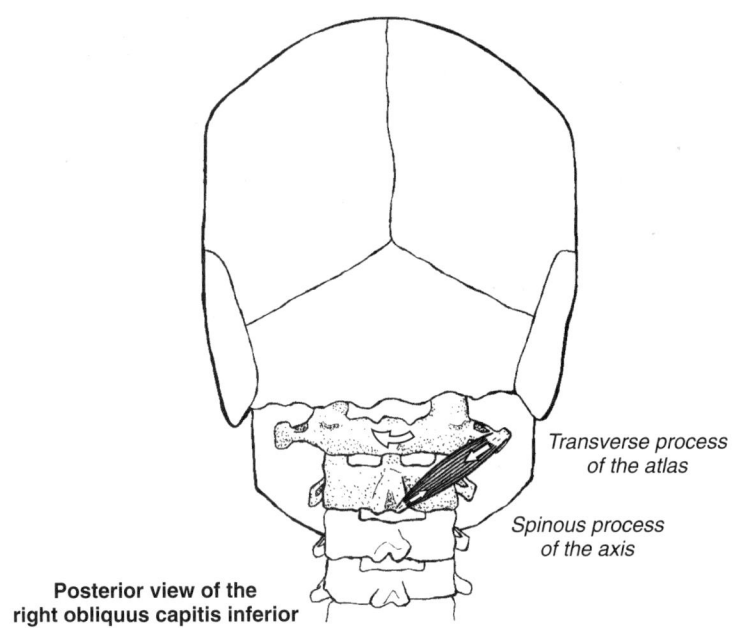

Posterior view of the right obliquus capitis inferior

OBLIQUUS CAPITIS SUPERIOR
(OF THE SUBOCCIPITAL GROUP)
ob-**lee**-kwus **kap**-i-tis sue-**pee**-ri-or

Actions
Protraction of the head at the atlanto-occipital joint
Extension of the head at the atlanto-occipital joint
Lateral flexion of the head at the atlanto-occipital joint

Innervation
The suboccipital nerve

Arterial Supply
The occipital artery and the deep cervical artery

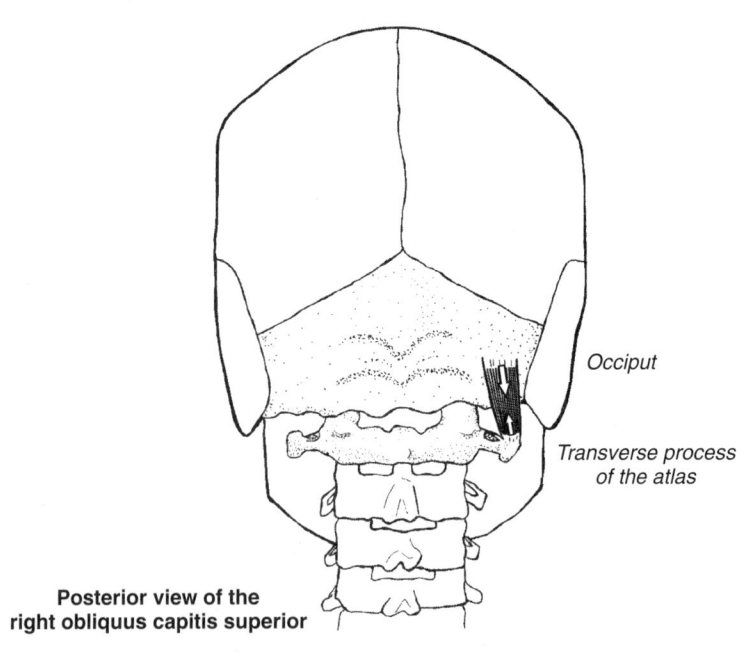

Posterior view of the right obliquus capitis superior

THE MUSCULAR SYSTEM Muscles of the Neck   81

The obliquus capitis inferior is the only one of the four suboccipital muscles that does not cross the atlanto-occipital joint to attach onto the head; therefore its name is a misnomer.

Of the four suboccipital muscles, the obliquus capitis superior attaches the most superiorly on the occiput.

PLATYSMA
pla-**tiz**-ma

Actions
Draws up the skin of the superior chest and neck, creating ridges of skin in the neck
Depresses and draws the lower lip laterally
Depression of the mandible at the temporomandibular joint

Innervation
Facial nerve (CN VII)

Arterial Supply
The facial artery

Anterior view of the right platysma

THE MUSCULAR SYSTEM Muscles of the Neck   83

DID YOU KNOW?

The platysma creates wrinkles on the neck that are reminiscent of the creature from the film, The Creature from the Black Lagoon.

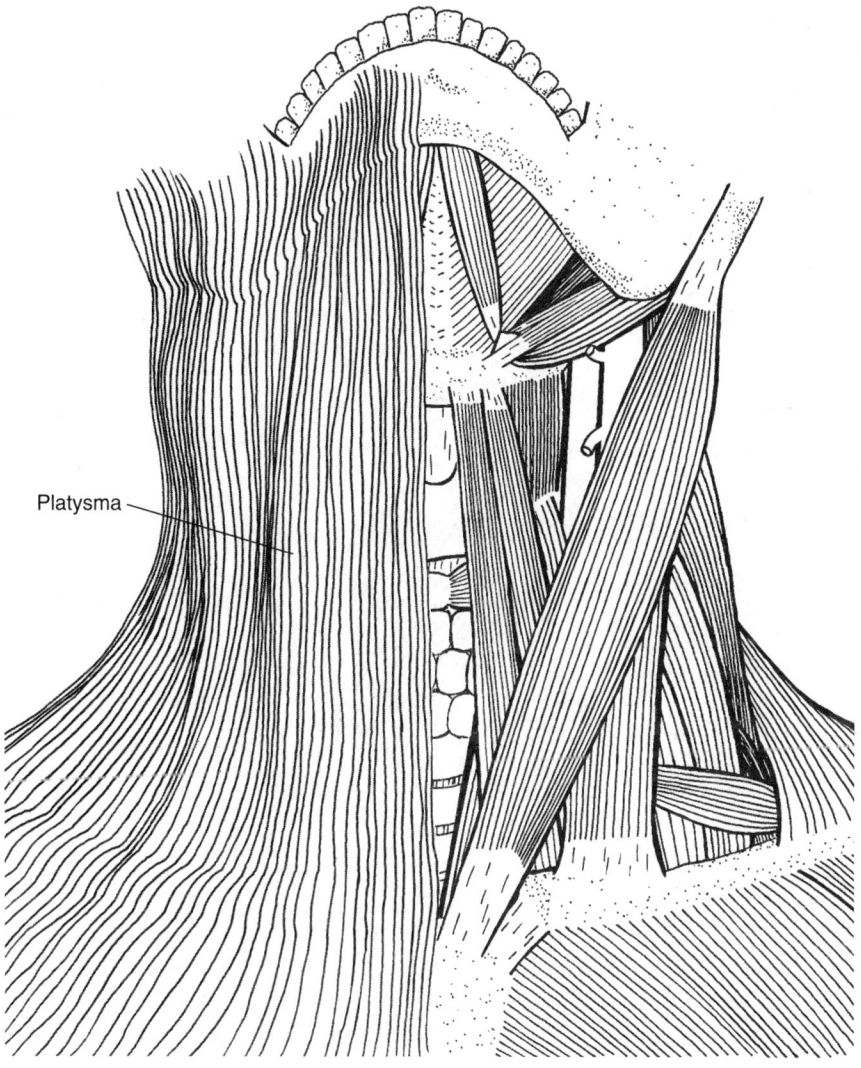

Platysma

STERNOCLEIDOMASTOID ("SCM")
ster-no-**kli**-do-**mas**-toyd

Actions
Flexion of the neck at the spinal joints
Lateral flexion of the neck and the head at the spinal joints
Contralateral rotation of the neck and the head at the spinal joints
Extension of the head at the atlanto-occipital joint
Elevation of the sternum and the clavicle

Innervation
Spinal accessory nerve (CN XI)

Arterial Supply
The occipital and posterior auricular arteries

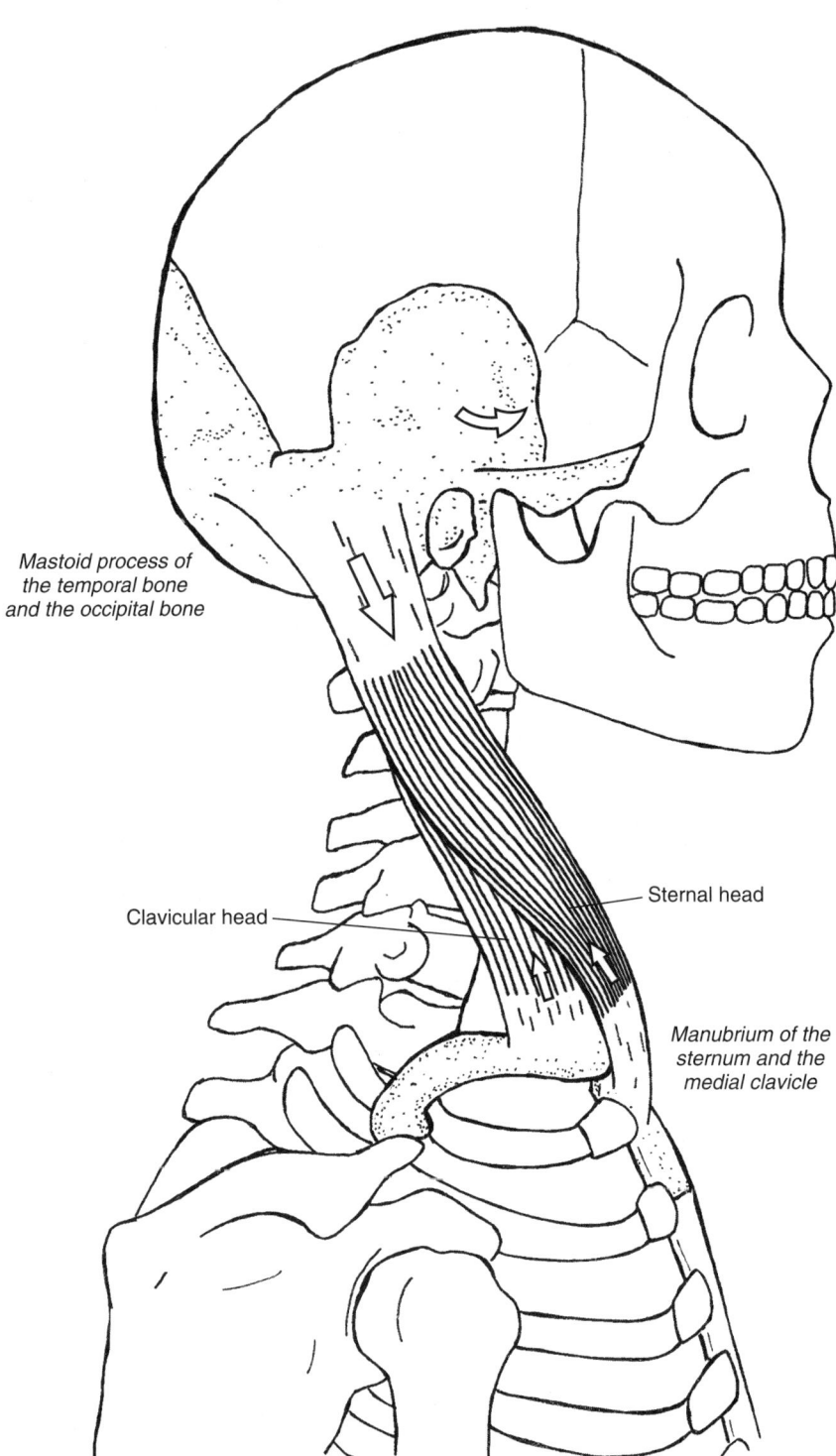

Mastoid process of the temporal bone and the occipital bone

Clavicular head — Sternal head

Manubrium of the sternum and the medial clavicle

Lateral view of the right sternocleidomastoid

THE MUSCULAR SYSTEM Muscles of the Neck

DID YOU KNOW

The sternocleidomastoid is unusual in that it flexes the neck at the spinal joints, but it extends the head at the atlanto-occipital joint.

Sternocleidomastoid

Sternocleidomastoid

Sternocleidomastoid

STERNOHYOID
(OF THE HYOID GROUP)

ster-no-**hi**-oyd

Action
Depression of the hyoid

Innervation
The cervical plexus

Arterial Supply
The superior thyroid artery

Anterior view of the right sternohyoid

STERNOTHYROID
(OF THE HYOID GROUP)

ster-no-**thi**-royd

Action
Depression of the thyroid cartilage

Innervation
The cervical plexus

Arterial Supply
The superior thyroid artery

Anterior view of the right sternothyroid

THE MUSCULAR SYSTEM Muscles of the Neck

The sternohyoid attaches to the posterior surface of both the manubrium of the sternum and the medial clavicle.

The sternothyroid attaches to the posterior surface of both the manubrium of the sternum and the costal cartilage of the 1st rib.

THYROHYOID
(OF THE HYOID GROUP)

thi-ro-hi-oyd

Actions
Depression of the hyoid
Elevation of the thyroid cartilage

Innervation
The hypoglossal nerve (CN XII)

Arterial Supply
The superior thyroid artery

Anterior view of the right thyrohyoid

OMOHYOID
(OF THE HYOID GROUP)

o-mo-hi-oyd

Action
Depression of the hyoid

Innervation
The cervical plexus

Arterial Supply
The superior thyroid artery and the transverse cervical artery

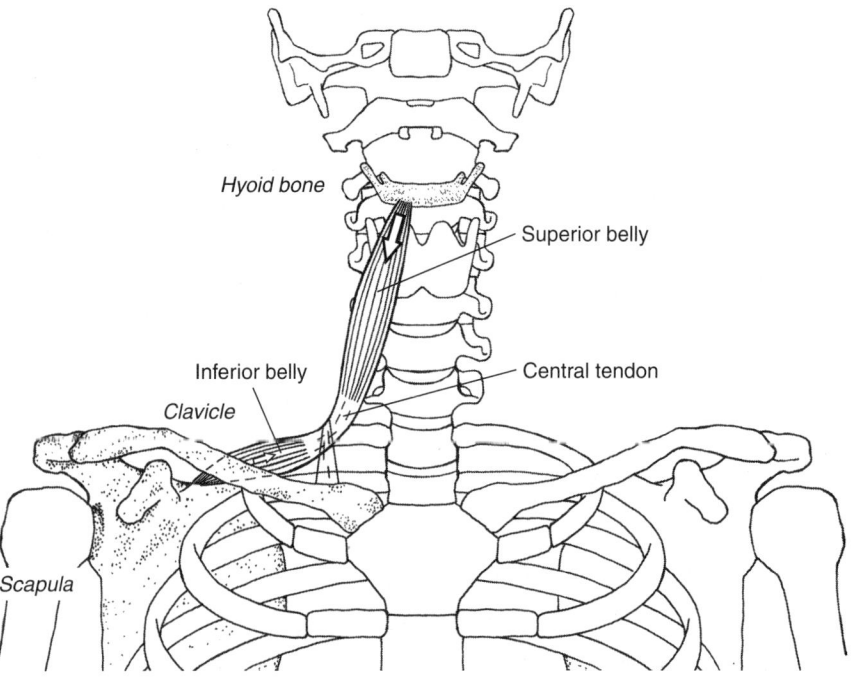

Anterior view of the right omohyoid

THE MUSCULAR SYSTEM Muscles of the Neck

The thyrohyoid can be considered to be an upward continuation of the sternothyroid muscle.

The omohyoid has two bellies separated by a central tendon that attaches to the clavicle by a fibrous sling of tissue.

DIGASTRIC
(OF THE HYOID GROUP)

di-**gas**-trik

Actions
Elevation of the hyoid
Depression of the mandible at the temporomandibular joints
Retraction of the mandible at the temporomandibular joints

Innervation
The trigeminal (CN V) and the facial nerve (CN VII)

Arterial Supply
The occipital, posterior auricular and facial arteries

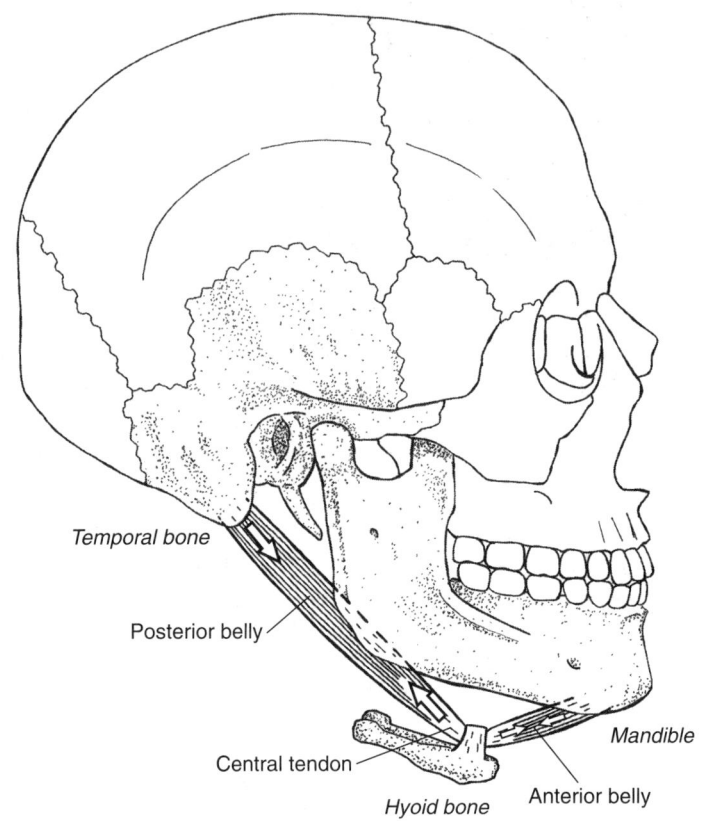

Lateral view of the right digastric

STYLOHYOID
(OF THE HYOID GROUP)

sti-lo-hi-oyd

Action
Elevation of the hyoid

Innervation
The facial nerve (CN VII)

Arterial Supply
The occipital, posterior auricular and facial arteries

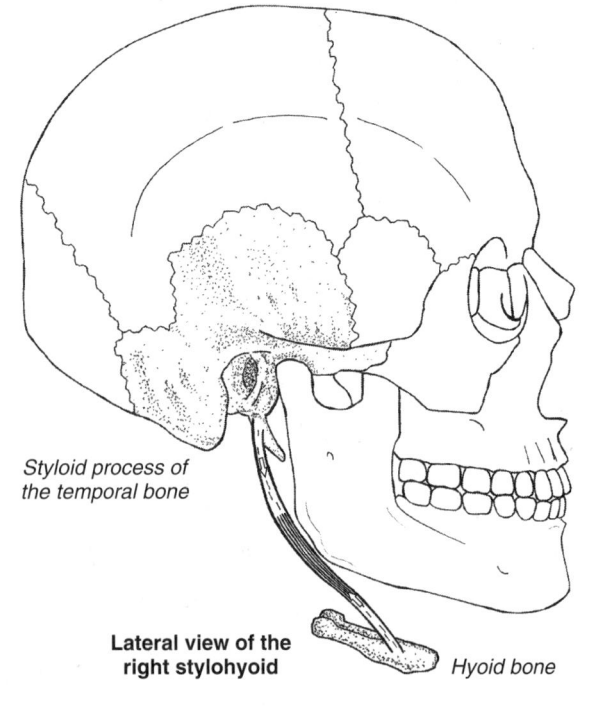

Lateral view of the right stylohyoid

THE MUSCULAR SYSTEM Muscles of the Neck   91

The digastric has two bellies that are separated by a central tendon that attaches to the hyoid bone by a fibrous sling of tissue. In fact, the name digastric means "two bellies" in Greek.

The attachment of the stylohyoid onto the hyoid bone is perforated by the central tendon of the digastric.

MYLOHYOID
(OF THE HYOID GROUP)

my-lo-**hi**-oyd

Actions
Elevation of the hyoid
Depression of the mandible at the temporomandibular joints

Innervation
The trigeminal nerve (CN V)

Arterial Supply
The inferior alveolar artery

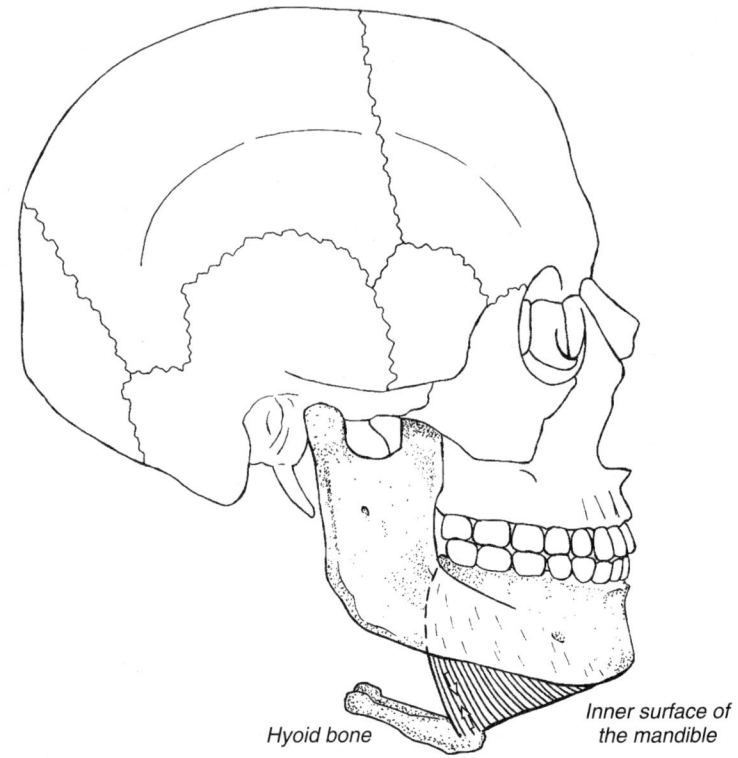

Hyoid bone — *Inner surface of the mandible*

Lateral view of the right mylohyoid

GENIOHYOID
(OF THE HYOID GROUP)

jee-nee-o-**hi**-oyd

Actions
Elevation of the hyoid
Depression of the mandible at the temporomandibular joints

Innervation
The hypoglossal nerve (CN XII)

Arterial Supply
The lingual artery

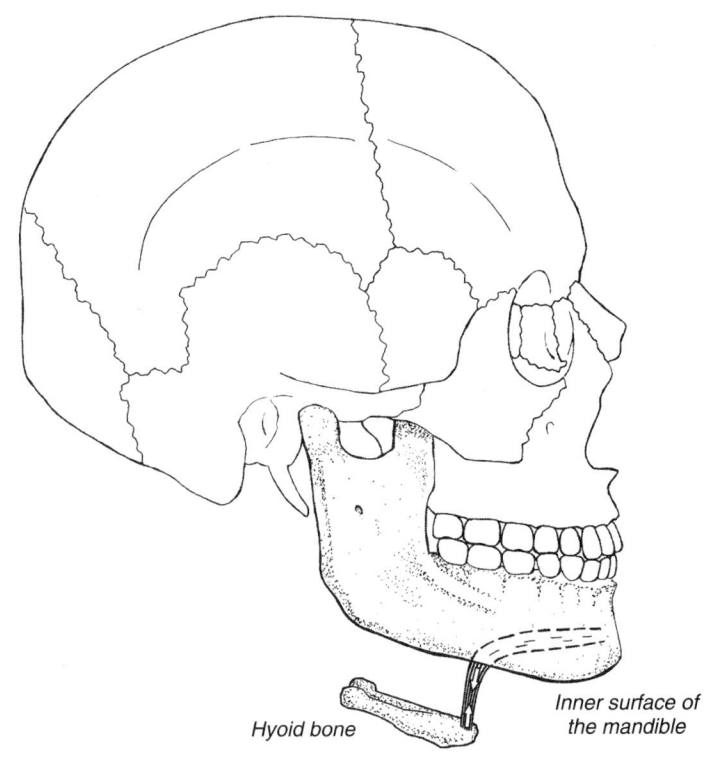

Hyoid bone — *Inner surface of the mandible*

Lateral view of the right geniohyoid

THE MUSCULAR SYSTEM Muscles of the Neck

Superior view of the floor of the mouth

> **DID YOU KNOW?**
> One function of the mylohyoid is to elevate the floor of the mouth during the first stage of swallowing.

> **DID YOU KNOW?**
> The geniohyoid muscles are two pencil-thin muscles located between the mylohyoids and the genioglossus muscles of the tongue.

ANTERIOR SCALENE
(OF THE SCALENE GROUP)

an-**tee**-ri-or **skay**-leen

Actions
Flexion of the neck at the spinal joints
Lateral flexion of the neck at the spinal joints
Elevation of the 1st rib at the sternocostal and costovertebral joints
Contralateral rotation of the neck at the spinal joints

Innervation
Cervical spinal nerves

Arterial Supply
The ascending cervical artery

Anterior view of the right anterior scalene

MIDDLE SCALENE
(OF THE SCALENE GROUP)

mi-dil **skay**-leen

Actions
Lateral flexion of the neck at the spinal joints
Flexion of the neck at the spinal joints
Elevation of the 1st rib at the sternocostal and costovertebral joints

Innervation
Cervical spinal nerves

Arterial Supply
The transverse cervical artery

Anterior view of the right middle scalene

THE MUSCULAR SYSTEM Muscles of the Neck   95

DID YOU KNOW?

The brachial plexus of nerves and subclavian artery run between the anterior and middle scalenes and can be compressed if these muscles are tight. When this occurs, it is called anterior scalene syndrome, a type of thoracic outlet syndrome.

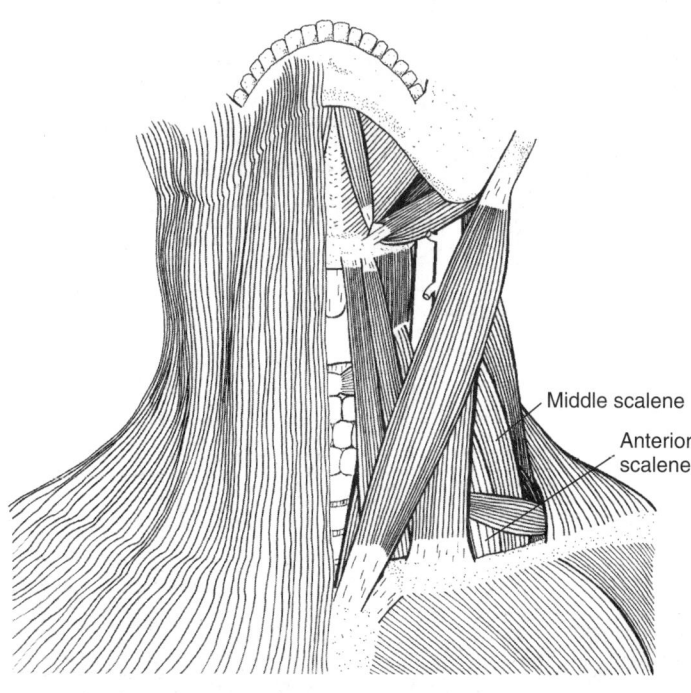

POSTERIOR SCALENE
(OF THE SCALENE GROUP)
pos-**tee**-ri-or **skay**-leen

Actions
Lateral flexion of the neck at the spinal joints
Elevation of the 2nd rib at the sternocostal and costovertebral joints

Innervation
Cervical spinal nerves

Arterial Supply
The transverse cervical artery

Transverse processes of the cervical spine

2nd rib

THE MUSCULAR SYSTEM Muscles of the Neck — 97

The posterior scalene is the smallest and shortest of the three scalenes.

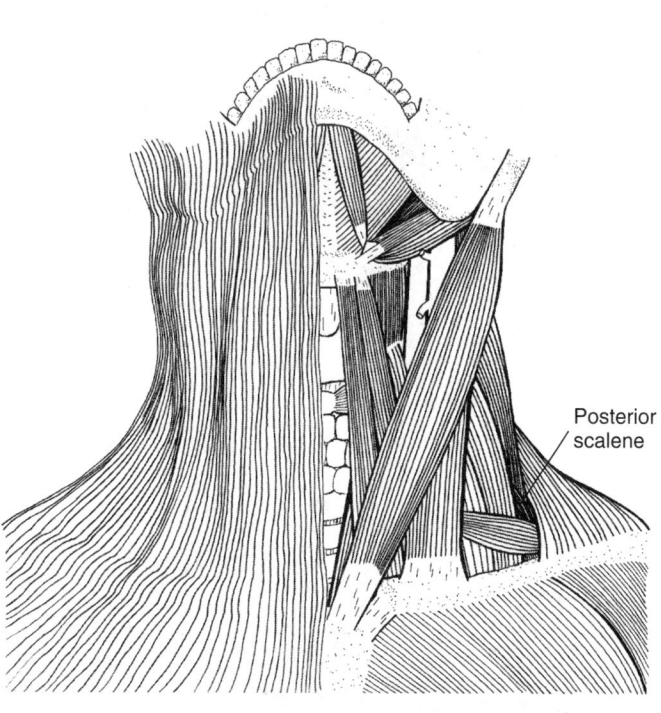

LONGUS COLLI
(OF THE PREVERTEBRAL GROUP)

long-us kol-eye

Actions
Flexion of the neck at the spinal joints
Lateral flexion of the neck at the spinal joints
Contralateral rotation of the neck at the spinal joints

Innervation
Cervical spinal nerves

Arterial Supply
The inferior thyroid artery and the vertebral artery

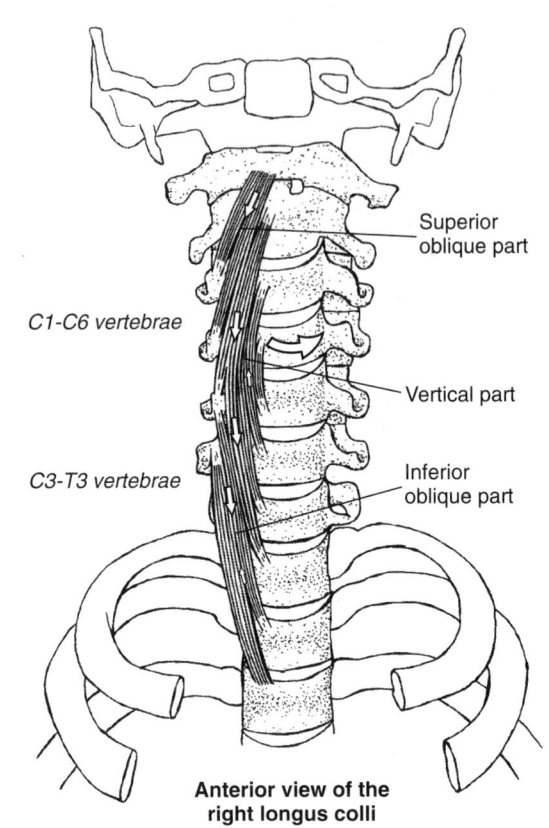

Anterior view of the right longus colli

LONGUS CAPITIS
(OF THE PREVERTEBRAL GROUP)

long-us kap-i-tis

Actions
Flexion of the head and the neck at the spinal joints
Lateral flexion of the head and the neck at the spinal joints

Innervation
Cervical spinal nerves

Arterial Supply
The inferior thyroid artery and the vertebral artery

Anterior view of the right longus capitis

THE MUSCULAR SYSTEM Muscles of the Neck

DID YOU KNOW

When the longus colli and longus capitis muscles are tight, it can hurt to swallow and feel like a sore throat.

RECTUS CAPITIS ANTERIOR
(OF THE PREVERTEBRAL GROUP)

rek-tus kap-i-tis an-tee-ri-or

Action
Flexion of the head at the atlanto-occipital joint

Innervation
Cervical spinal nerves

Arterial Supply
The vertebral artery

Anterior view of the right rectus capitis anterior

RECTUS CAPITIS LATERALIS
(OF THE PREVERTEBRAL GROUP)

rek-tus kap-i-tis la-ter-a-lis

Action
Lateral flexion of the head at the atlanto-occipital joint

Innervation
Cervical spinal nerves

Arterial Supply
The vertebral artery and the occipital artery

Anterior view of the right rectus capitis lateralis

THE MUSCULAR SYSTEM Muscles of the Neck

DID YOU KNOW?

The rectus capitis anterior and rectus capitis lateralis are generally considered to be more important as postural stabilization muscles of the head than as movers.

102 THE MUSCULAR SYSTEM Muscles of the Neck

ANTERIOR VIEW OF THE NECK (SUPERFICIAL)

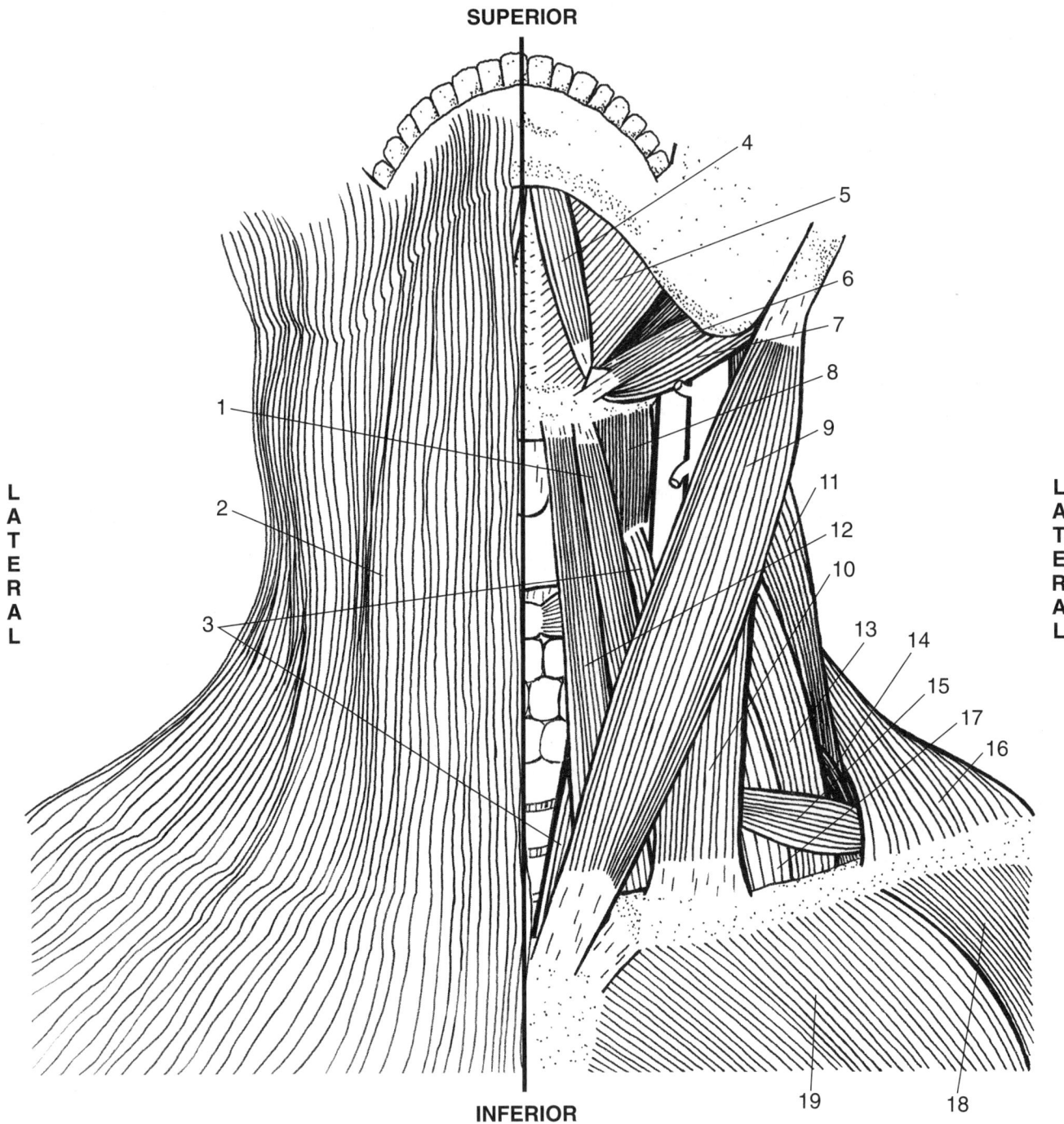

Answers to labeling exercises are on p. 463.

THE MUSCULAR SYSTEM Muscles of the Neck

ANTERIOR VIEW OF THE NECK (INTERMEDIATE)

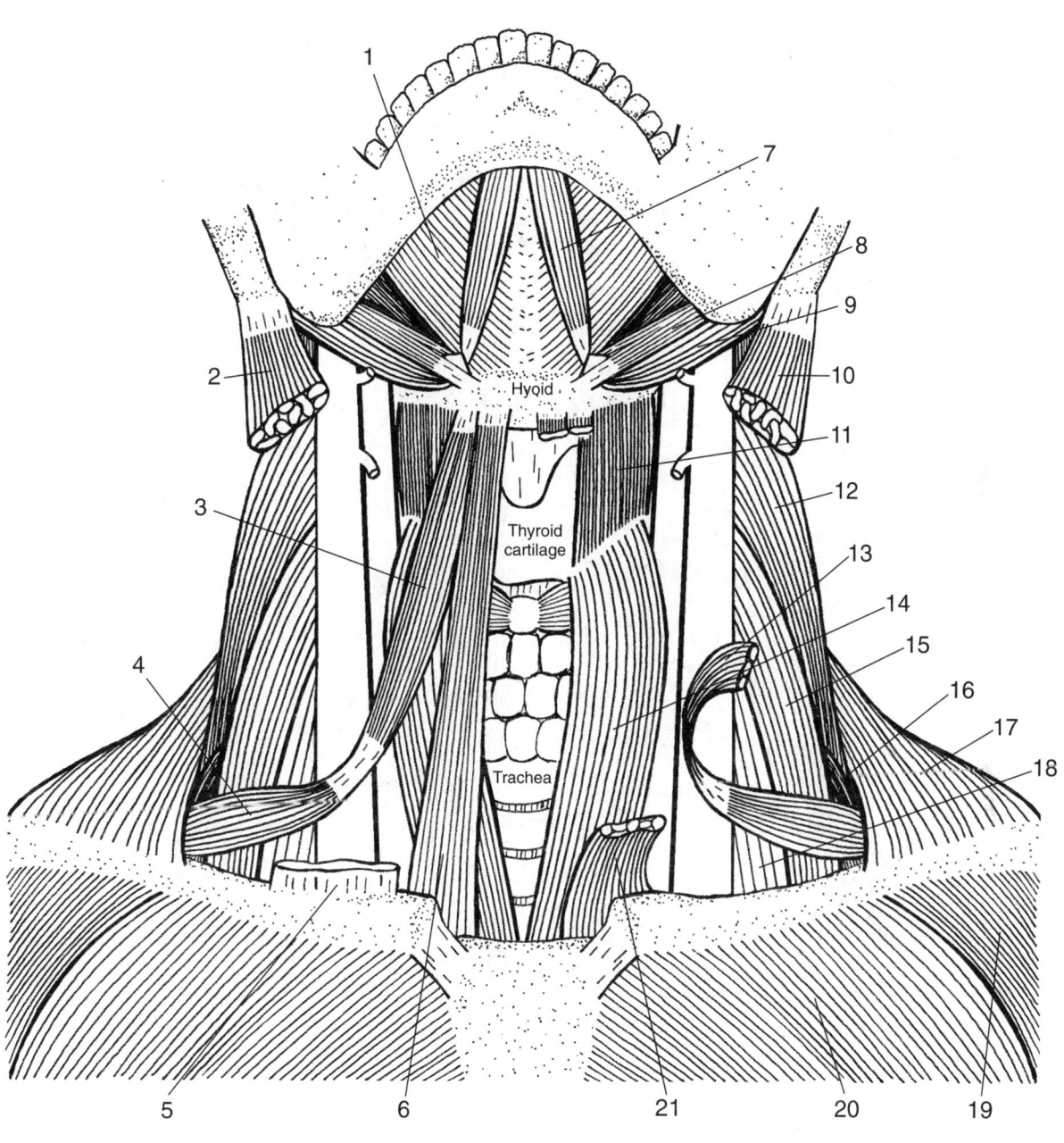

THE MUSCULAR SYSTEM: Muscles of the Neck

ANTERIOR VIEW OF THE NECK (DEEP)

SUPERIOR

LATERAL

LATERAL

Aorta

INFERIOR

THE MUSCULAR SYSTEM Muscles of the Neck

LATERAL VIEW OF THE NECK

THE MUSCULAR SYSTEM — Muscles of the Neck

POSTERIOR VIEW OF THE NECK
(SUPERFICIAL AND INTERMEDIATE)

Superficial — Intermediate

THE MUSCULAR SYSTEM Muscles of the Neck

POSTERIOR VIEW OF THE NECK (INTERMEDIATE AND DEEP)

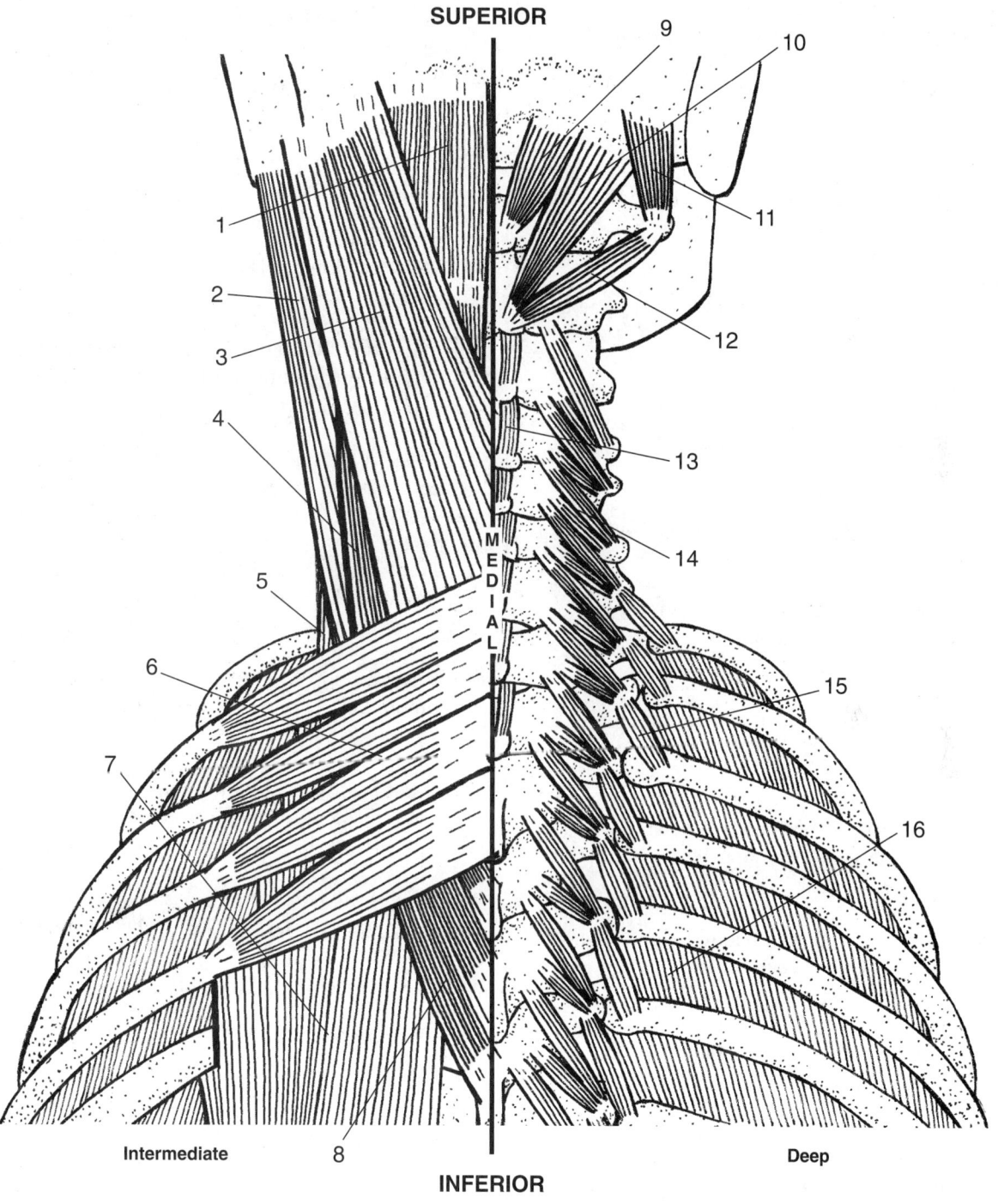

Review Questions

Muscles of the Neck
Answers to these questions are found on page 464.

1. What type of neck and head rotation does the right upper trapezius do?

2. What muscle is immediately superficial to the rectus capitis posterior major and minor?

3. At its scapular attachment, the levator scapulae is deep to what muscle?

4. What passive joint action of the mandible would shorten and slacken the mylohyoid?

5. What does the name *digastric* literally mean?

6. What muscle perforates the attachment of the stylohyoid onto the hyoid bone?

7. What action would lengthen and stretch the sternohyoid?

8. What muscle can be considered to be an upward extension of the sternothyroid?

9. How are the right and left obliquus capitis inferior muscles antagonistic to each other?

10. What are the names of the two bellies of the omohyoid?

11. If the left posterior scalene is eccentrically contracting, what spinal joint motion is occurring?

12. What muscles are immediately deep to the middle trapezius in the interscapular region?

13. What muscle is superficial to the sternocleidomastoid?

14. Why is the stylohyoid antagonistic to the sternohyoid?

15. What effect would right rotation of the neck at the spinal joints have upon the right sternocleidomastoid?

16. What two suboccipital muscles attach to the inferior nuchal line of the occiput?

17. What is the only hyoid muscle that does not attach to the hyoid bone?

18. From underneath the mandible, what muscle is immediately superficial to the mylohyoid?

19. What motion would lengthen and stretch the omohyoid?

20. What passive ranges of motion would shorten and slacken the right splenius capitis?

21. Besides the rectus capitis posterior major, what other suboccipital muscle attaches to the spinous process of C2?

22. What muscles attach to the medial border of the scapula?

23. From underneath the mandible, which suprahyoid muscle is deeper, the mylohyoid or the geniohyoid?

24. Name a muscle that is antagonistic to the scapular downward rotation action of the levator scapulae.

25. What four muscles comprise the suprahyoid group?

26. What happens to the length of the right posterior scalene if the neck is left laterally flexed?

27. How are the left upper trapezius and the left posterior scalene synergistic with each other?

28. What three muscles comprise the scalene group?

29. Which muscle attaches to cervical transverse processes and is directly posterior to the posterior scalene?

30. Which scalene is the largest?

31. What happens to the length of the longus colli muscles if the neck is thrown back into extension?

32. What passive joint motion would shorten and slacken both longus colli muscles?

33. How are the right longus colli and the left sternocleidomastoid muscles synergistic with each other?

34. Which muscle attaches more superiorly, the longus colli or the longus capitis?

35. What muscle group is directly lateral to the longus colli?

36. At what spinal levels do the longus colli and capitis overlap?

37. What passive joint motion would lengthen and stretch the right rectus capitis lateralis?

38. What four muscles comprise the prevertebral group?

39. If the rectus capitis anterior concentrically contracts, what joint motion would occur?

40. What inferior attachment is shared by the rectus capitis anterior and lateralis?

41. What muscle is directly medial to the rectus capitis anterior?

42. What superior attachment is shared by the rectus capitis anterior and lateralis?

43. What attachment is shared by the sternothyroid and the thyrohyoid?

44. How is the left sternocleidomastoid synergistic with the left upper trapezius?

45. How are the digastric and masseter antagonistic to each other?

46. What joint actions would lengthen and stretch the right splenius cervicis?

47. What four muscles comprise the suboccipital group?

48. What effect would passive depression of the mandible at the temporomandibular joints have upon the platysma?

THE MUSCULAR SYSTEM — Muscles of the Neck

49. Which one of the following passive joint motions of the head would shorten and slacken the right rectus capitis posterior major? left lateral flexion / right lateral flexion

50. What joint action is common to all three scalenes?

51. What joint motion of the head is occurring if both rectus capitis posterior major muscles are eccentrically contracting at the same time?

52. What four muscles comprise the infrahyoid group?

53. Which scalene muscle attaches the highest on the cervical spine?

54. What two muscles attach to the lateral clavicle, acromion process, and spine of the scapula?

55. If both anterior scalene muscles contract at the same time, what spinal joint action would occur?

56. Which two suboccipital muscles attach to the transverse process of the atlas?

57. Name a synergistic to the digastric with respect to motion of the hyoid bone?

58. What muscle is superficial to nearly the entire splenius capitis?

59. What effect would right rotation of the neck at the spinal joints have upon the right sternocleidomastoid?

60. What action is common to all four infrahyoid muscles?

61. What muscle is immediately deep to the superior attachment of the sternocleidomastoid?

62. How are the right sternocleidomastoid and upper trapezius muscles synergistic with each other?

63. What happens to the length of the mylohyoid if the temporalis muscle contracts and shortens?

64. What two muscles are immediately deep to the inferior aspect of the sternocleidomastoid's clavicular head?

65. What joint actions would lengthen and stretch the digastric?

66. What passive motion would shorten and slacken the omohyoid?

67. What muscles have the same superior attachment as the splenius capitis?

68. Besides the digastric, what other hyoid muscle has a central tendon?

69. Name a synergist to the scapular elevation action of the levator scapulae?

70. Which scalene muscle is the smallest?

71. What happens to the length of the right anterior scalene if the left posterior scalene contracts and shortens?

72. Which one of the following joint actions of the neck would lengthen and stretch the left levator scapulae? extension / right lateral flexion / left rotation

THE MUSCULAR SYSTEM Muscles of the Neck

73. What type of neck and head rotation does the left splenius capitis do?

74. How many hyoid muscles attach onto the mandible?

75. Which two suboccipital muscles attach to the spinous process of the axis?

76. What is the only suboccipital muscle that does not attach to the head?

77. Which is more superficial, the omohyoid or the scalenes?

78. What joint actions would lengthen and stretch the left lower trapezius?

79. What joint action is shared by all three parts of the trapezius?

80. What is the nickname for the splenius capitis muscles?

81. How are the omohyoid and sternohyoid synergistic with each other?

82. What joint action would lengthen and stretch the left obliquus capitis inferior?

83. From a posterior perspective, what muscle is superficial to the levator scapulae at its spinal attachment?

84. Where is the brachial plexus of nerves found relative to the scalene muscles?

THE MUSCULAR SYSTEM — Muscles of the Trunk

POSTERIOR VIEW OF THE TRUNK (SUPERFICIAL AND INTERMEDIATE)

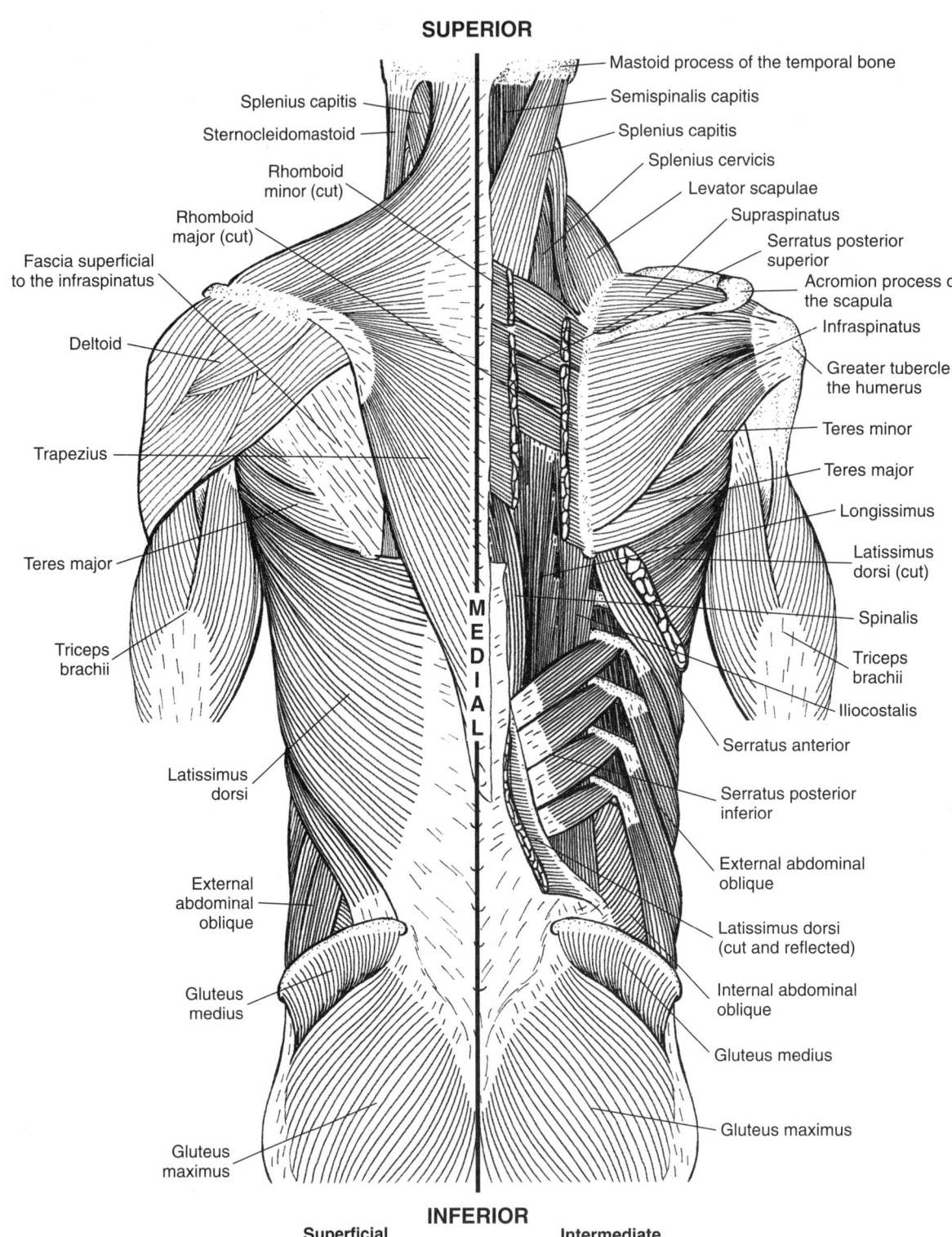

THE MUSCULAR SYSTEM Muscles of the Trunk

POSTERIOR VIEW OF THE TRUNK (DEEP LAYERS)

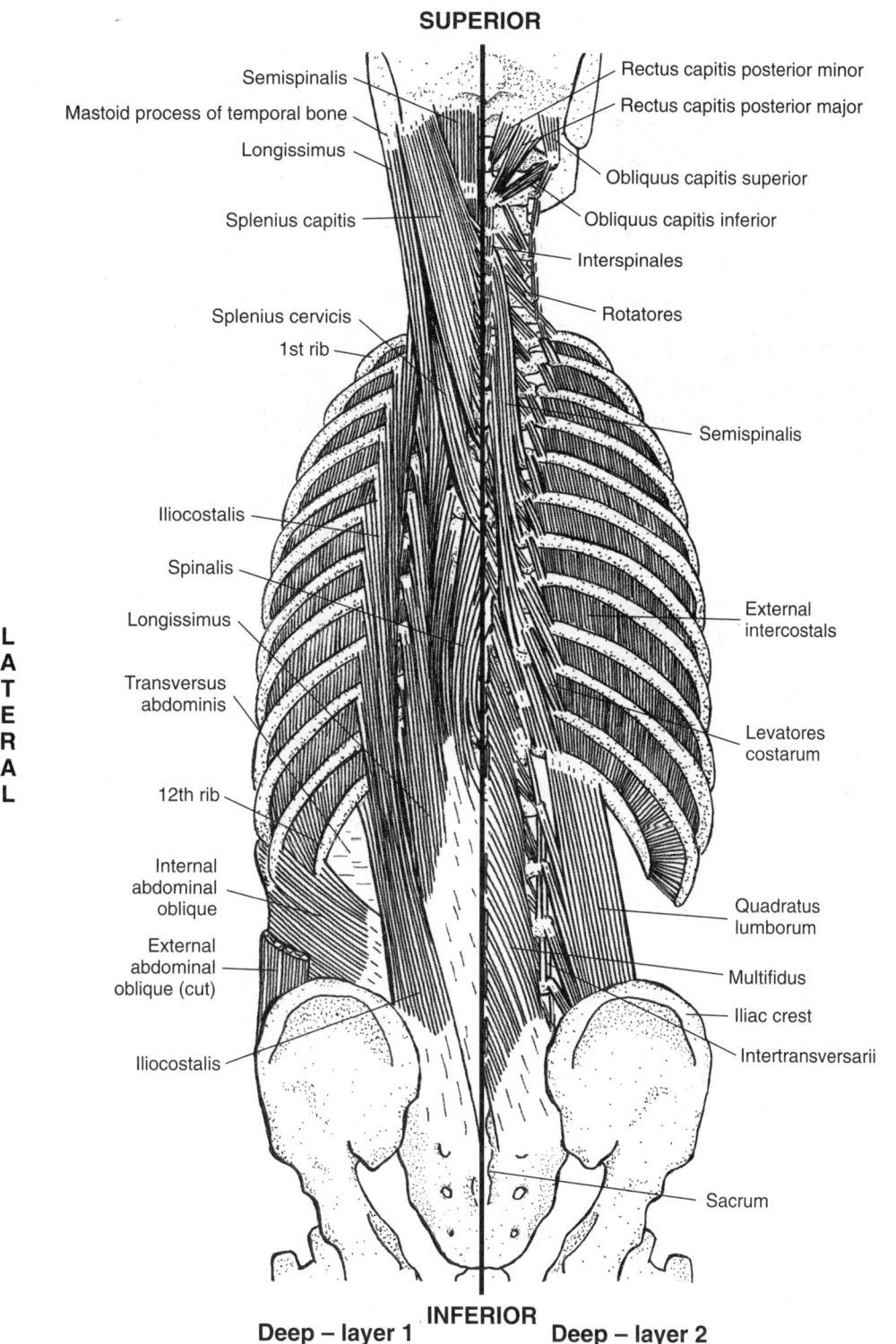

THE MUSCULAR SYSTEM — Muscles of the Trunk

ANTERIOR VIEW OF THE TRUNK
(SUPERFICIAL AND INTERMEDIATE)

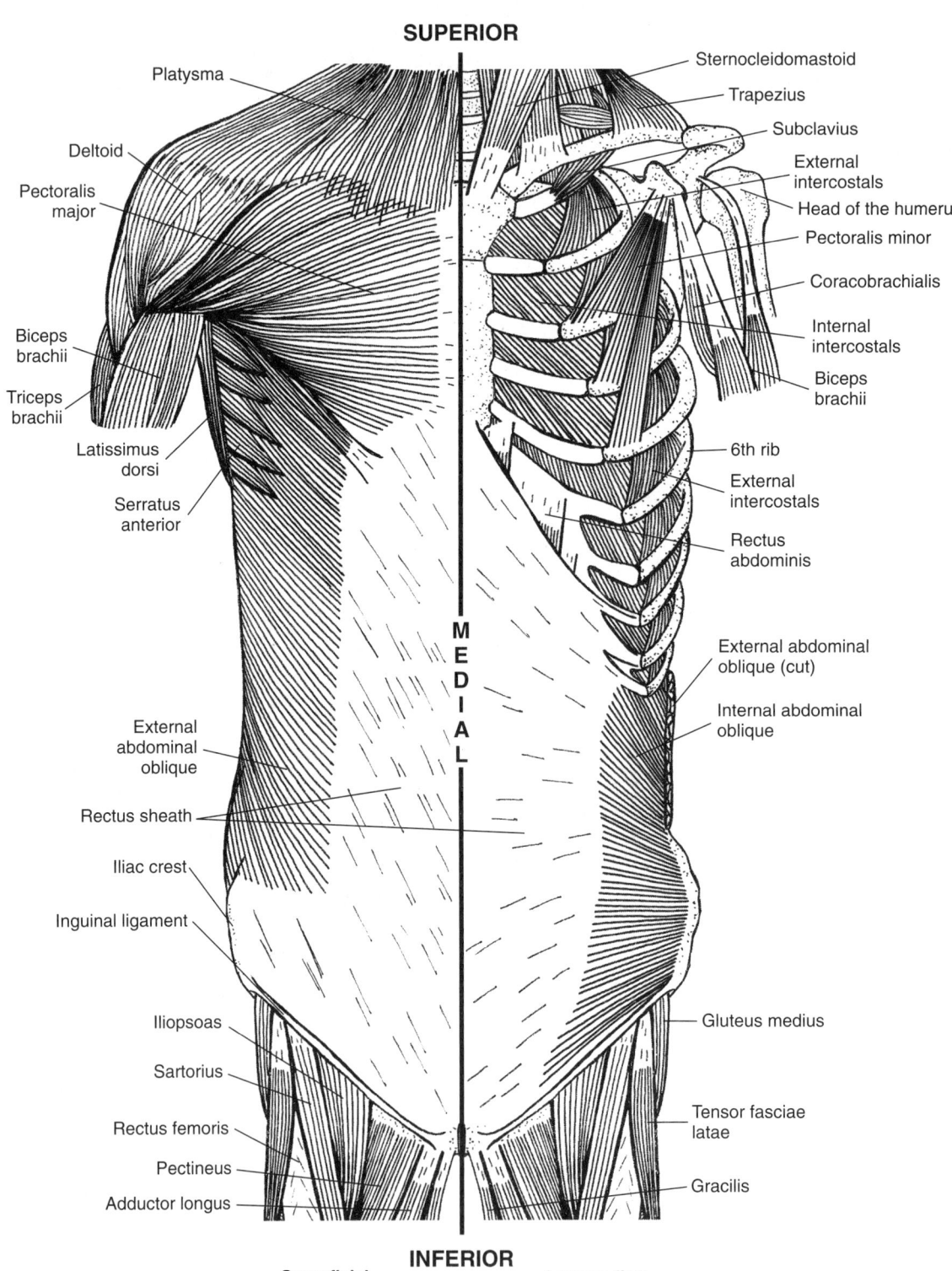

THE MUSCULAR SYSTEM Muscles of the Trunk

ANTERIOR VIEW OF THE TRUNK (INTERMEDIATE AND DEEP)

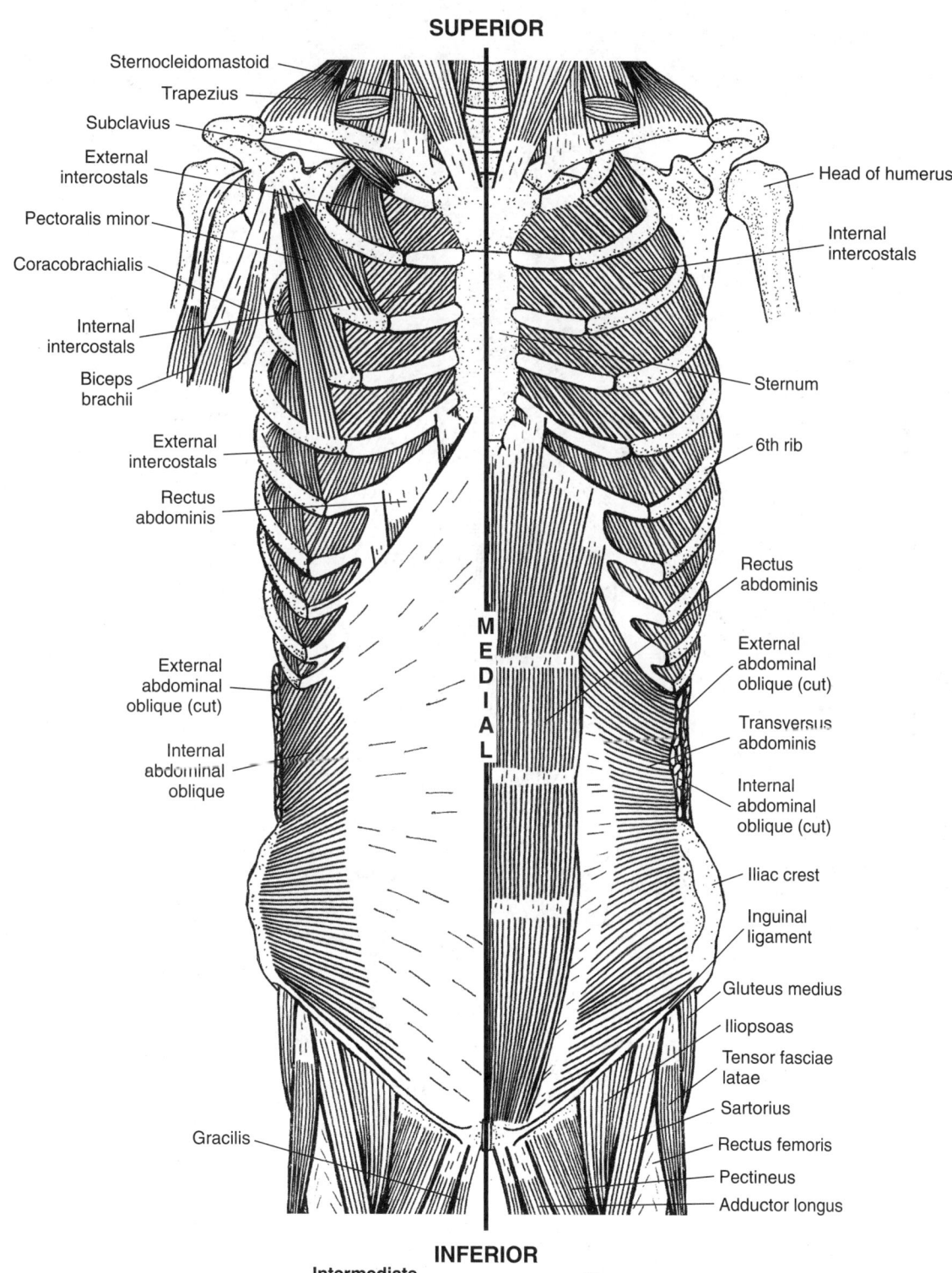

THE MUSCULAR SYSTEM — Muscles of the Trunk

LATERAL VIEW OF THE TRUNK

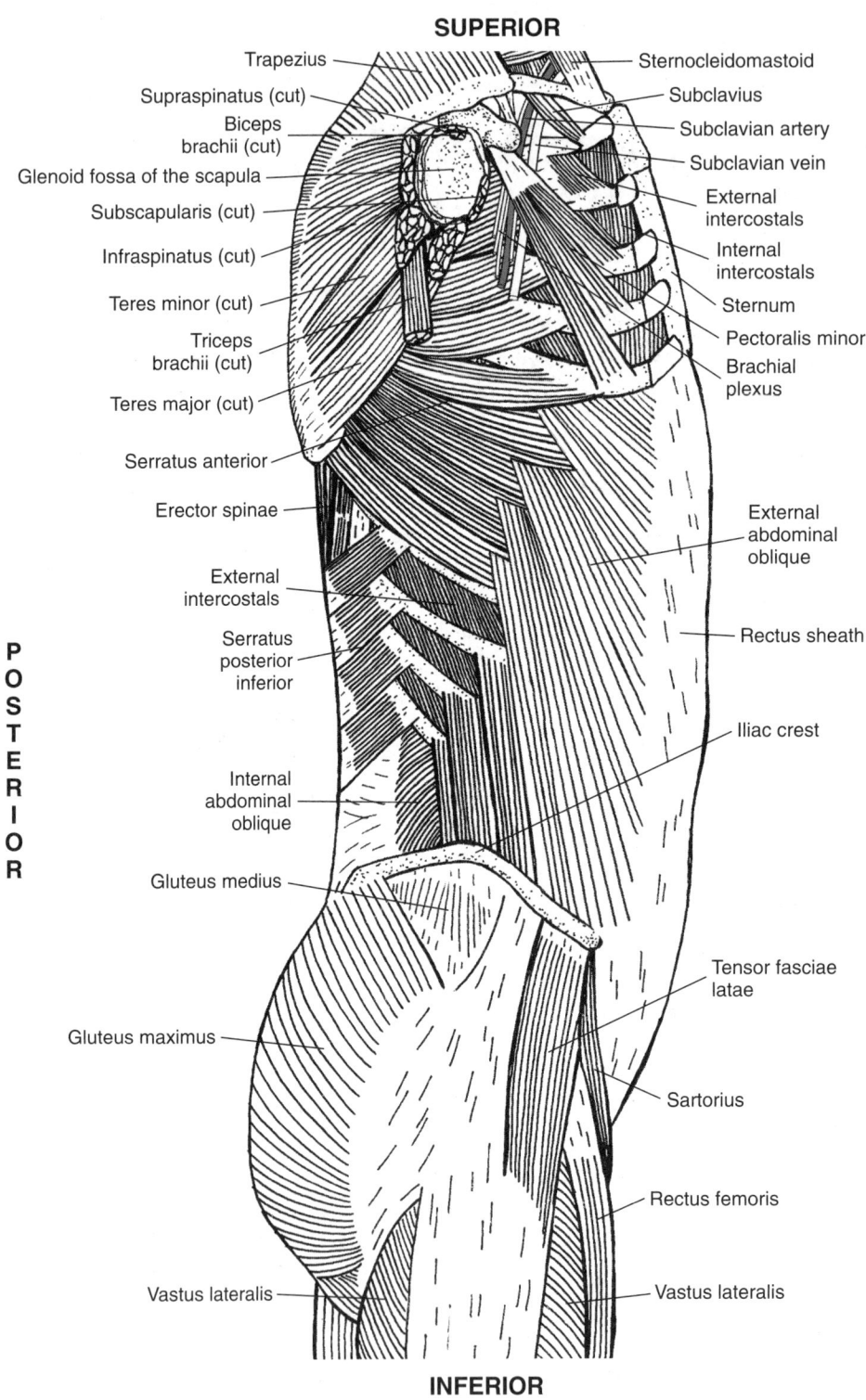

THE MUSCULAR SYSTEM Muscles of the Trunk

CROSS SECTION VIEWS OF THE TRUNK

Thoracic cross section

Lumbar cross section

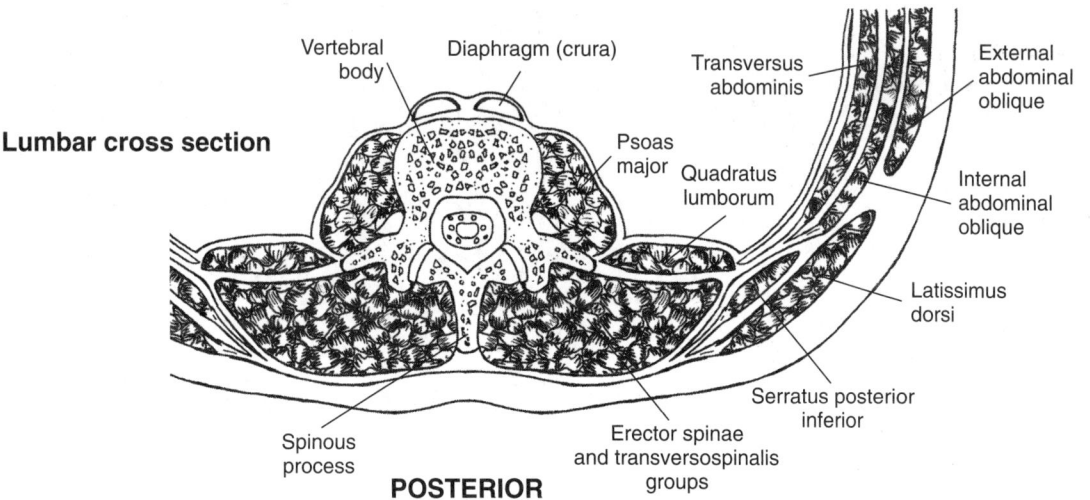

LATISSIMUS DORSI ("LAT")
la-**tis**-i-mus **door**-si

Actions
Medial rotation of the arm at the shoulder joint
Adduction of the arm at the shoulder joint
Extension of the arm at the shoulder joint
Anterior tilt of the pelvis at the lumbosacral joint
Depression of the scapula at the scapulocostal joint
Lateral deviation of the trunk at the scapulocostal joint
Elevation of the trunk at the scapulocostal joint
Contralateral rotation of the trunk at the scapulocostal joint
Elevation of the pelvis at the lumbosacral joint

Innervation
The thoracodorsal nerve

Arterial Supply
The thoracodorsal artery and the dorsal branches of the posterior intercostal arteries

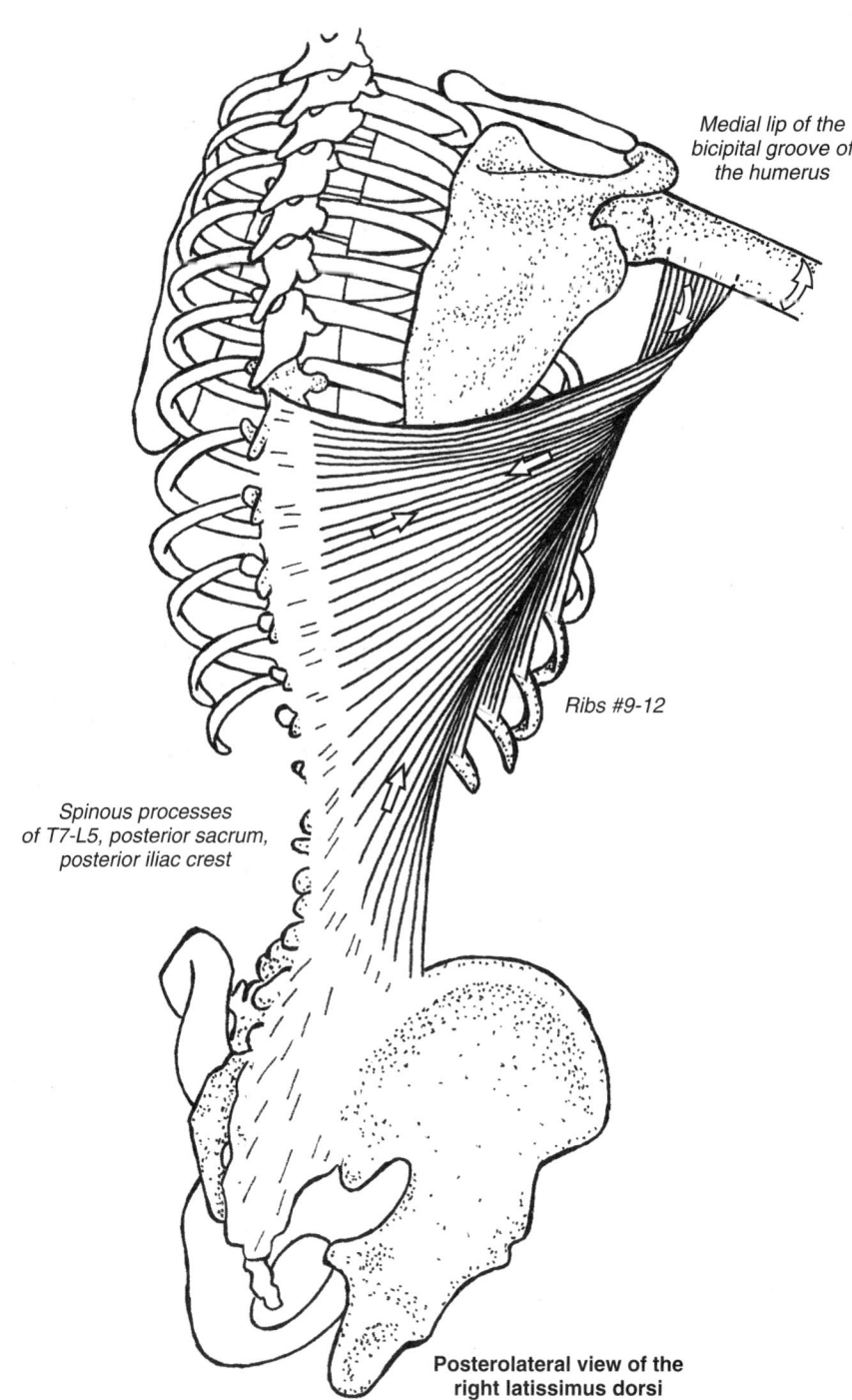

Posterolateral view of the right latissimus dorsi

THE MUSCULAR SYSTEM Muscles of the Trunk

DID YOU KNOW? The latissimus dorsi (and the teres major) make up the majority of the posterior axillary fold of tissue, which borders the armpit posteriorly.

RHOMBOIDS MAJOR AND MINOR

rom-boyd may-jor, my-nor

Actions
Retraction (adduction) of the scapula at the scapulocostal joint
Elevation of the scapula at the scapulocostal joint
Downward rotation of the scapula at the scapulocostal joint
Contralateral rotation of the trunk at the spinal joints

Innervation
The dorsal scapular nerve

Arterial Supply
The dorsal scapular artery

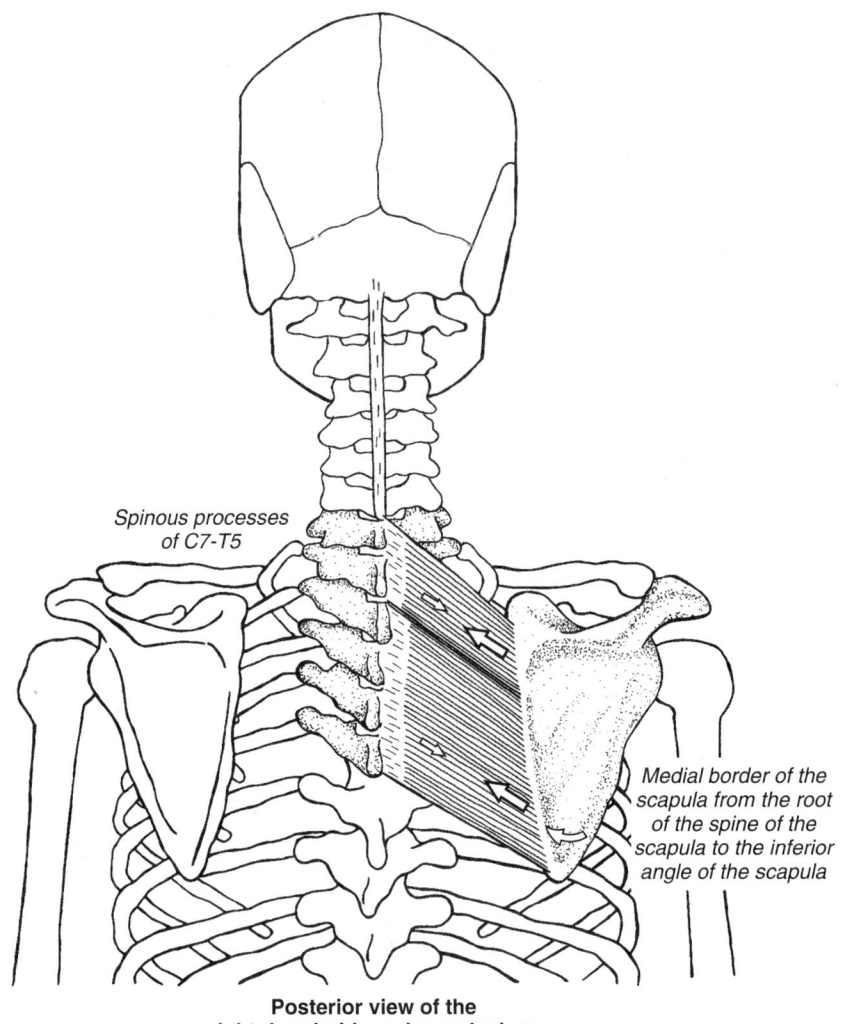

Spinous processes of C7-T5

Medial border of the scapula from the root of the spine of the scapula to the inferior angle of the scapula

Posterior view of the right rhomboids major and minor

THE MUSCULAR SYSTEM Muscles of the Trunk

The rhomboids are sometimes known as the "Christmas tree" muscles. When you look at them bilaterally with the spine between them, they look like a Christmas tree.

SERRATUS ANTERIOR
ser-**a**-tus an-**tee**-ri-or

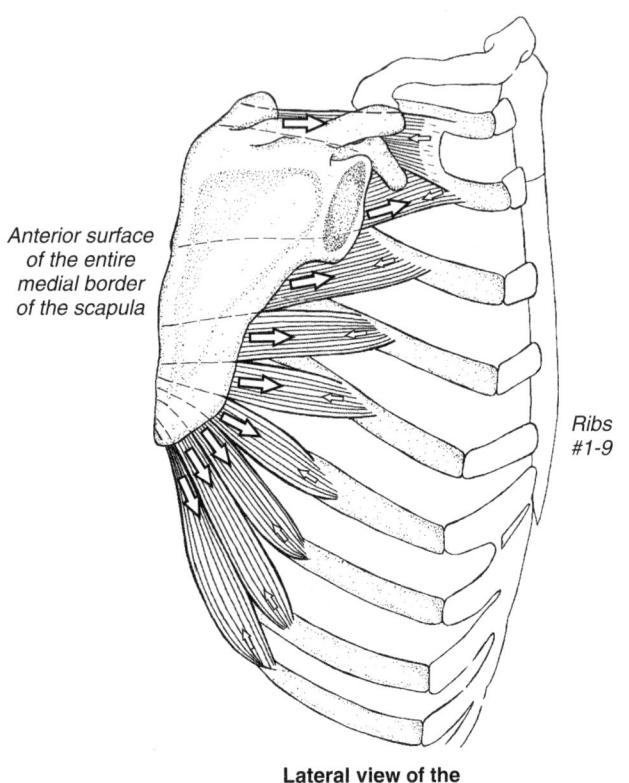

Lateral view of the
right serratus anterior

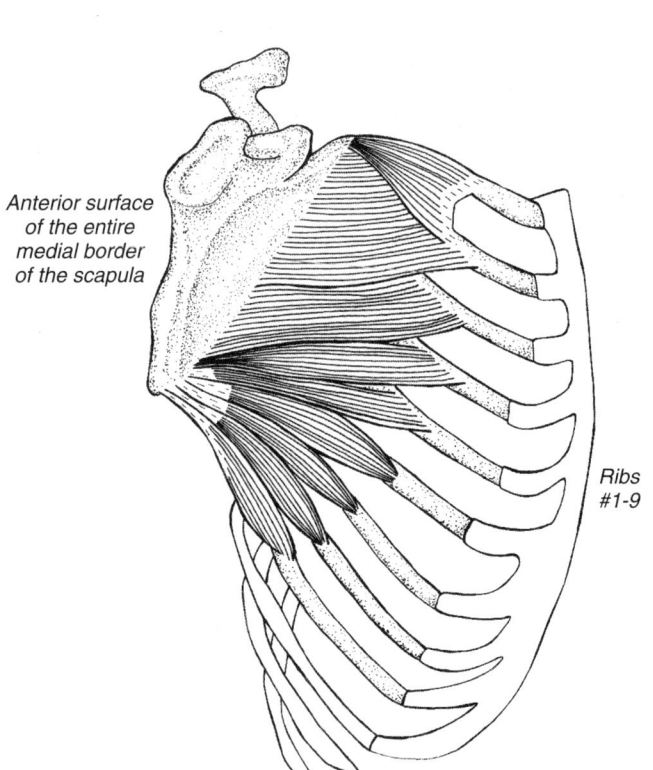

Lateral view of the
right serratus anterior
(with the lateral border of the scapula
pulled away from the trunk
to view the scapular attachment
of the serratus anterior)

Actions
Protraction (abduction) of the scapula at the scapulocostal joint
Upward rotation of the scapula at the scapulocostal joint
Elevation of the scapula at the scapulocostal joint
Depression of the scapula at the scapulocostal joint

Innervation
The long thoracic nerve

Arterial Supply
The dorsal scapular artery and the lateral thoracic artery

THE MUSCULAR SYSTEM Muscles of the Trunk   123

DID YOU KNOW?

In very well-developed individuals, the serratus anterior looks like ribs standing out in the anterolateral trunk.

SERRATUS POSTERIOR SUPERIOR

ser-**a**-tus pos-**tee**-ri-or sue-**pee**-ri-or

Action
Elevation of ribs #2-5 at the sternocostal and costovertebral joints

Innervation
Intercostal nerves

Arterial Supply
The dorsal branches of the posterior intercostal arteries

Posterior view of the right serratus posterior superior

SERRATUS POSTERIOR INFERIOR

ser-**a**-tus pos-**tee**-ri-or in-**fee**-ri-or

Actions
Depression of ribs #9-12 at the sternocostal and costovertebral joints

Innervation
Subcostal nerve and intercostal nerves

Arterial Supply
The dorsal branches of the posterior intercostal arteries

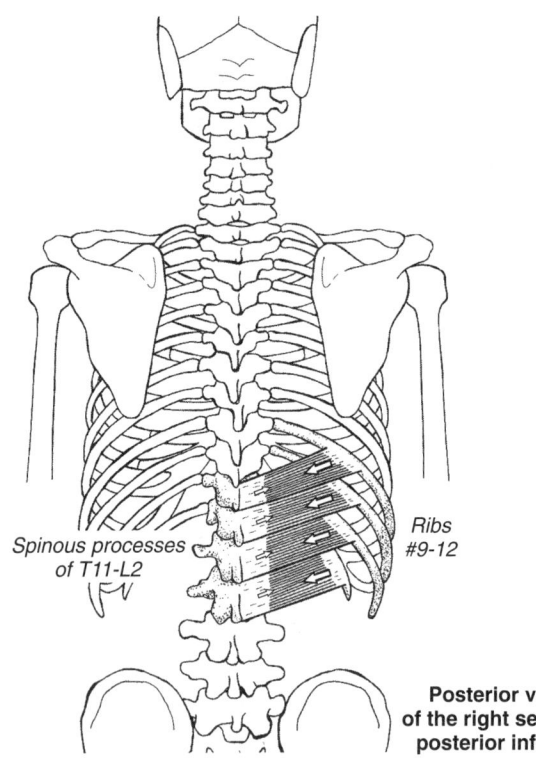

Posterior view of the right serratus posterior inferior

THE MUSCULAR SYSTEM Muscles of the Trunk 125

By their action of moving the ribs, the serratus posterior superior and inferior muscles are primarily important as muscles of respiration.

THE ERECTOR SPINAE GROUP
ee-**rek**-tor **spee**-nee

Actions
Extension of the trunk and the neck and the head at the spinal joints
Lateral flexion of the trunk and the neck and the head at the spinal joints
Ipsilateral rotation of the trunk and the neck and the head at the spinal joints
Anterior tilt of the pelvis at the lumbosacral joint
Elevation of the pelvis at the lumbosacral joint
Contralateral rotation of the pelvis at the lumbosacral joint

Innervation
Spinal nerves

Arterial Supply
The dorsal branches of the posterior intercostal and lumbar arteries

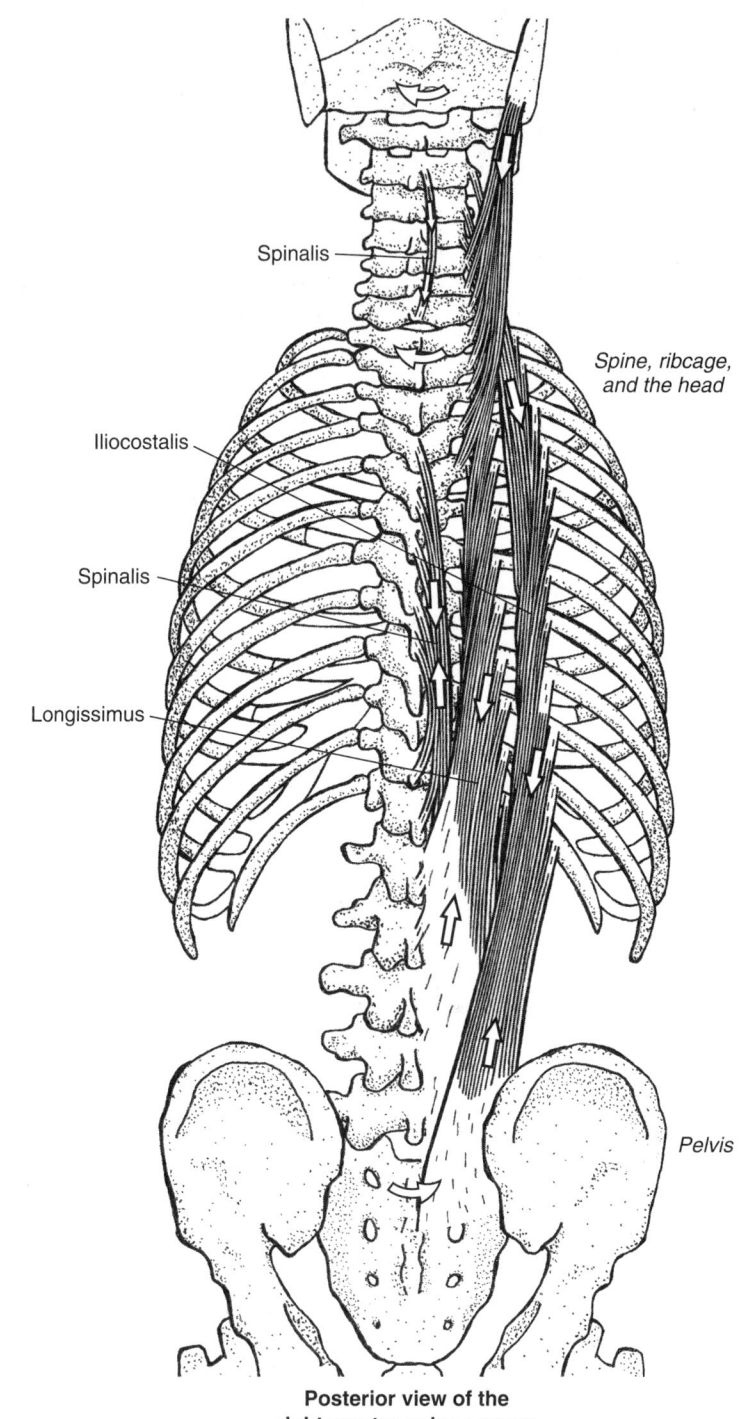

Posterior view of the right erector spinae group

THE MUSCULAR SYSTEM: Muscles of the Trunk

DID YOU KNOW?
The erector spinae group, as its name implies, makes the spine erect, i.e., it does extension of the spine.

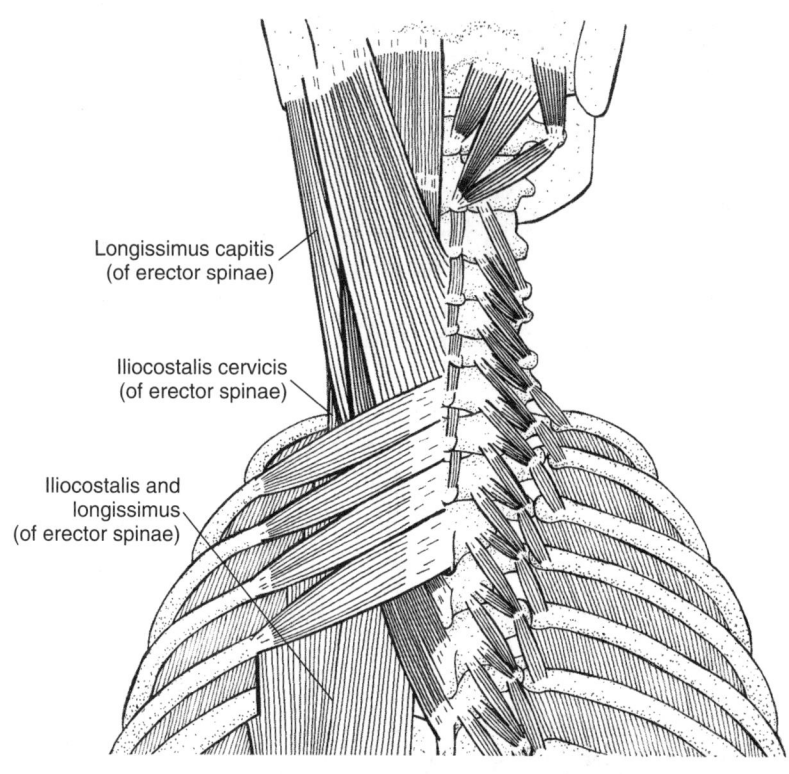

ILIOCOSTALIS
(OF THE ERECTOR SPINAE GROUP)
il-ee-o-kos-**ta**-lis

Actions
Extension of the trunk and the neck at the spinal joints
Lateral flexion of the trunk and the neck at the spinal joints
Ipsilateral rotation of the trunk and the neck at the spinal joints
Anterior tilt of the pelvis at the lumbosacral joint
Elevation of the pelvis at the lumbosacral joint
Contralateral rotation of the pelvis at the lumbosacral joint

Innervation
Spinal nerves

Arterial Supply
The dorsal branches of the posterior intercostal and lumbar arteries

Posterior view of the right iliocostalis

LONGISSIMUS
(OF THE ERECTOR SPINAE GROUP)
lon-**jis**-i-mus

Actions
Extension of the trunk and the neck and the head at the spinal joints
Lateral flexion of the trunk and the neck and the head at the spinal joints
Ipsilateral rotation of the trunk and the neck and the head at the spinal joints
Anterior tilt of the pelvis at the lumbosacral joint
Elevation of the pelvis at the lumbosacral joint
Contralateral rotation of the pelvis at the lumbosacral joint

Innervation
Spinal nerves

Arterial Supply
The dorsal branches of the posterior intercostal and lumbar arteries

Posterior view of the right longissimus

THE MUSCULAR SYSTEM Muscles of the Trunk

The iliocostalis, as its name implies, attaches from the ilium to the ribs

The longissimus, as its name implies, is the longest of the three subgroups of the erector spinae.

SPINALIS
(OF THE ERECTOR SPINAE GROUP)
spy-**na**-lis

Actions
Extension of the trunk and the neck and the head at the spinal joints
Lateral flexion of the trunk and the neck and the head at the spinal joints
Ipsilateral rotation of the trunk and the neck and the head at the spinal joints

Innervation
Spinal nerves

Arterial Supply
The dorsal branches of the posterior inter-costal and lumbar arteries

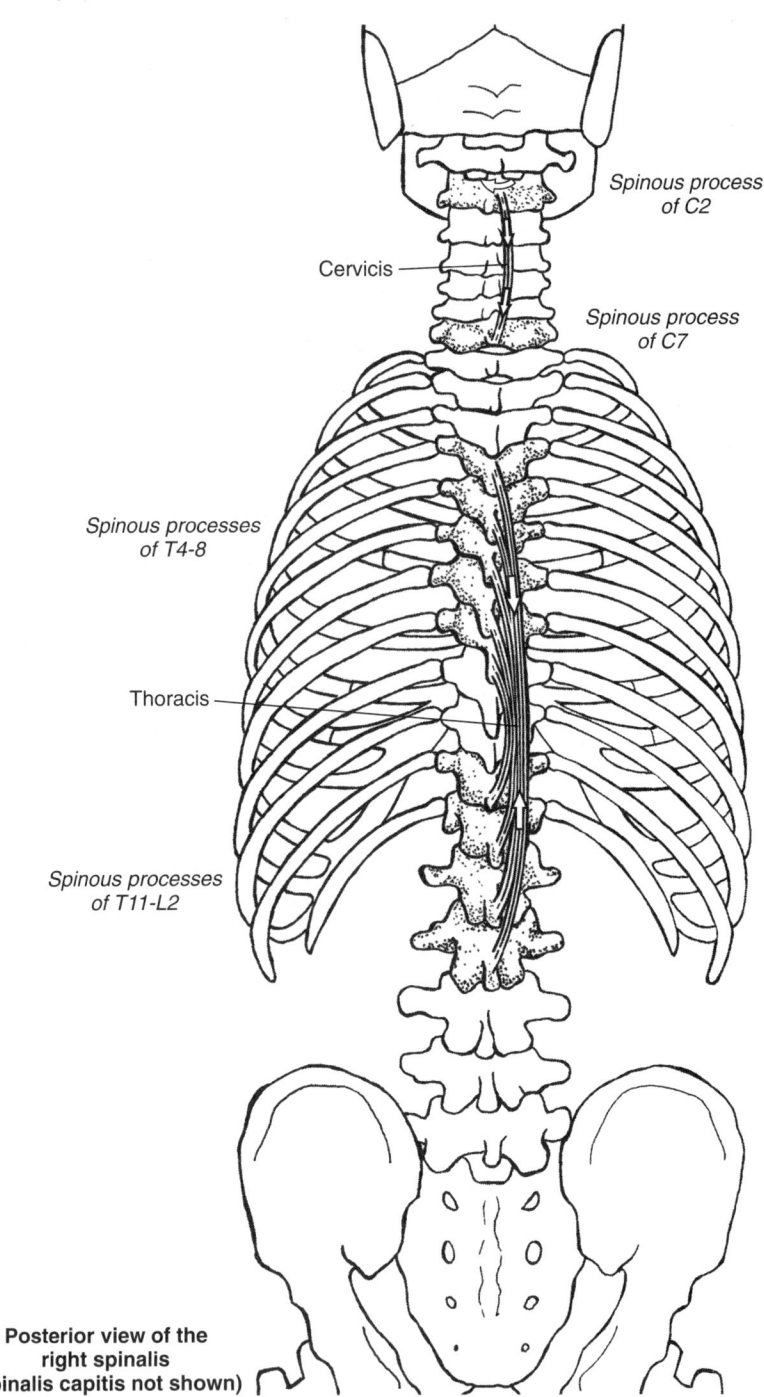

Posterior view of the right spinalis
(spinalis capitis not shown)

THE MUSCULAR SYSTEM Muscles of the Trunk

Spinalis

Longissimus

Iliocostalis

The spinalis, as its name implies, attaches from spinous processes to spinous processes.

THE TRANSVERSOSPINALIS GROUP
trans-**ver**-so-spy-**na**-lis

Actions
Extension of the trunk and the neck and the head at the spinal joints
Lateral flexion of the trunk and the neck and the head at the spinal joints
Contralateral rotation of the trunk and the neck at the spinal joints
Anterior tilt of the pelvis at the lumbosacral joint
Elevation of the pelvis at the lumbosacral joint
Ipsilateral rotation of the pelvis at the lumbosacral joint

Innervation
Spinal nerves

Arterial Supply
The occipital artery and the dorsal branches of the posterior intercostal and lumbar arteries

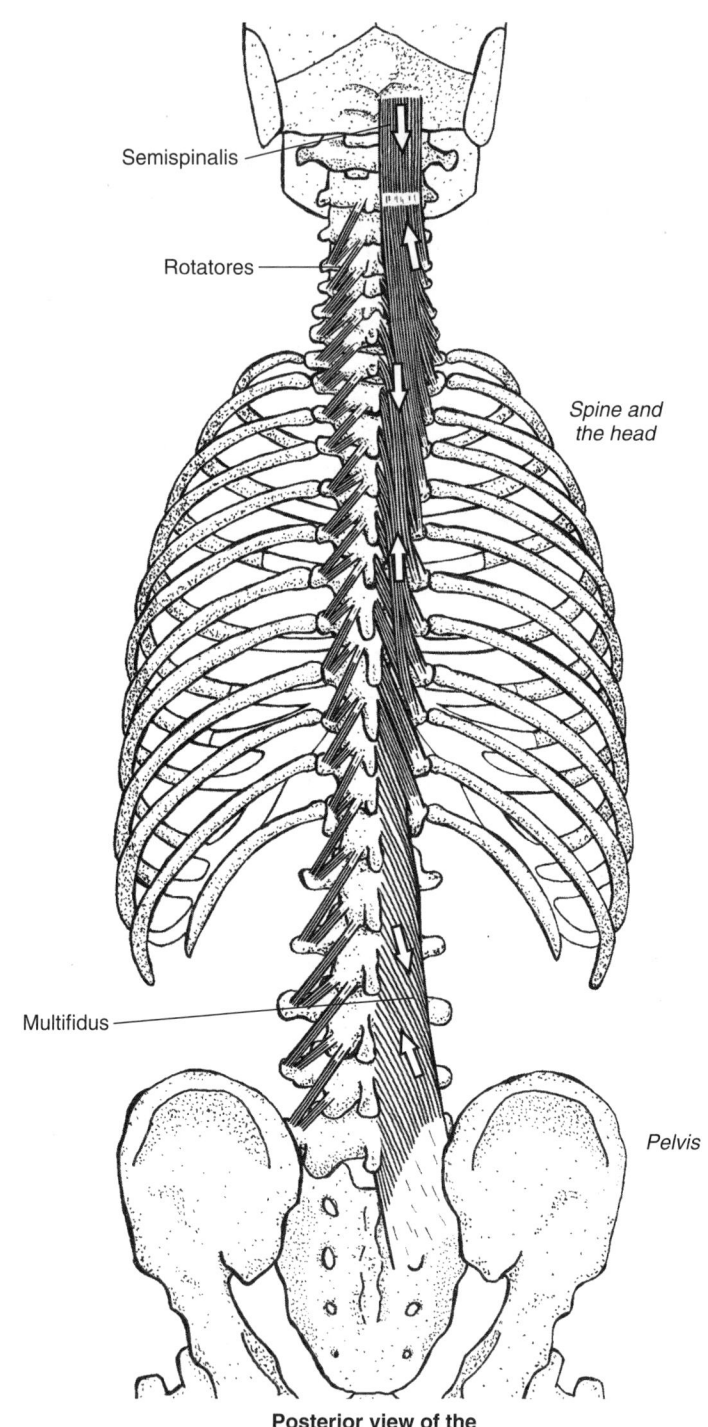

Posterior view of the transversospinalis group
(semispinalis and multifidus on the right)
(rotatores on the left)

THE MUSCULAR SYSTEM Muscles of the Trunk

The transversospinalis group, as its name implies, attaches from transverse processes to spinous processes.

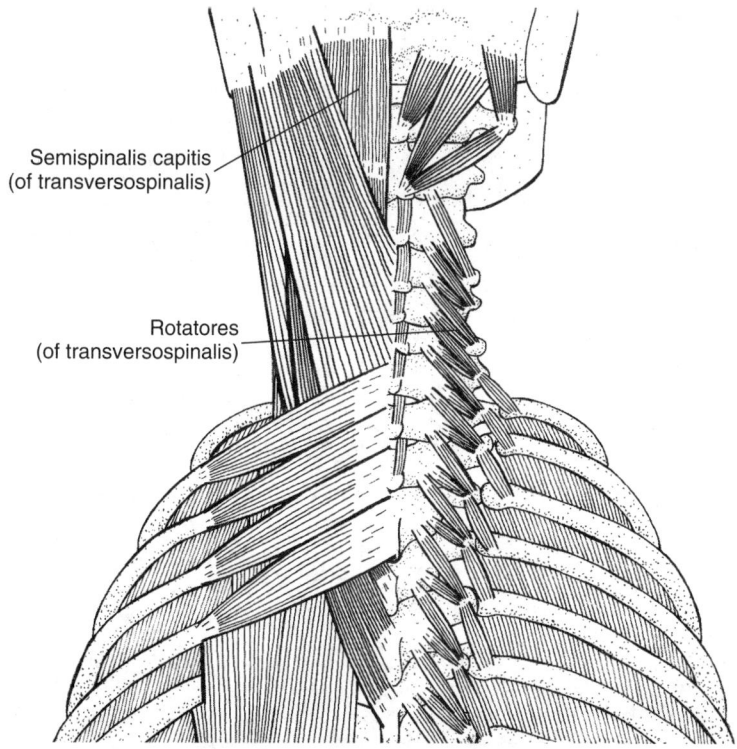

SEMISPINALIS
(OF THE TRANSVERSOSPINALIS GROUP)

sem-ee-spy-na-lis

Actions
Extension of the trunk and the neck and the head at the spinal joints
Lateral flexion of the trunk and the neck and the head at the spinal joints
Contralateral rotation of the trunk and the neck at the spinal joints

Innervation
Spinal nerves

Arterial Supply
The occipital artery and the dorsal branches of the posterior intercostal arteries

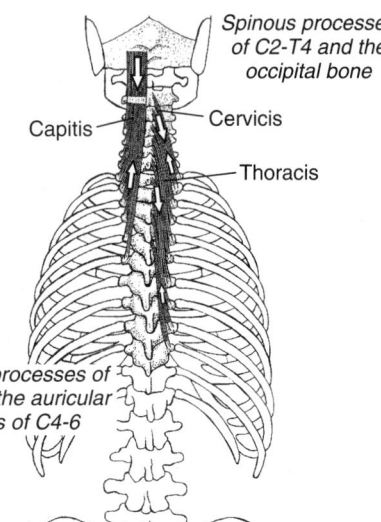

Spinous processes of C2-T4 and the occipital bone
Capitis — Cervicis — Thoracis
Transverse processes of C7-T10 and the auricular processes of C4-6

Posterior view of the semispinalis (semispinalis thoracis and cervicis on the right) (semispinalis capitis on the left)

MULTIFIDUS
(OF THE TRANSVERSOSPINALIS GROUP)

mul-tif-id-us

Actions
Extension of the trunk and the neck at the spinal joints
Lateral flexion of the trunk and the neck at the spinal joints
Contralateral rotation of the trunk and the neck at the spinal joints
Anterior tilt of the pelvis at the lumbosacral joint
Elevation of the pelvis at the lumbosacral joint
Ipsilateral rotation of the pelvis at the lumbosacral joint

Innervation
Spinal nerves

Arterial Supply
The dorsal branches of the posterior intercostal and lumbar arteries

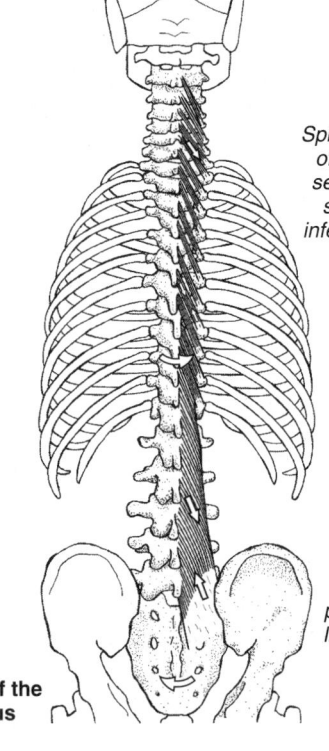

Spinous processes of vertebrae 3-4 segmental levels superior to the inferior attachment

Posterior sacrum, posterior superior iliac spine (PSIS), posterior sacro-iliac ligament and L5-C4 vertebrae

Posterior view of the right multifidus

THE MUSCULAR SYSTEM Muscles of the Trunk   135

The semispinalis capitis is the largest muscle in the posterior neck.

The multifidus is the largest muscle in the low back.

ROTATORES
(OF THE TRANSVERSOSPINALIS GROUP)

ro-ta-**to**-reez

Actions
Contralateral rotation of the trunk and the neck at the spinal joints
Extension of the trunk and the neck at the spinal joints

Innervation
Spinal nerves

Arterial Supply
The dorsal branches of the posterior intercostal and lumbar arteries

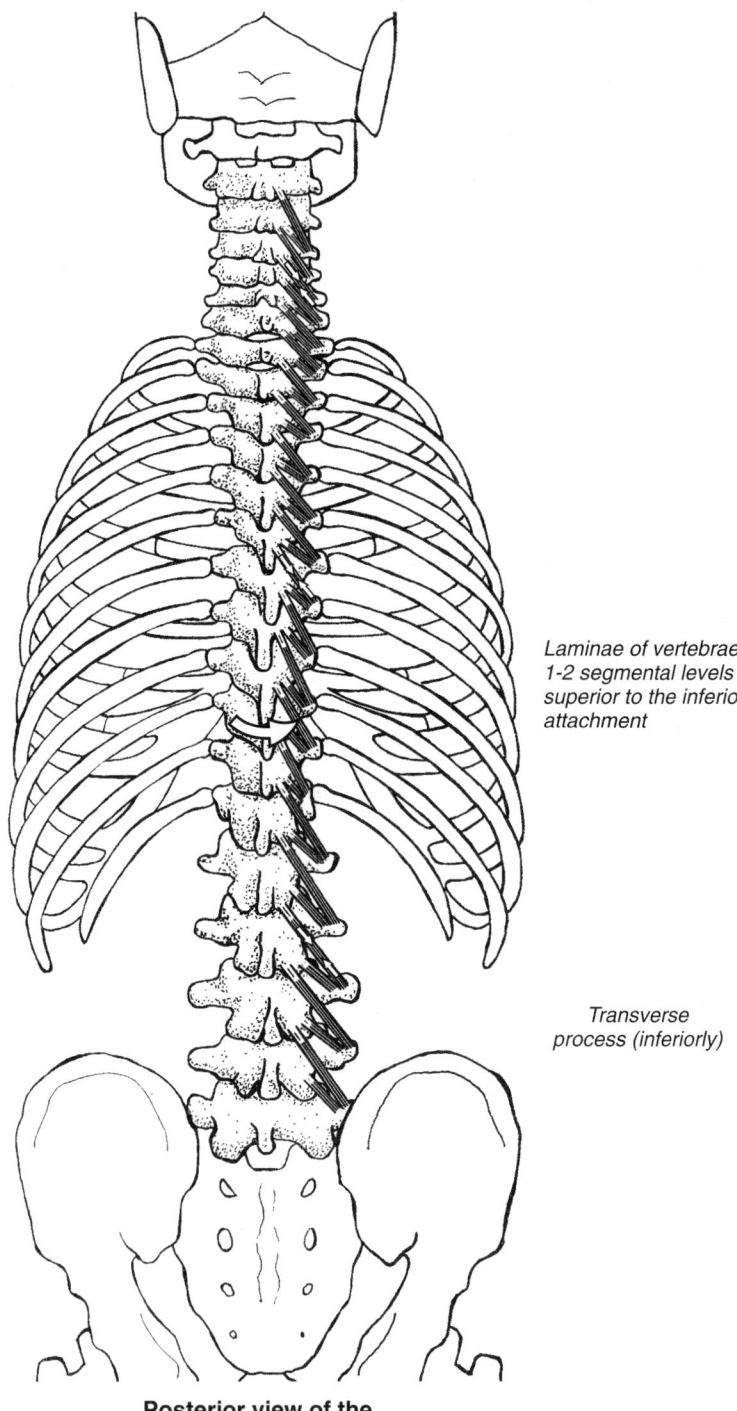

Laminae of vertebrae 1-2 segmental levels superior to the inferior attachment

Transverse process (inferiorly)

Posterior view of the right rotatores

THE MUSCULAR SYSTEM Muscles of the Trunk

DID YOU KNOW?

The rotatores, as their name implies, are best at rotation (contralaterally) of the spine.

QUADRATUS LUMBORUM ("QL")
kwod-**ray**-tus lum-**bor**-um

Actions
Elevation of the pelvis at the lumbosacral joint
Anterior tilt of the pelvis at the lumbosacral joint
Lateral flexion of the trunk at the spinal joints
Extension of the trunk at the spinal joints
Depression of the 12th rib at the costovertebral joints

Innervation
Lumbar plexus

Arterial Supply
Branches of the subcostal and lumbar arteries

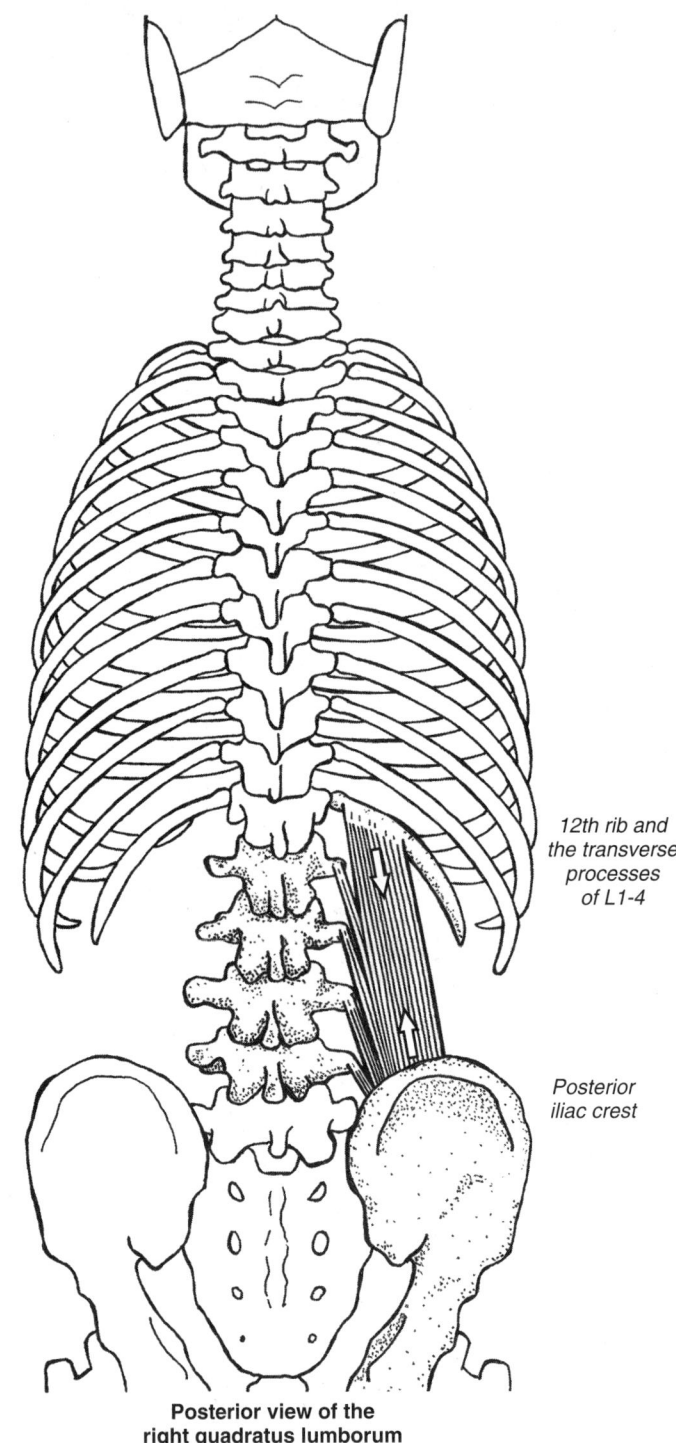

12th rib and the transverse processes of L1-4

Posterior iliac crest

Posterior view of the right quadratus lumborum

THE MUSCULAR SYSTEM   Muscles of the Trunk   139

When palpating the quadratus lumborum, it must be accessed from the side.

INTERSPINALES
in-ter-spy-na-leez

Action
Extension of the neck and the trunk at the spinal joints

Innervation
Spinal nerves

Arterial Supply
The dorsal branches of the posterior intercostal arteries

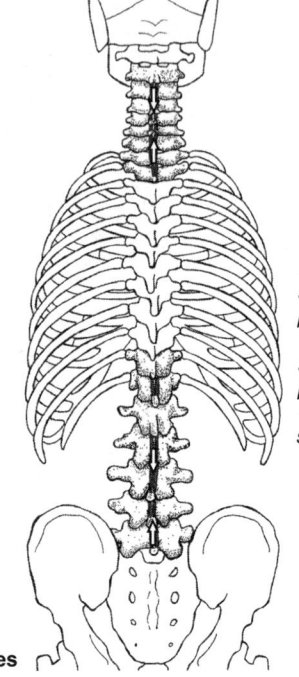

From a spinous process to the spinous process directly superior

Posterior view of the right and left interspinales

INTERTRANSVERSARII
in-ter-trans-ver-sa-ri-eye

Action
Lateral flexion of the neck and the trunk at the spinal joints

Innervation
Spinal nerves

Arterial Supply
The dorsal branches of the posterior intercostal arteries

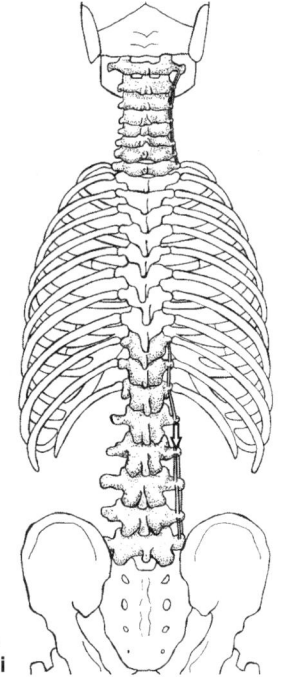

From a transverse process to the transverse process directly superior

Posterior view of the right intertransversarii

THE MUSCULAR SYSTEM Muscles of the Trunk

DID YOU KNOW

The interspinales are small, paired muscles located between spinous processes. The intertransversarii are small muscles located between transverse processes. Both of these muscle groups are poorly developed in the thoracic region.

LEVATORES COSTARUM

le-va-**to**-rez (singular: le-**vay**-tor) kos-**tar**-um

Actions
Elevation of the ribs at the sternocostal and costovertebral joints
Extension of the trunk at the spinal joints
Lateral flexion of the trunk at the spinal joints
Contralateral rotation of the trunk at the spinal joints

Innervation
Spinal nerves

Arterial Supply
The dorsal branches of the posterior intercostal arteries

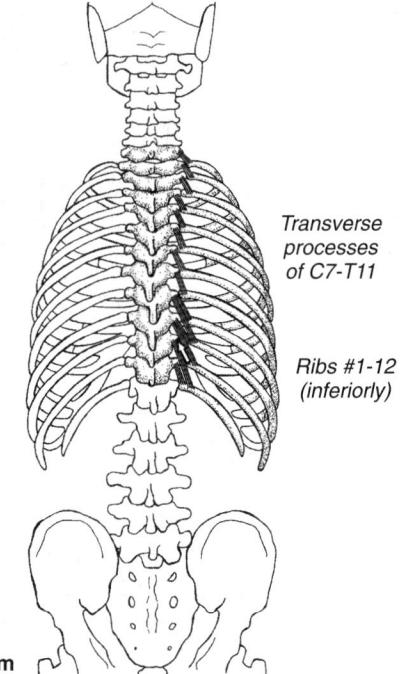

Transverse processes of C7-T11

Ribs #1-12 (inferiorly)

Posterior view of the right levatores costarum

SUBCOSTALES

sub-kos-**tal**-eez

Action
Depression of ribs #8-10 at the sternocostal and costovertebral joints

Innervation
Intercostal nerves

Arterial Supply
The dorsal branches of the posterior inter-costal arteries

Ribs #8-10

Ribs #10-12

Posterior view of the right subcostales

THE MUSCULAR SYSTEM Muscles of the Trunk   143

As their name implies, the levatores costarum elevate the ribs.

Anterior view

There are usually three subcostales muscles and they are located deep to the ribcage from the posterior perspective.

PECTORALIS MAJOR
pek-to-ra-lis **may**-jor

Actions
Adduction of the arm at the shoulder joint
Medial rotation of the arm at the shoulder joint
Flexion of the arm at the shoulder joint (clavicular head)
Extension of the arm at the shoulder joint (sternocostal head)
Abduction of the arm at the shoulder joint (clavicular head, above 90°)
Depression of the scapula at the scapulocostal joint
Elevation of the trunk at the scapulocostal joint
Lateral deviation of the trunk at the scapulocostal joint
Ipsilateral rotation of the trunk at the scapulocostal joint

Innervation
The medial and lateral pectoral nerves

Arterial Supply
The pectoral branches of the thoracoacromial trunk

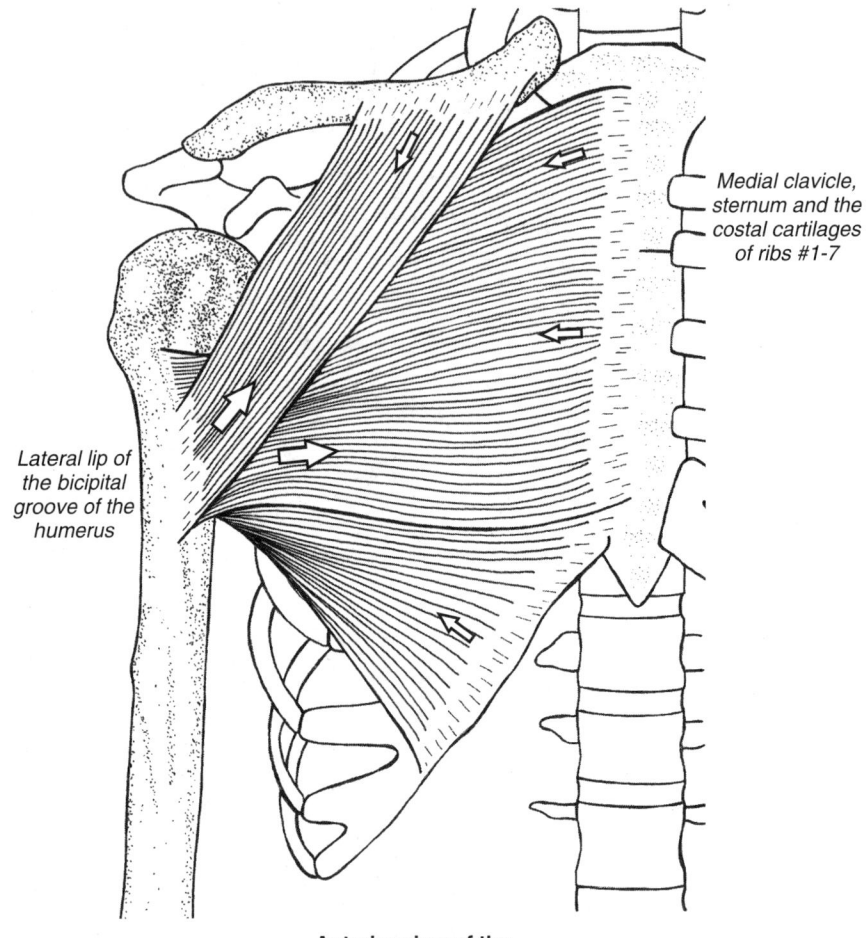

Anterior view of the right pectoralis major

THE MUSCULAR SYSTEM Muscles of the Trunk

DID YOU KNOW?

The pectoralis major makes up the vast majority of the anterior axillary fold of tissue, which borders the armpit anteriorly.

PECTORALIS MINOR
pek-to-**ra**-lis **my**-nor

Actions
Protraction (abduction) of the scapula at the scapulocostal joint
Depression of the scapula at the scapulocostal joint
Downward rotation of the scapula at the scapulocostal joint
Elevation of ribs #3-5 at the sternocostal and costovertebral joints

Innervation
The medial and lateral pectoral nerves

Arterial Supply
The pectoral branches of the thoracoacromial trunk

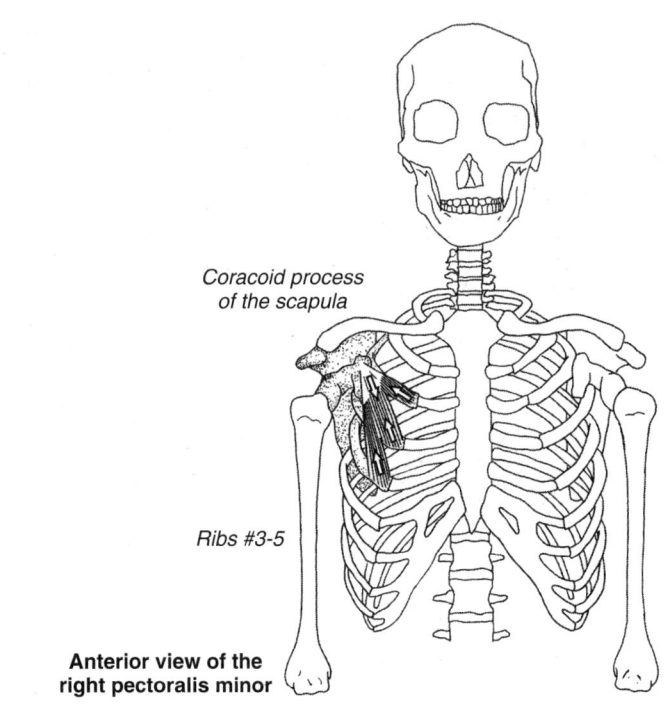

Anterior view of the right pectoralis minor

SUBCLAVIUS
sub-**klay**-vee-us

Actions
Depression of the clavicle at the sternoclavicular joint
Elevation of the 1st rib at the sternocostal and costovertebral joints
Protraction of the clavicle at the sternoclavicular joint
Downward rotation of the clavicle at the sternoclavicular joint

Innervation
A nerve from the brachial plexus

Arterial Supply
The clavicular branch of the thoracoacromial trunk and the suprascapular artery

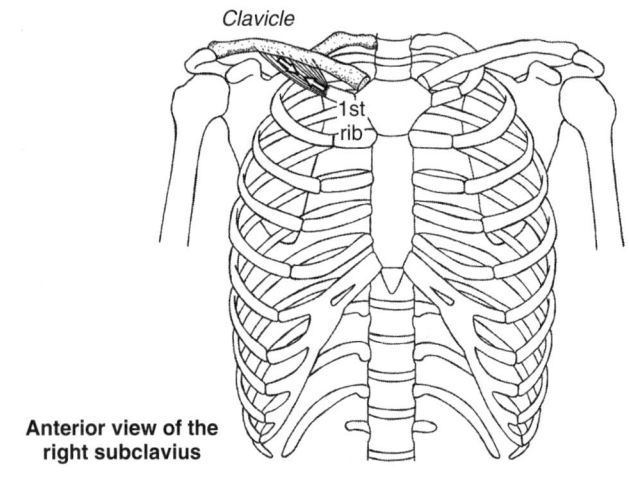

Anterior view of the right subclavius

THE MUSCULAR SYSTEM Muscles of the Trunk   147

If the pectoralis minor is tight, it may compress the brachial plexus of nerves and/or the subclavian artery and vein against the ribcage. This condition is called pectoralis minor syndrome, a type of thoracic outlet syndrome.

If the subclavius is tight, the brachial plexus of nerves and/or the subclavian artery and vein can be compressed between the 1st rib and the clavicle; this condition is called costoclavicular syndrome, a type of thoracic outlet syndrome.

EXTERNAL INTERCOSTALS
eks-turn-al in-ter-**kos**-tals

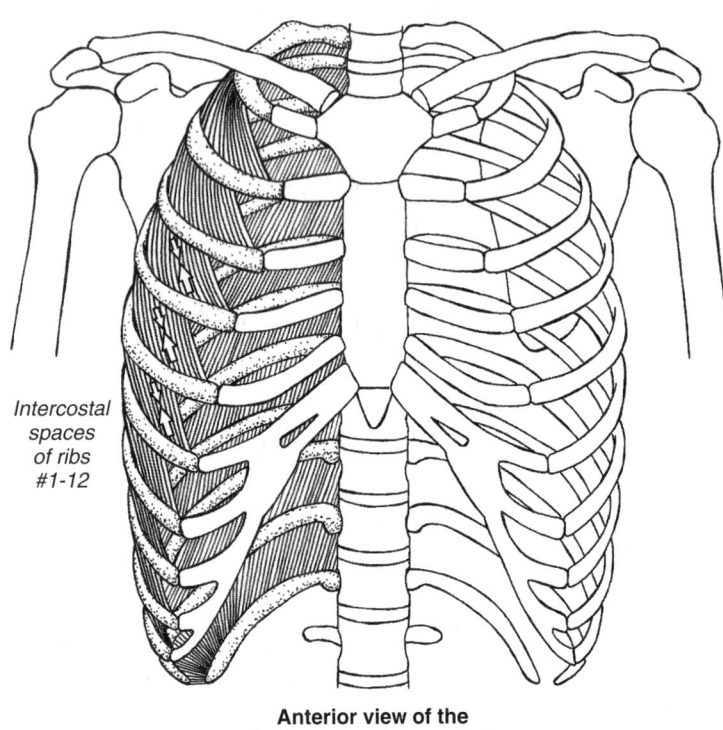

Intercostal spaces of ribs #1-12

Anterior view of the right external intercostals

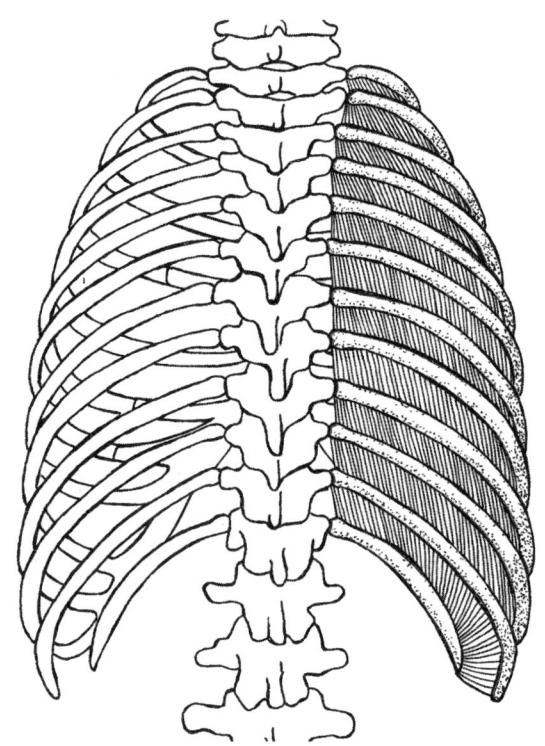

Posterior view of the right external intercostals

Actions
Elevation of ribs #2-12 at the sternocostal and costoclavicular joints
Depression of ribs #1-11 at the sternocostal and costoclavicular joints

Innervation
Intercostal nerves

Arterial Supply
Anterior intercostal arteries and the posterior intercostal arteries

THE MUSCULAR SYSTEM Muscles of the Trunk

Given their attachments to and movement of ribs, the external and internal intercostals are primarily muscles of respiration.

INTERNAL INTERCOSTALS
in-turn-al in-ter-kos-tals

Intercostal spaces of ribs #1-12

Anterior view of the right internal intercostals

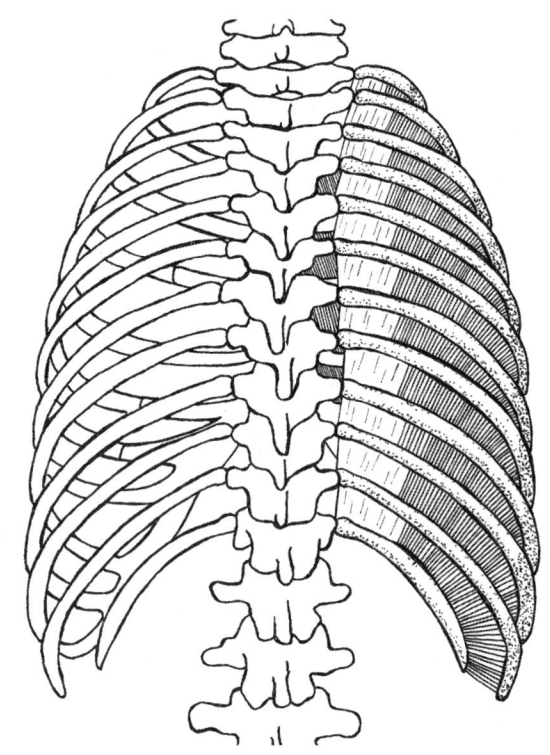

Posterior view of the right internal intercostals

Actions
Depression of ribs #1-11 at the sternocostal and costoclavicular joints
Elevation of ribs #2-12 at the sternocostal and costoclavicular joints

Innervation
Intercostal nerves

Arterial Supply
Anterior intercostal arteries and the posterior intercostal arteries

THE MUSCULAR SYSTEM Muscles of the Trunk

 DID YOU KNOW

Given their attachments to and movement of ribs, the external and internal intercostals are primarily muscles of respiration.

RECTUS ABDOMINIS
rek-tus ab-dom-i-nis

Actions
Flexion of the trunk at the spinal joints
Posterior tilt of the pelvis at the lumbosacral joint
Lateral flexion of the trunk at the spinal joints
Compression of the abdominal contents

Innervation
Intercostal nerves

Arterial Supply
The superior epigastric artery and the inferior epigastric artery

Xiphoid process and the cartilage of ribs #5-7

Pubis

Anterior view of the right rectus abdominis

THE MUSCULAR SYSTEM Muscles of the Trunk

DID YOU KNOW

Because of its separate compartments, the rectus abdominis is often called the 6-pack muscle. Given that there are 8 compartments, a better name would be the 8-pack muscle ☺.

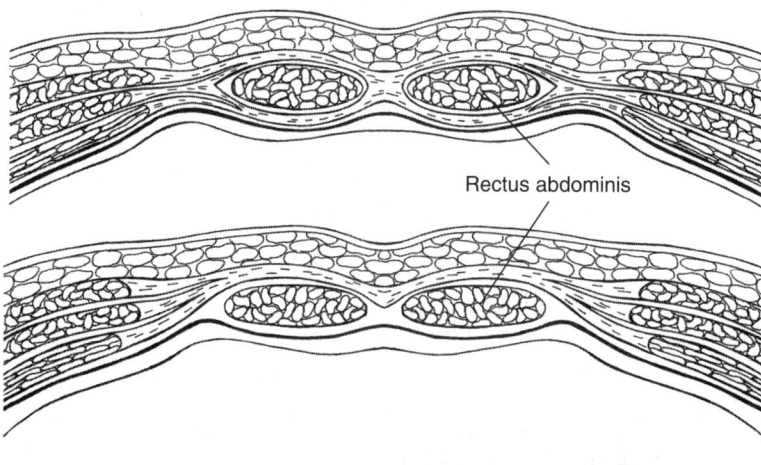

Anterior abdominal wall cross section superior to the arcuate line

Anterior abdominal wall cross section inferior to the arcuate line

EXTERNAL ABDOMINAL OBLIQUE

eks-turn-al
ab-**dom**-in-al
o-**bleek**

Actions
Flexion of the trunk at the spinal joints
Lateral flexion of the trunk at the spinal joints
Contralateral rotation of the trunk at the spinal joints
Posterior tilt of the pelvis at the lumbosacral joint
Ipsilateral rotation of the pelvis at the lumbosacral joint
Compression of the abdominal contents

Innervation
Intercostal nerves

Arterial Supply
The subcostal and posterior intercostal arteries and the deep circumflex iliac artery

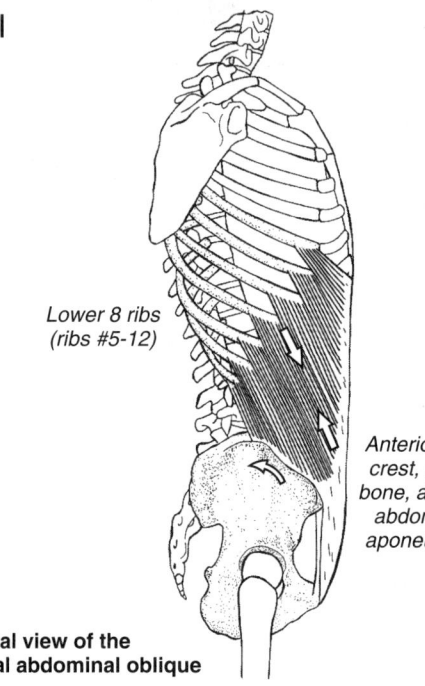

Lower 8 ribs (ribs #5-12)

Anterior iliac crest, pubic bone, and the abdominal aponeurosis

Lateral view of the right external abdominal oblique

INTERNAL ABDOMINAL OBLIQUE

in-**turn**-al
ab-**dom**-in-al
o-**bleek**

Actions
Flexion of the trunk at the spinal joints
Lateral flexion of the trunk at the spinal joints
Ipsilateral rotation of the trunk at the spinal joints
Posterior tilt of the pelvis at the lumbosacral joint
Contralateral rotation of the pelvis at the lumbosacral joint
Compression of the abdominal contents

Innervation
Intercostal nerves

Arterial Supply
The subcostal and posterior intercostal arteries and the deep circumflex iliac artery

Lower 3 ribs (#10-12) and the abdominal aponeurosis

Inguinal ligament, iliac crest and the thoracolumbar fascia

Lateral view of the right internal abdominal oblique

THE MUSCULAR SYSTEM Muscles of the Trunk

DID YOU KNOW?
The direction of fibers of the external abdominal obliques is the same as coat pockets. For this reason, these muscles are sometimes called the pocket muscles.

DID YOU KNOW?
The fiber direction of the internal abdominal oblique is opposite, i.e., perpendicular to the fiber direction of the external abdominal oblique on the same side of the body.

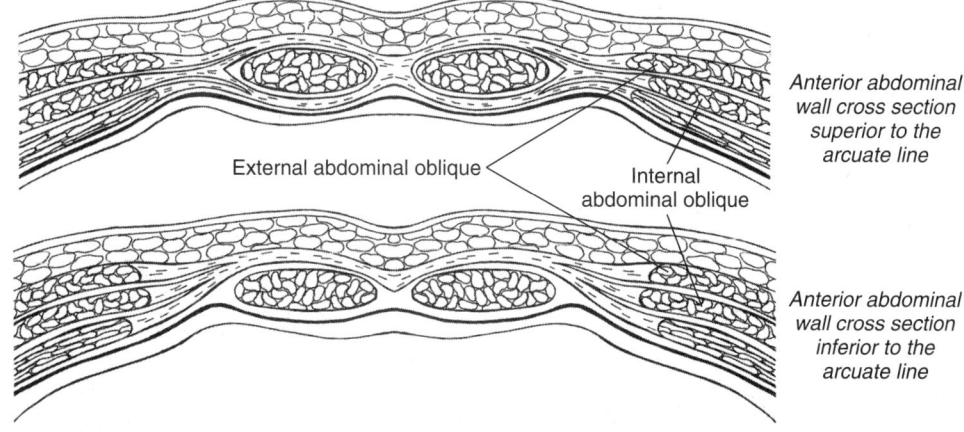

TRANSVERSUS ABDOMINIS
trans-**ver**-sus ab-**dom**-i-nis

Action
Compression of the abdominal contents

Innervation
Intercostal nerves

Arterial Supply
The subcostal and posterior intercostal arteries and the deep circumflex iliac artery

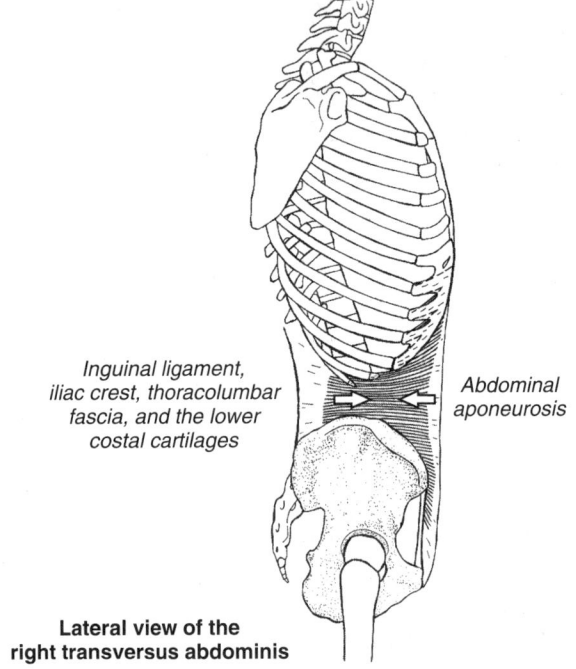

Inguinal ligament, iliac crest, thoracolumbar fascia, and the lower costal cartilages

Abdominal aponeurosis

Lateral view of the right transversus abdominis

TRANSVERSUS THORACIS
trans-**ver**-sus thor-**as**-is

Action
Depression of ribs #2-6 at the sternocostal and costovertebral joints

Innervation
Intercostal nerves

Arterial Supply
The anterior intercostal arteries

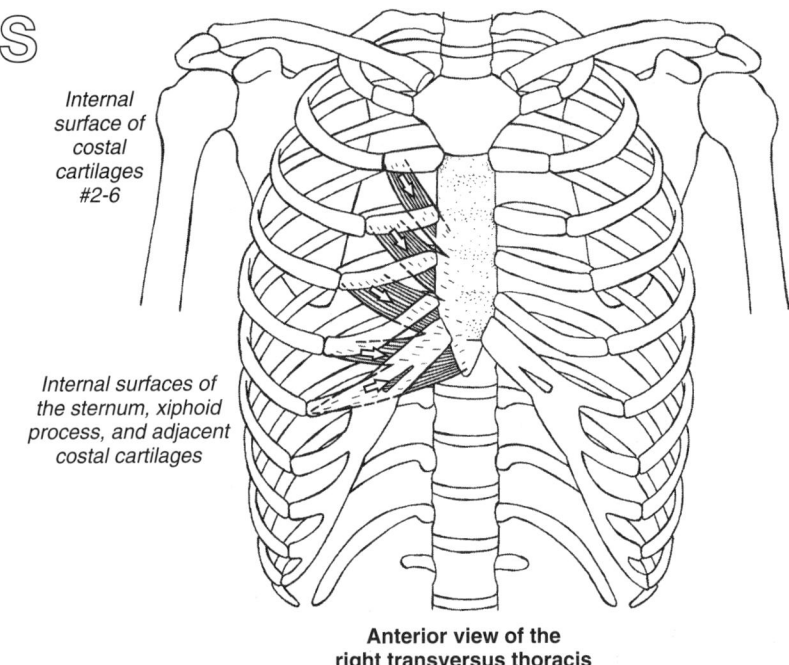

Internal surface of costal cartilages #2-6

Internal surfaces of the sternum, xiphoid process, and adjacent costal cartilages

Anterior view of the right transversus thoracis

THE MUSCULAR SYSTEM Muscles of the Trunk 157

DID YOU KNOW?

The transversus abdominis is sometimes called the corset muscle because it wraps around the abdomen like a corset, and like a corset, it functions to hold in the abdomen.

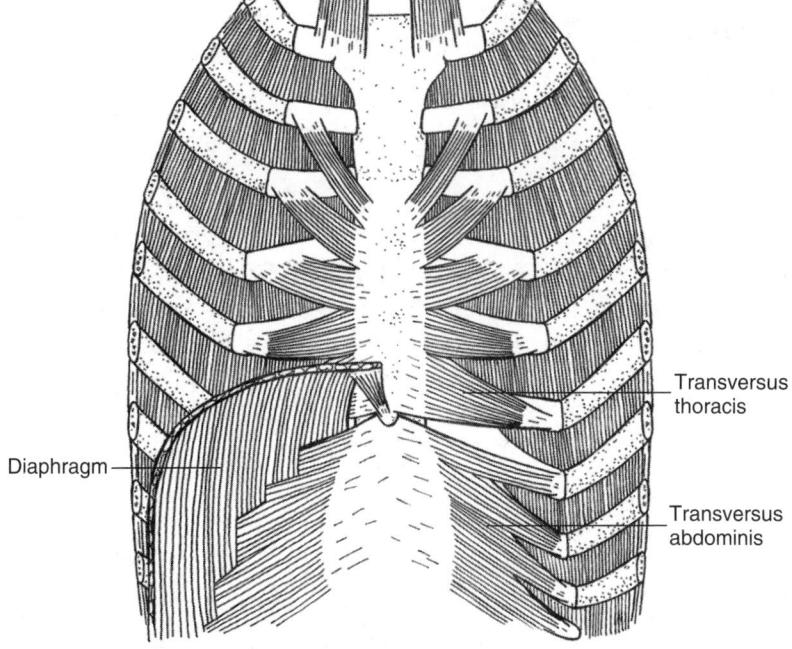

Posterior view of the anterior ribcage

DID YOU KNOW?

The transversus thoracis is located deep to the ribcage.

DIAPHRAGM
di-a-fram

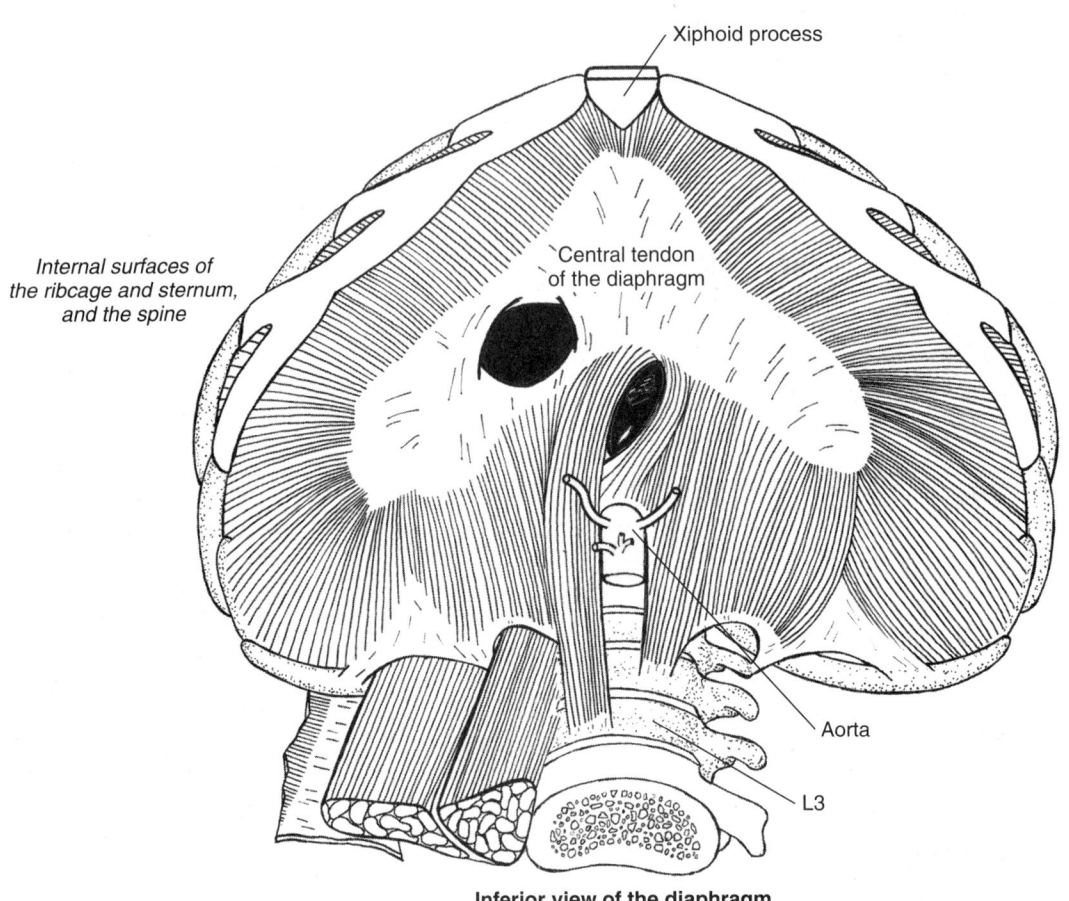

Inferior view of the diaphragm

Action	Innervation	Arterial Supply
Increases the volume of the thoracic cavity	The phrenic nerve	Branches of the aorta and the internal thoracic artery

THE MUSCULAR SYSTEM Muscles of the Trunk

DID YOU KNOW

The diaphragm is an unusual muscle in that it is under both conscious and unconscious control by the nervous system.

Transversus thoracis

Transversus abdominis

Diaphragm

Posterior view

THE MUSCULAR SYSTEM — Muscles of the Trunk

POSTERIOR VIEW OF THE TRUNK (SUPERFICIAL AND INTERMEDIATE)

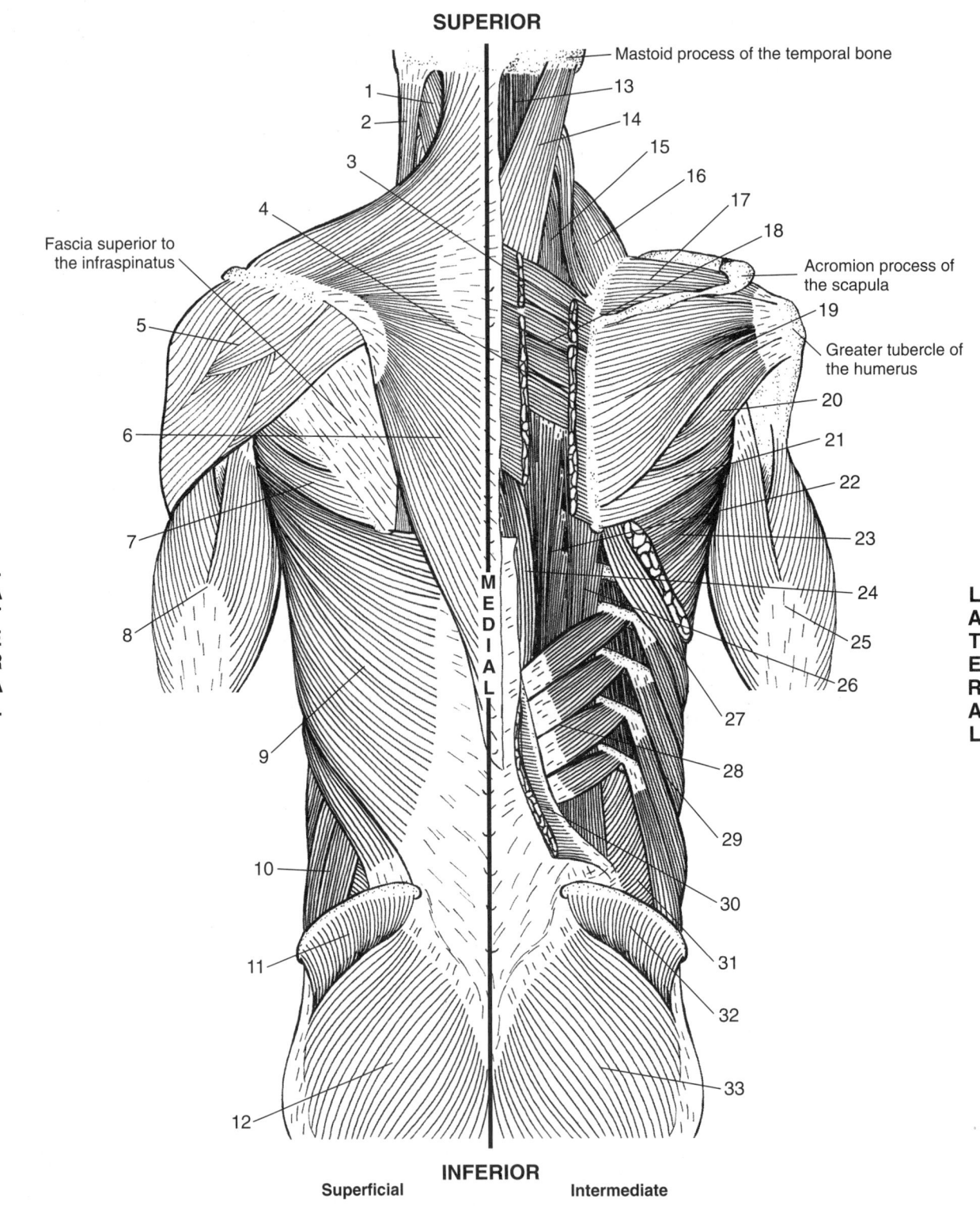

THE MUSCULAR SYSTEM Muscles of the Trunk

POSTERIOR VIEW OF THE TRUNK (DEEP LAYERS)

Deep – layer 1   Deep – layer 2

162 THE MUSCULAR SYSTEM Muscles of the Trunk

ANTERIOR VIEW OF THE TRUNK
(SUPERFICIAL AND INTERMEDIATE)

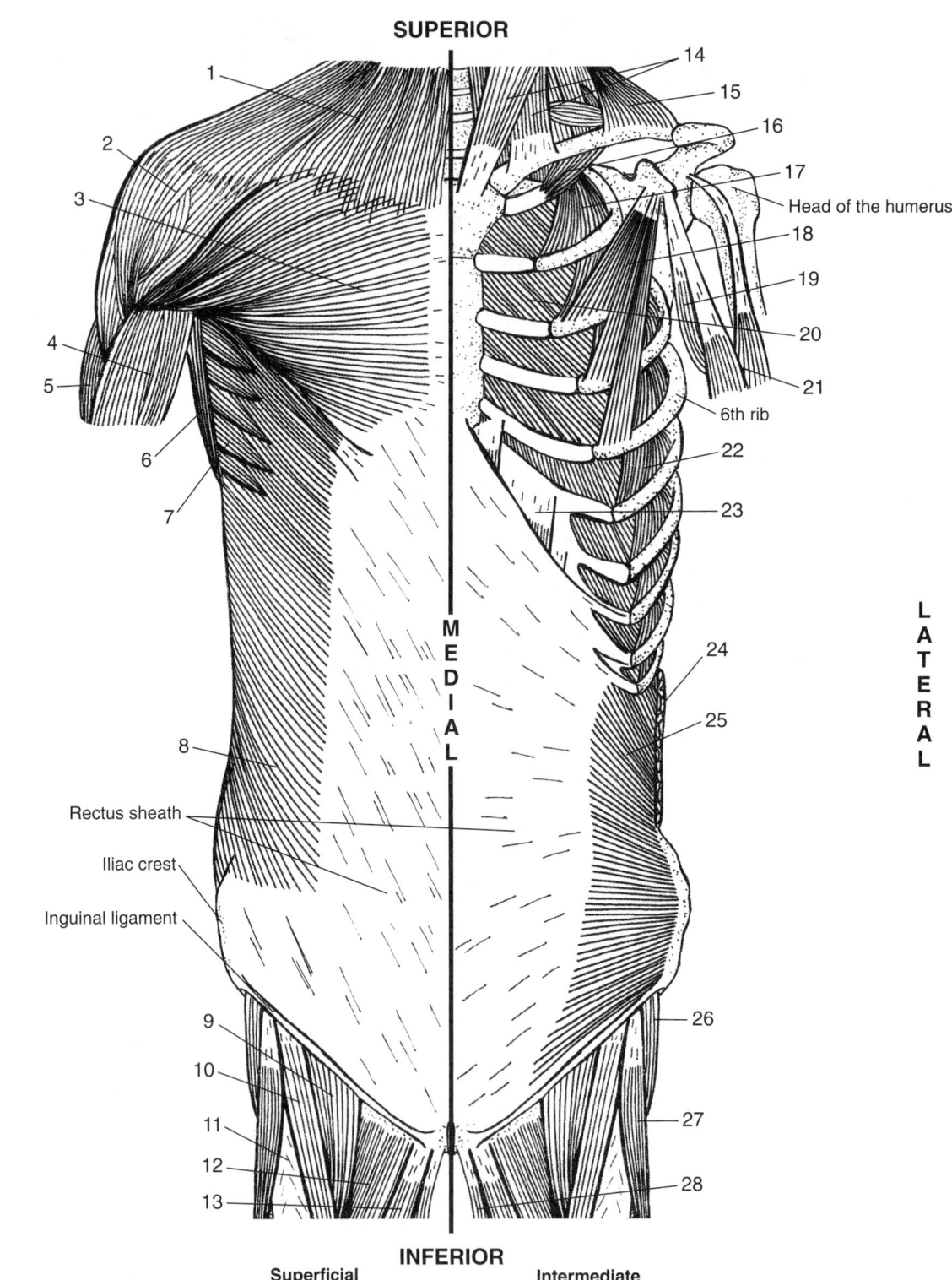

Superficial / Intermediate

THE MUSCULAR SYSTEM Muscles of the Trunk

ANTERIOR VIEW OF THE TRUNK (INTERMEDIATE AND DEEP)

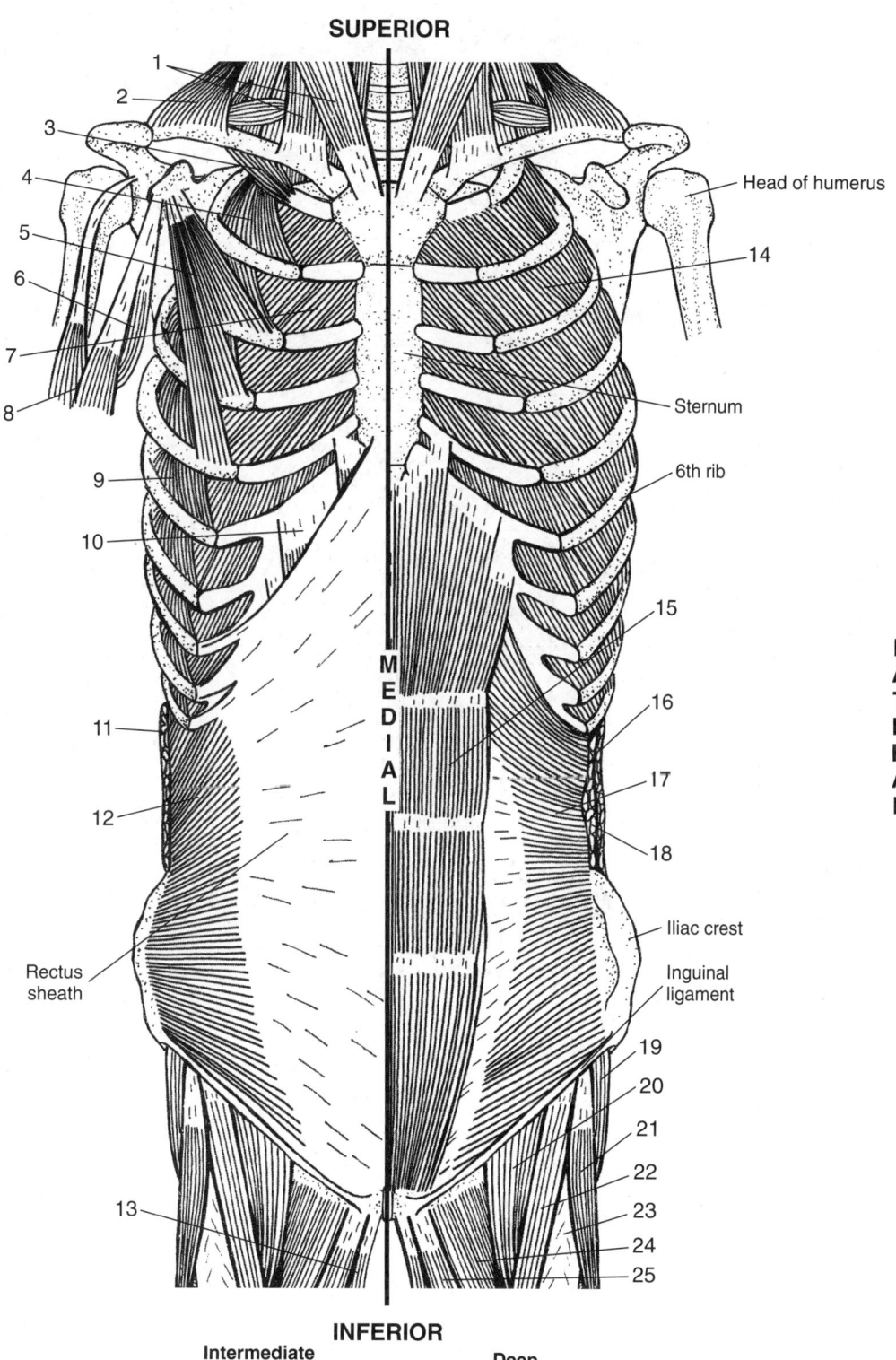

164 THE MUSCULAR SYSTEM Muscles of the Trunk

LATERAL VIEW OF THE TRUNK

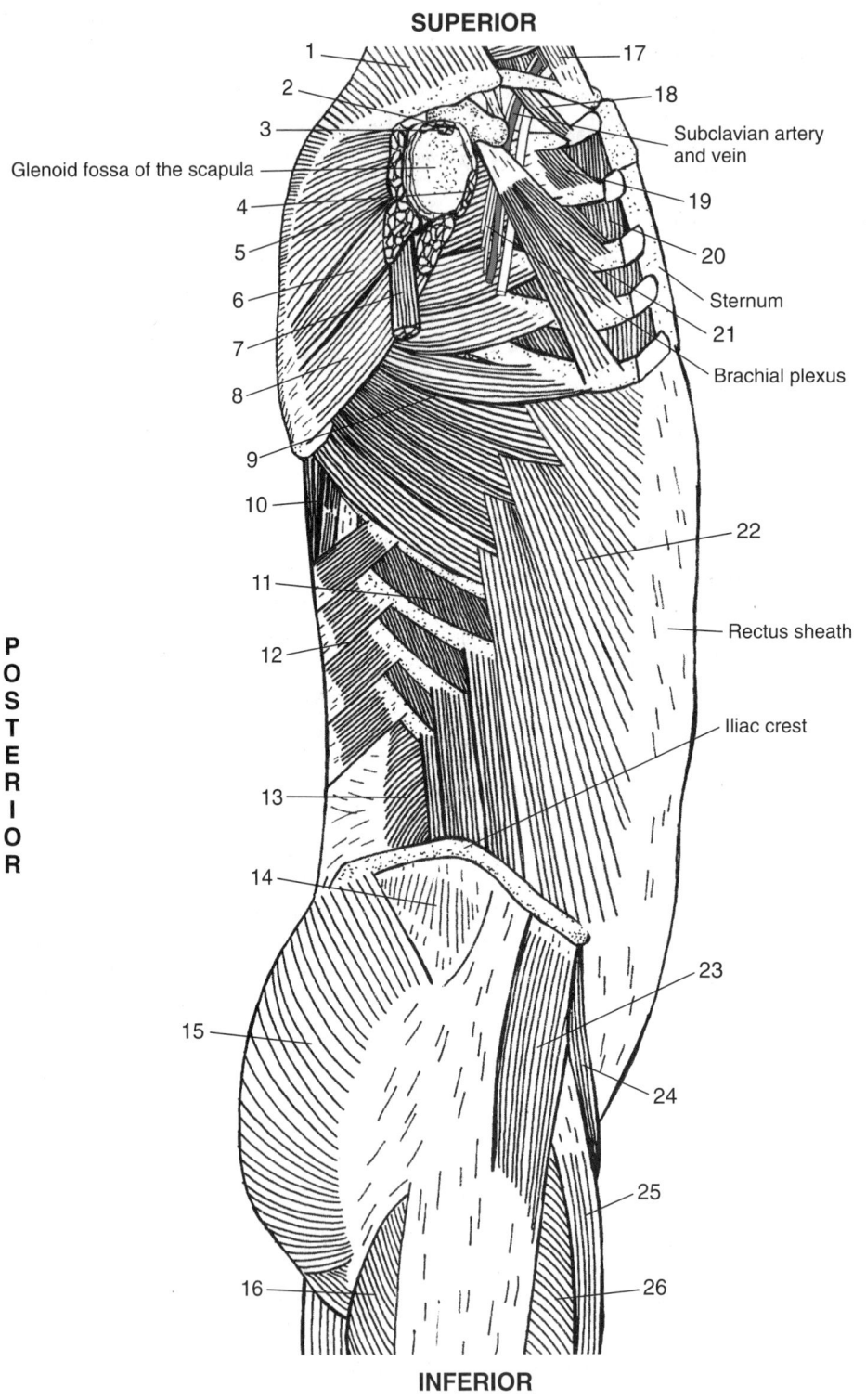

THE MUSCULAR SYSTEM Muscles of the Trunk

CROSS SECTION VIEWS OF THE TRUNK

Thoracic cross section

Lumbar cross section

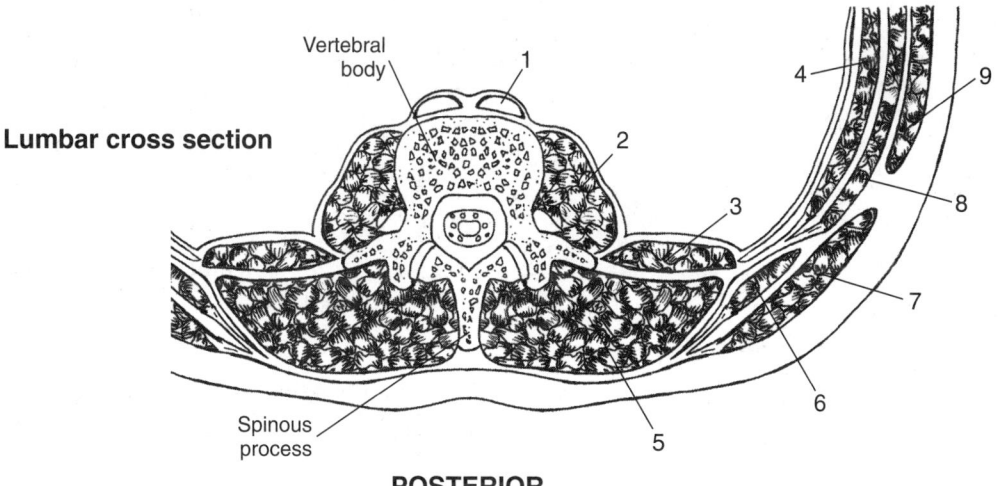

Review Questions

Muscles of the Trunk
Answers to these questions are found on page 465.

1. What subgroup of the transversospinalis is immediately superficial to the rotatores?

2. What muscle makes up the vast majority of the anterior axillary fold of tissue?

3. What muscles sit the deepest in the laminar groove of the spine?

4. What are the two heads of the pectoralis major?

5. With regard to flexion of the trunk at the spinal joints, what two abdominal wall muscles are synergistic with the rectus abdominis?

6. What joint action is occurring when the right sided intertransversarii are eccentrically contracting?

7. Name two actions of the serratus anterior that are synergistic with actions of the pectoralis minor?

8. What muscle is immediately superficial to the pectoralis minor?

9. True or false: the diaphragm is under both conscious and unconscious control.

10. What is the direction of fibers of the external abdominal oblique compared to the internal abdominal oblique on the same side?

11. What two muscles make up the vast majority of the posterior axillary fold of tissue?

12. What structures can the pectoralis minor compress against the ribcage?

13. What joint action is occurring when the interspinales are lengthening?

14. If the pelvis is anteriorly tilting at the lumbosacral joint, what is happening to the length of the erector spinae group?

15. What two muscles pierce the diaphragm posteriorly?

16. What muscle attaches to the underside of the clavicle?

17. Would left lateral flexion of the trunk at the spinal joints lengthen or shorten the right sided levatores costarum?

18. Which subgroup of the erector spinae goes from spinous processes to spinous processes?

19. The serratus anterior interdigitates (blends) with what muscle anteriorly?

20. What muscle group is immediately superficial to the levatores costarum?

21. The upper fibers on the ribcage of the serratus anterior are deep to what two muscles?

22. If the superior rib attachment of an external intercostal muscle is fixed, what action will occur?

23. What muscles are often called the *coat pocket muscles*?

24. What is happening to the length of the left quadratus lumborum when the pelvis is posteriorly tilting at the lumbosacral joint?

25. What two abdominal wall muscles attach into the thoracolumbar fascia?

26. What happens to the length of the rhomboids as the scapula protracts [abducts] at the scapulocostal joint?

27. What muscles are known as the "Christmas Tree" muscles?

28. What muscle is located deep (posterior) to the anterior ribcage and is analogous to the transversus abdominis?

29. If the inferior rib attachment of an external intercostal muscle is fixed, what action will occur?

30. What two muscles can upwardly rotate the scapula at the scapulocostal joint?

31. How are the serratus posterior inferior and quadratus lumborum synergistic with each other?

32. Where the latissimus dorsi and trapezius overlap, which muscle is superficial?

33. What happens to the length of the rectus abdominis as the pelvis anteriorly tilts at the lumbosacral joint?

34. The serratus posterior inferior is immediately deep to what muscle?

35. If the right-sided rotatores are concentrically contracting, what type of rotation of the spine is occurring?

36. Where are intercostal muscles not deep to external intercostals?

37. If the pectoralis minor is eccentrically contracting, is the scapula protracting or retracting at the scapulocostal joint?

38. Which subgroup of the erector spinae is the most lateral?

39. What is the only subgroup of the transversospinalis that attaches to the pelvis?

40. The direction of fibers of the external intercostals is similar to what muscle?

41. How is the right external abdominal oblique synergistic with and also antagonistic to the right internal abdominal oblique?

42. Which subgroup of the erector spinae is the longest?

43. What happens to the length of the left rectus abdominis as the trunk is passively left laterally flexed at the spinal joints?

44. If the latissimus dorsi eccentrically contracts as the pelvis moves, how is the pelvis moving?

45. What three muscles are located lateral to the rectus abdominis?

46. If the arm medially rotates at the shoulder joint, what happens to the length of the latissimus dorsi?

47. What happens to the length of the right-sided rotatores if the spine is rotated to the right?

48. Name a muscle that is antagonistic to the elevation of the twelfth rib action of the internal intercostals.

49. Which subgroup of the transversospinalis is deepest?

50. If the right-sided rotatores are eccentrically contracting, what type of rotation of the spine is occurring?

51. Which subgroup of the erector spinae is the most medial?

52. Which subgroup of the erector spinae goes from the pelvis to ribs?

53. Which subgroup of the transversospinalis is most superficial?

54. What is happening to the length of the left quadratus lumborum when the spine is laterally flexing to the left?

55. What muscle is superficial to the rhomboids?

56. As a rule, transversospinalis musculature attaches from where to where?

57. Which muscle attaches farther posteriorly, the external or internal abdominal oblique?

58. How are the serratus posterior superior and scalenes synergistic with each other?

59. What muscle is immediately deep to the internal abdominal oblique?

60. What happens to the length of the transversus abdominis as a person breathes in and their belly rises?

61. When the diaphragm concentrically contracts, what happens to its dome (central tendon)?

62. In what region is the multifidus of the transversospinalis group the largest?

63. What muscle is deep to the rhomboids and has the same direction of fibers?

64. What muscle attaches from the pelvis to the lumbar spine and twelfth rib and is deep to the erector spinae group?

65. What is the name of the connective tissue that envelops the rectus abdominis?

66. In the thoracic region, the transversospinalis musculature is deep to which muscle of the erector spinae group?

67. Name a synergist to the pectoralis minor's action of protraction of the scapula at the scapulocostal joint?

68. What happens to the length of the pectoralis major if the arm laterally rotates at the shoulder joint?

69. What muscle is immediately superficial to the transversus abdominis?

70. What muscle group is immediately superficial to the quadratus lumborum?

71. If the subclavius is tight, what condition might be caused?

72. Which subgroup of the transversospinalis is best suited for rotation of the spine and why?

73. What is the superior attachment of the rotatores?

74. From a posterior perspective, which is deeper, the intercostals or the subcostales?

75. What muscle is immediately deep to the external intercostals?

76. How are the rhomboids synergistic with the middle trapezius?

77. What muscle is immediately superficial to the semispinalis in the suboccipital region?

78. If the serratus posterior inferior is eccentrically contracting, what joint motion is occurring?

79. What spinal rotation is created by the transversospinalis musculature on the right side of the body?

80. In what region is the semispinalis of the transversospinalis group the largest?

81. If the trunk is passively flexing at the spinal joints, what is happening to the length of the erector spinae group?

82. What muscle group is deep to the rhomboids and has a vertical direction to its fibers?

83. What is the superior attachment of the diaphragm?

84. Which head of the pectoralis major is better suited to create flexion of the arm at the shoulder joint?

85. Are the right and left side intertransversarii synergistic with or antagonistic to each other?

86. What muscle has the same humeral actions as the latissimus dorsi?

87. Where they overlap, which is deeper, the erector spinae group or the transversospinalis group?

88. What muscle is known as the *corset muscle*?

89. What muscle is immediately deep to the distal attachment of the pectoralis major?

90. If a person's trunk is actively rotated to the right, what happens to the length of the transversospinalis musculature on the right?

91. The direction of fibers of the internal intercostals is similar to what muscle?

92. What region of the spine is mostly missing interspinales?

93. What is the action upon the spine if both quadratus lumborum muscles contract together?

94. What muscle is immediately superficial to the internal intercostals?

95. Why are the levatores costarum and subcostales antagonistic to each other?

170 THE MUSCULAR SYSTEM Muscles of the Pelvis

ANTERIOR VIEW OF THE RIGHT PELVIS

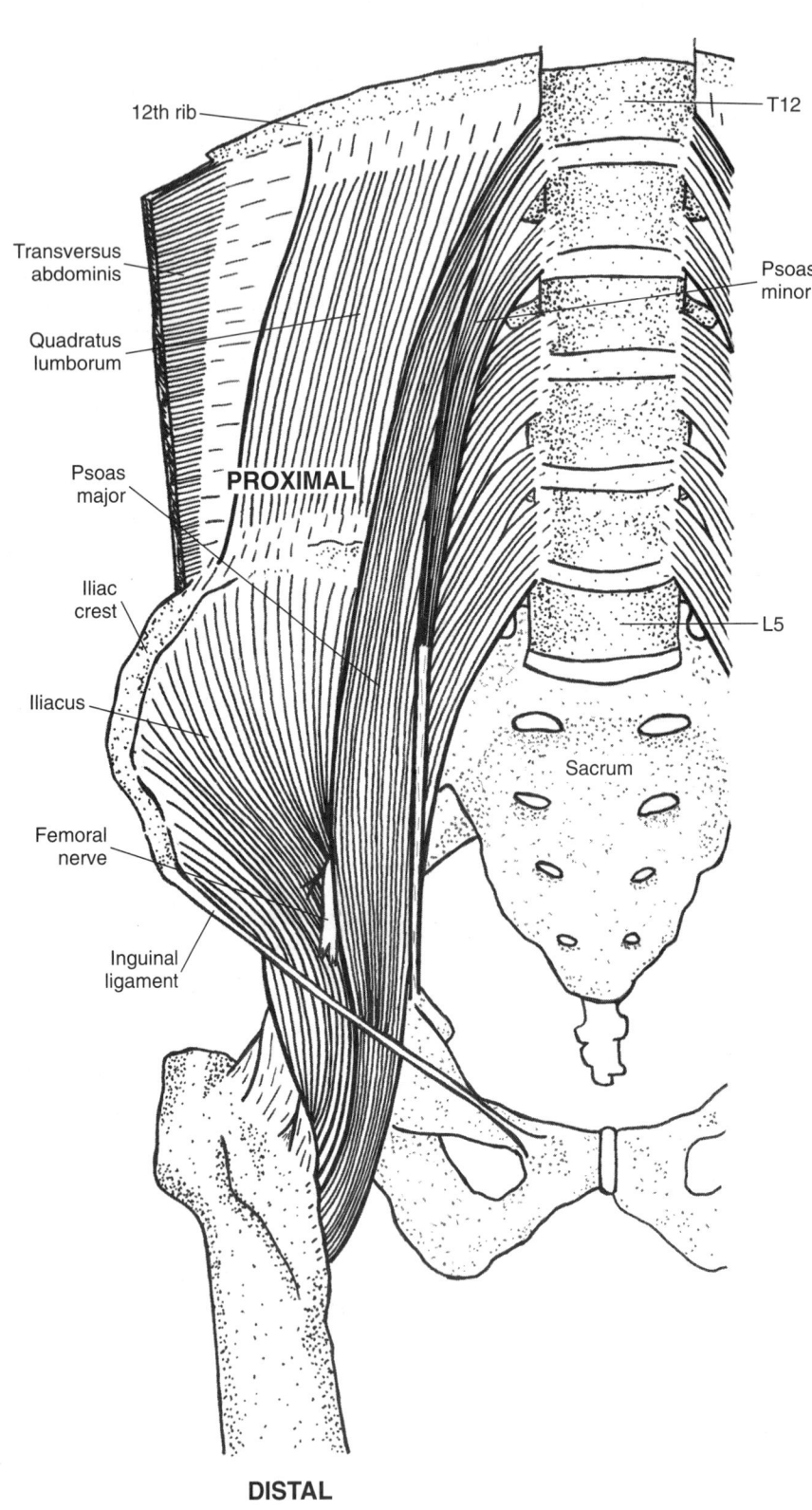

THE MUSCULAR SYSTEM Muscles of the Pelvis

LATERAL VIEW OF THE RIGHT PELVIS

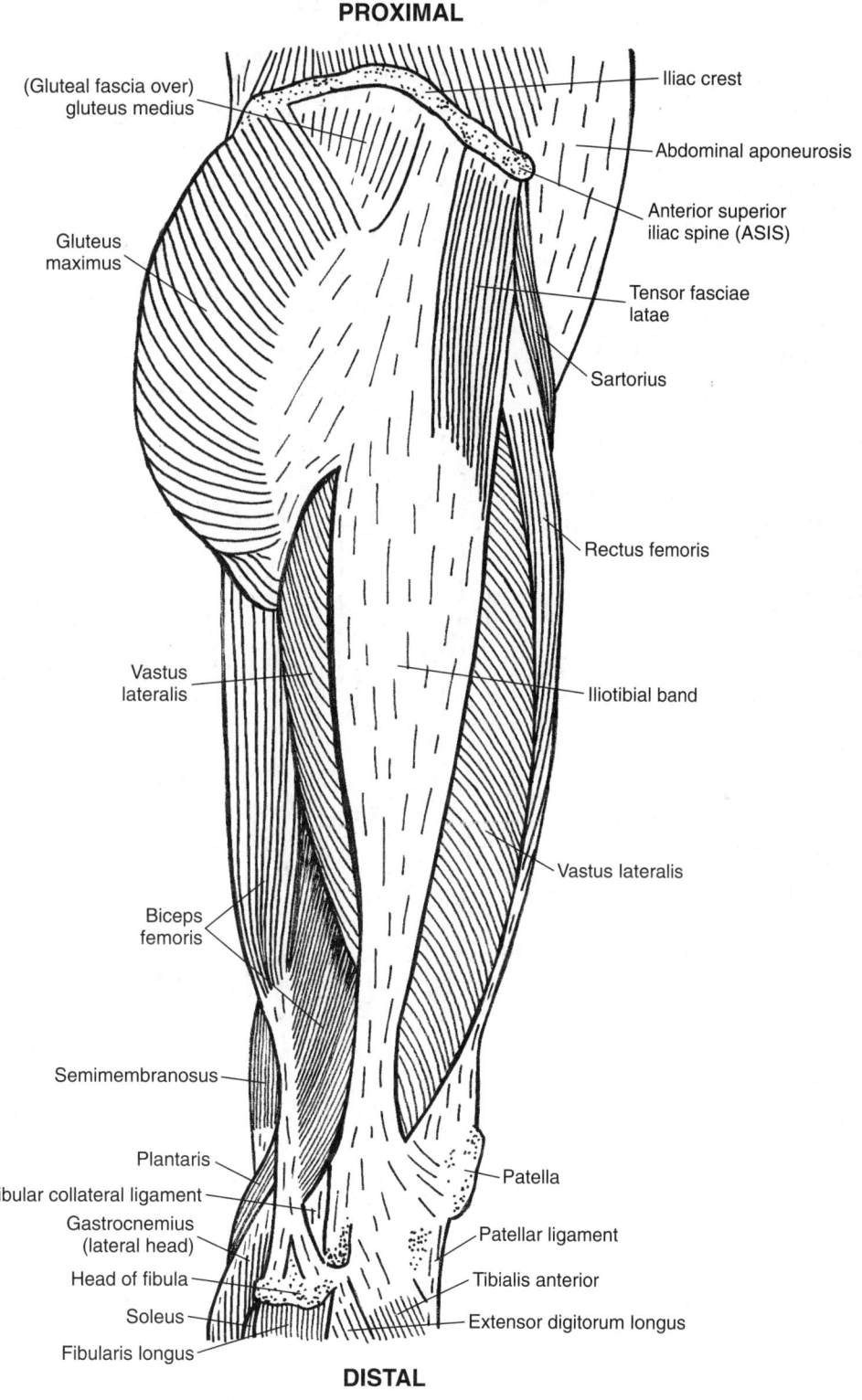

172 THE MUSCULAR SYSTEM Muscles of the Pelvis

POSTERIOR VIEW OF THE RIGHT PELVIS (SUPERFICIAL)

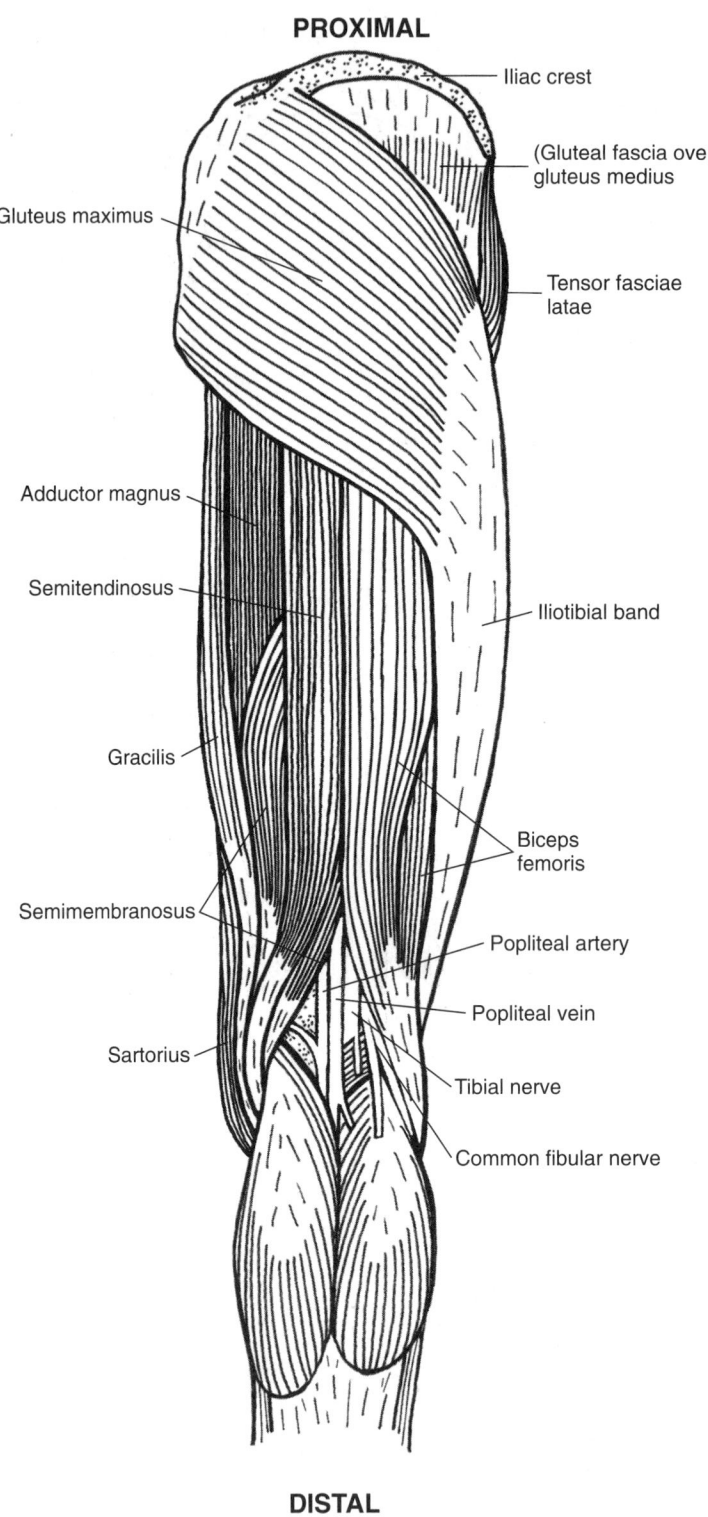

THE MUSCULAR SYSTEM Muscles of the Pelvis

POSTERIOR VIEW OF THE RIGHT PELVIS (DEEP)

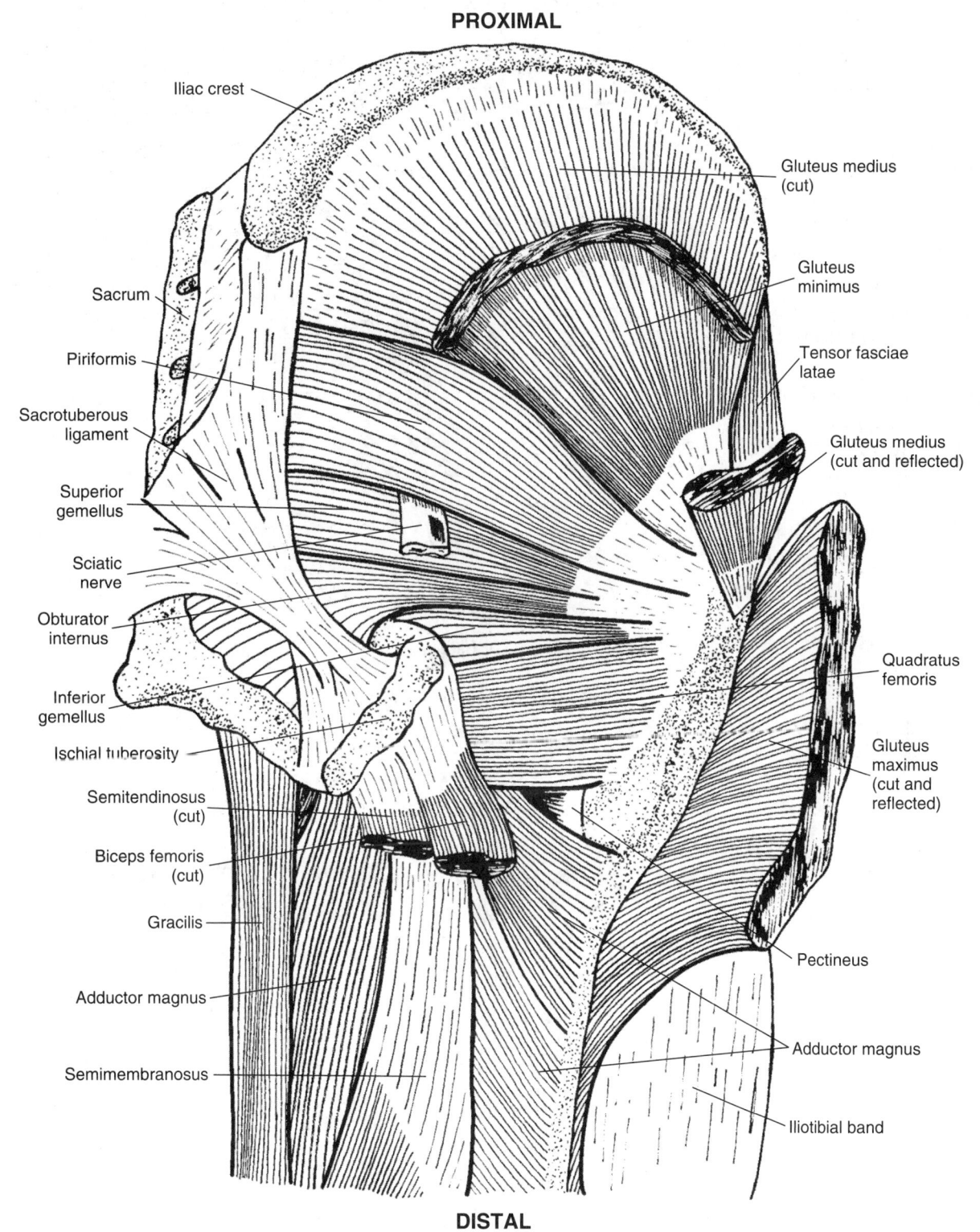

PSOAS MAJOR
(OF THE ILIOPSOAS)
so-as may-jor

Actions
Flexion of the thigh at the hip joint
Lateral rotation of the thigh at the hip joint
Flexion of the trunk at the spinal joints
Lateral flexion of the trunk at the spinal joints
Anterior tilt of the pelvis at the hip joint
Contralateral rotation of the trunk at the spinal joints
Contralateral rotation of the pelvis at the hip joint

Innervation
Lumbar plexus

Arterial Supply
The lumbar arteries

Anterolateral lumbar spine

Lesser trochanter of the femur

Anterior view of the right psoas major

THE MUSCULAR SYSTEM Muscles of the Pelvis

DID YOU KNOW

The reason that old-fashioned sit-ups have been replaced by abdominal curl-ups or crunches is to avoid creating an overly strengthened and perhaps overly tight psoas major.

ILIACUS
(OF THE ILIOPSOAS)
i-lee-**ak**-us

Actions
Flexion of the thigh at the hip joint
Lateral rotation of the thigh at the hip joint
Anterior tilt of the pelvis at the hip joint
Contralateral rotation of the pelvis at the hip joint

Innervation
The femoral nerve

Arterial Supply
The iliolumbar artery

Internal ilium

Lesser trochanter of the femur

Anterior view of the right iliacus

THE MUSCULAR SYSTEM Muscles of the Pelvis

DID YOU KNOW?

The distal tendon of the iliacus joins into the distal tendon of the psoas major; together, these two muscles are often called the iliopsoas muscle.

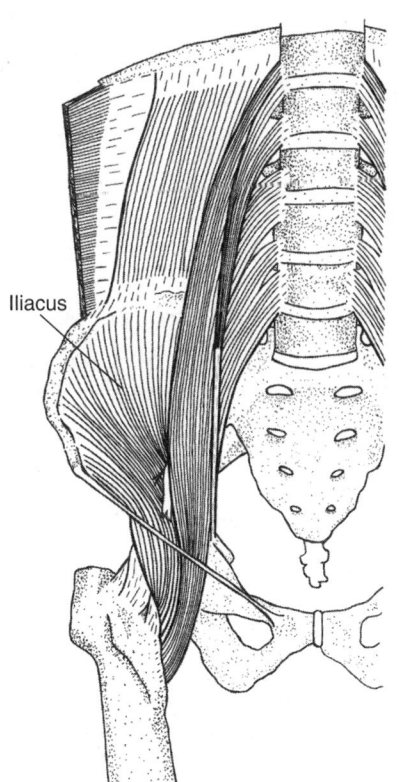

PSOAS MINOR
so-as my-nor

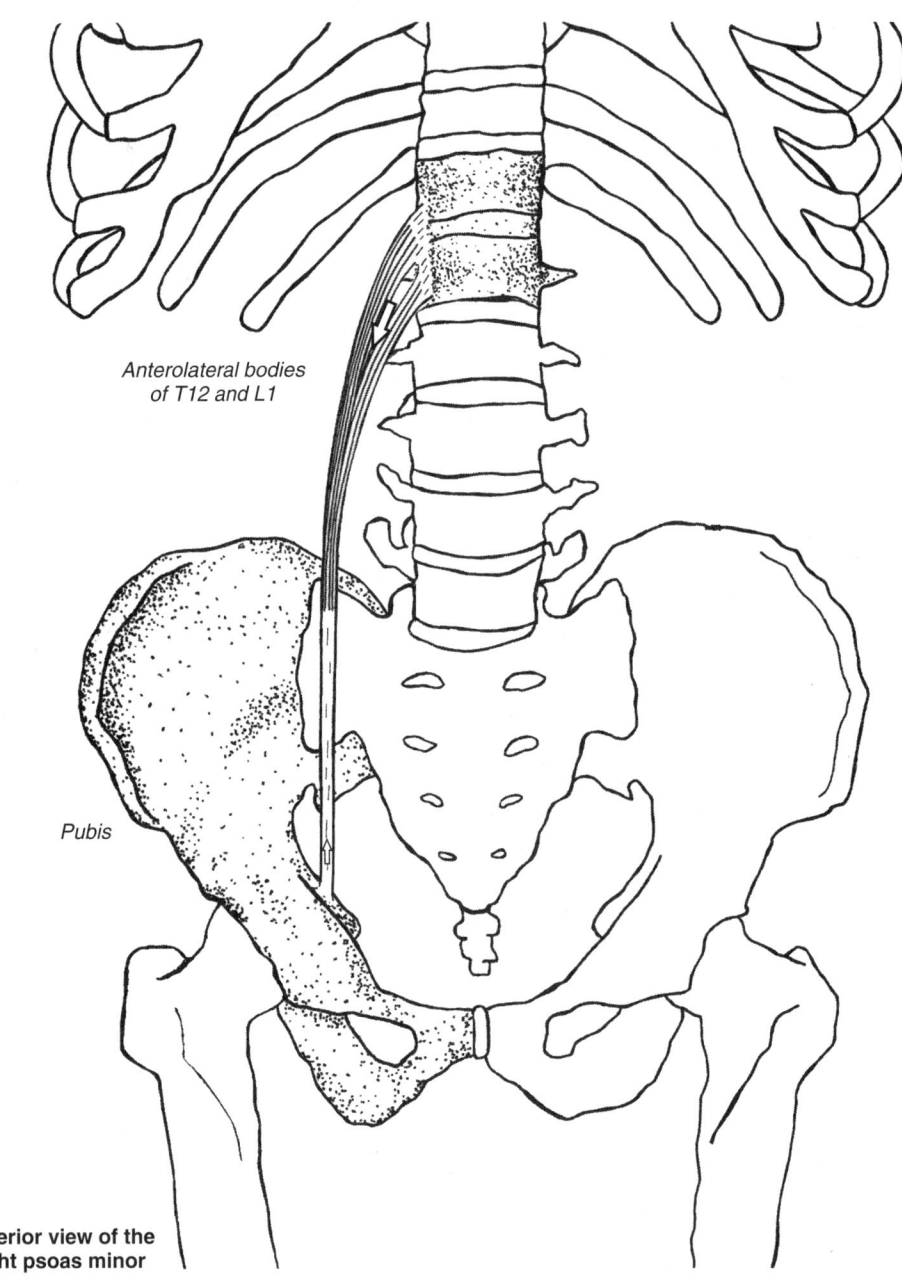

Anterolateral bodies of T12 and L1

Pubis

Anterior view of the right psoas minor

Actions	Innervation	Arterial Supply
Flexion of the trunk at the spinal joints Posterior tilt of the pelvis at the lumbosacral joint	L1 spinal nerve	Lumbar arteries

THE MUSCULAR SYSTEM Muscles of the Pelvis

Psoas minor

DID YOU KNOW

The psoas minor is absent in up to 40% of individuals.

GLUTEUS MAXIMUS
gloo-tee-us max-i-mus

Actions
Extension of the thigh at the hip joint
Lateral rotation of the thigh at the hip joint
Abduction of the thigh at the hip joint (upper 1/3)
Adduction of the thigh at the hip joint (lower 2/3)
Posterior tilt of the pelvis at the hip joint
Contralateral rotation of the pelvis at the hip joint
Extension of the leg at the knee joint

Innervation
The inferior gluteal nerve (L5, S1, 2)

Arterial Supply
The superior gluteal artery and the inferior gluteal artery

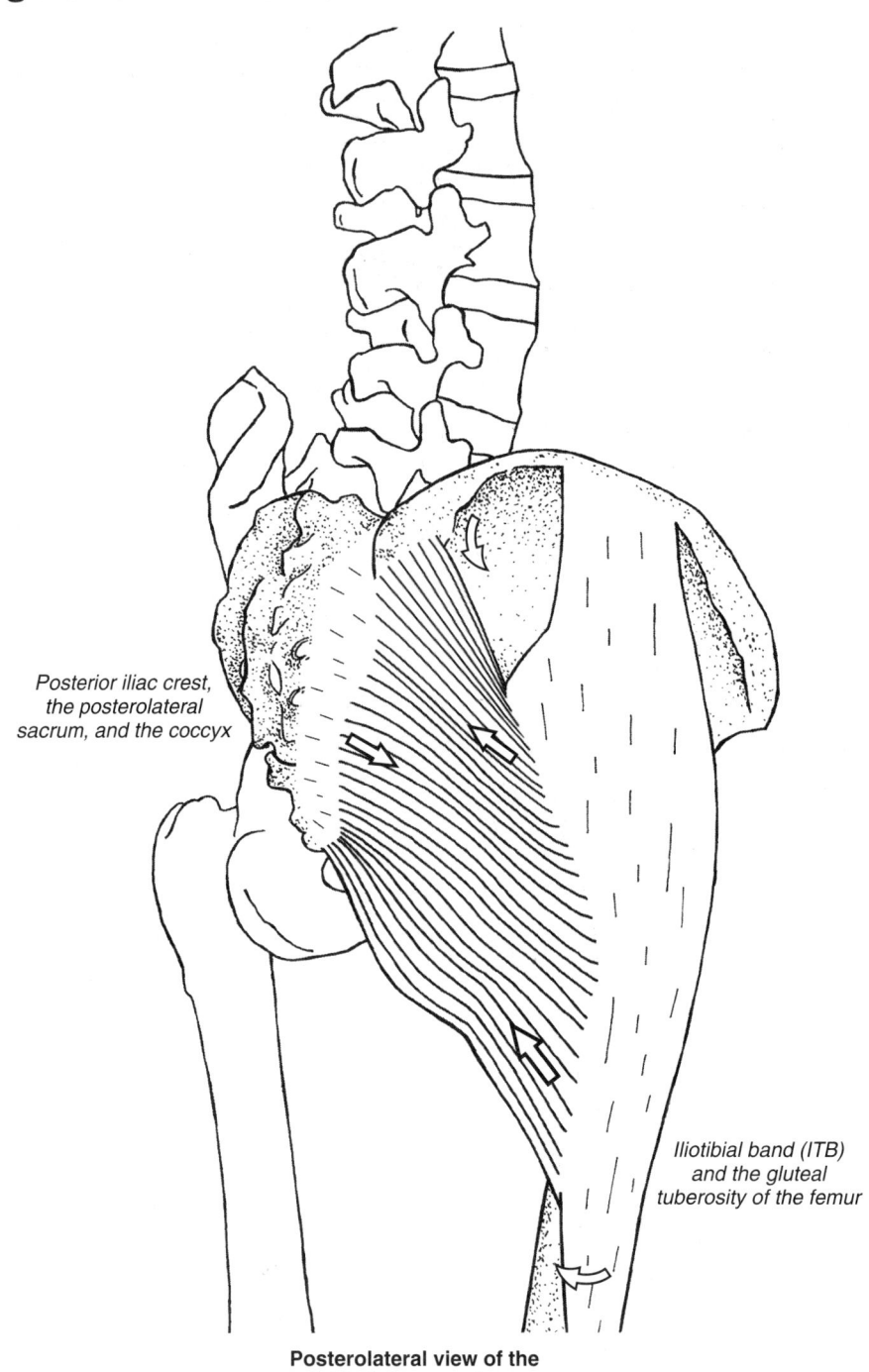

Posterior iliac crest, the posterolateral sacrum, and the coccyx

Iliotibial band (ITB) and the gluteal tuberosity of the femur

Posterolateral view of the right gluteus maximus

THE MUSCULAR SYSTEM Muscles of the Pelvis

The gluteus maximus is the largest muscle in the human body.

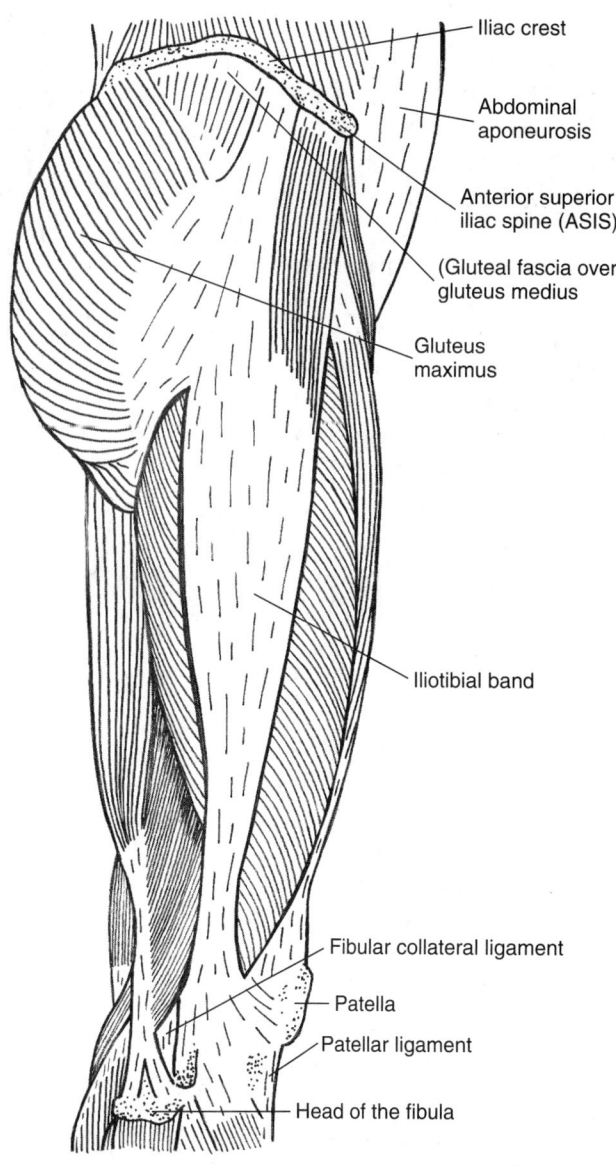

GLUTEUS MEDIUS
gloo-tee-us **meed**-ee-us

Actions
Abduction of the thigh at the hip joint (entire muscle)
Flexion of the thigh at the hip joint (anterior fibers)
Medial rotation of the thigh at the hip joint (anterior fibers)
Extension of the thigh at the hip joint (posterior fibers)
Lateral rotation of the thigh at the hip joint (posterior fibers)
Posterior tilt of the pelvis at the hip joint (posterior fibers)
Anterior tilt of the pelvis at the hip joint (anterior fibers)
Depression (lateral tilt) of the pelvis at the hip joint (entire muscle)
Ipsilateral rotation of the pelvis at the hip joint (anterior fibers)
Contralateral rotation of the pelvis at the hip joint (posterior fibers)

Innervation
The superior gluteal nerve

Arterial Supply
The superior gluteal artery

Posterolateral view of the right gluteus medius

THE MUSCULAR SYSTEM Muscles of the Pelvis

DID YOU KNOW?

Depression of the pelvis at the hip joint during walking is actually the most important action of the gluteus medius.

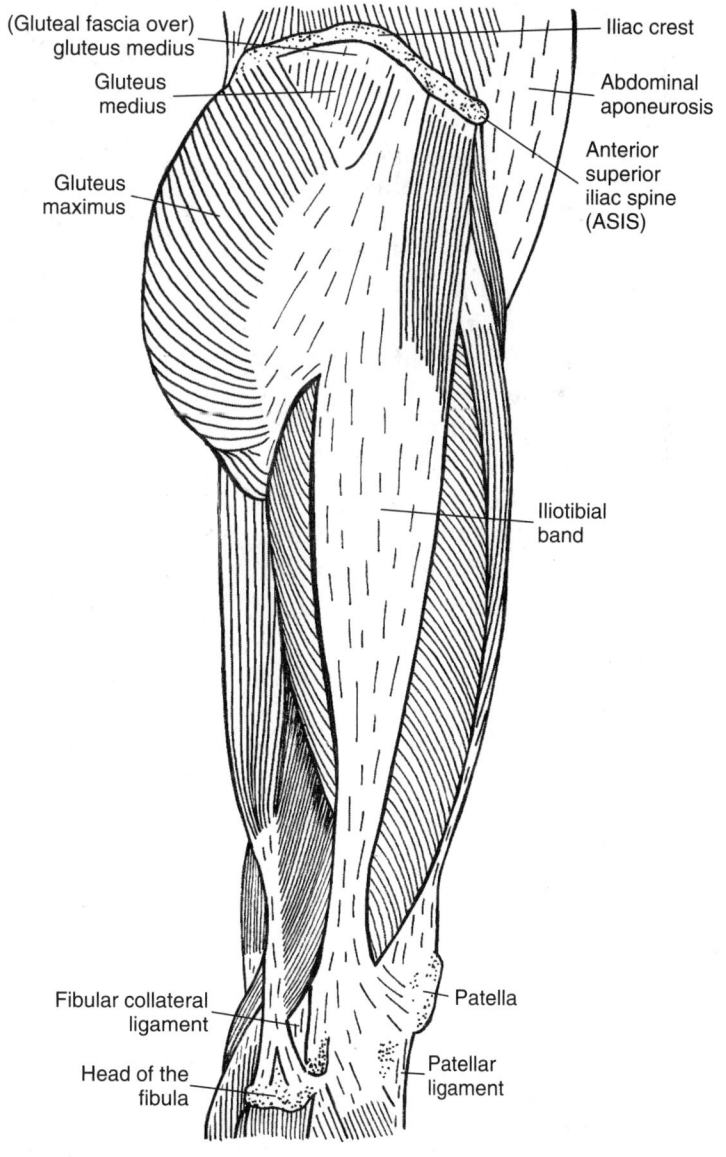

GLUTEUS MINIMUS
gloo-tee-us min-i-mus

Actions
Abduction of the thigh at the hip joint (entire muscle)
Flexion of the thigh at the hip joint (anterior fibers)
Medial rotation of the thigh at the hip joint (anterior fibers)
Extension of the thigh at the hip joint (posterior fibers)
Lateral rotation of the thigh at the hip joint (posterior fibers)
Posterior tilt of the pelvis at the hip joint (posterior fibers)
Anterior tilt of the pelvis at the hip joint (anterior fibers)
Depression (lateral tilt) of the pelvis at the hip joint (entire muscle)
Ipsilateral rotation of the pelvis at the hip joint (anterior fibers)
Contralateral rotation of the pelvis at the hip joint (posterior fibers)

Innervation
The superior gluteal nerve

Arterial Supply
The superior gluteal artery

Posterolateral view of the right gluteus minimus

THE MUSCULAR SYSTEM Muscles of the Pelvis

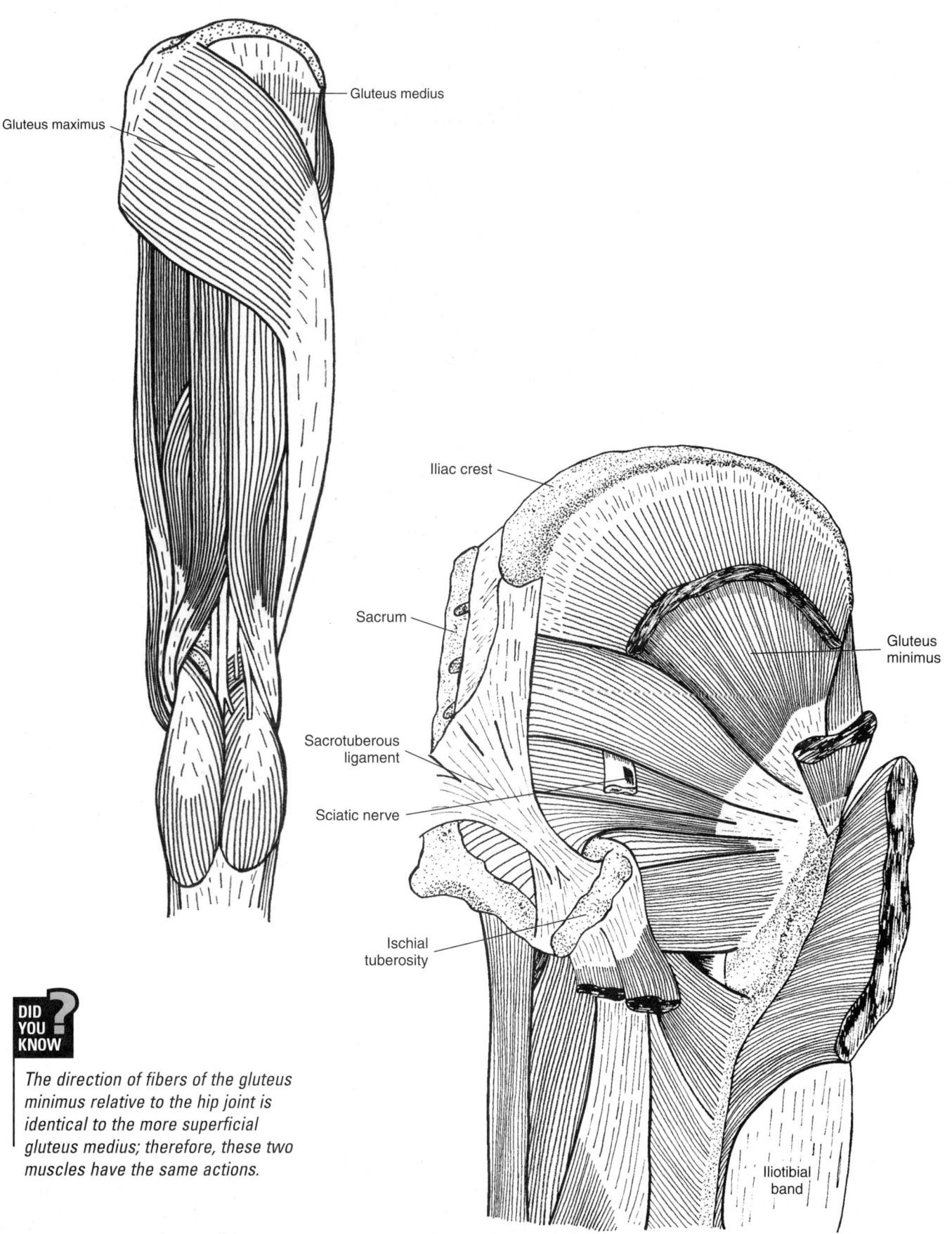

DID YOU KNOW?

The direction of fibers of the gluteus minimus relative to the hip joint is identical to the more superficial gluteus medius; therefore, these two muscles have the same actions.

PIRIFORMIS
(OF THE DEEP LATERAL ROTATORS OF THE THIGH)

pi-ri-**for**-mis

Posterior view of the
right piriformis
(sacrotuberous ligament not shown)

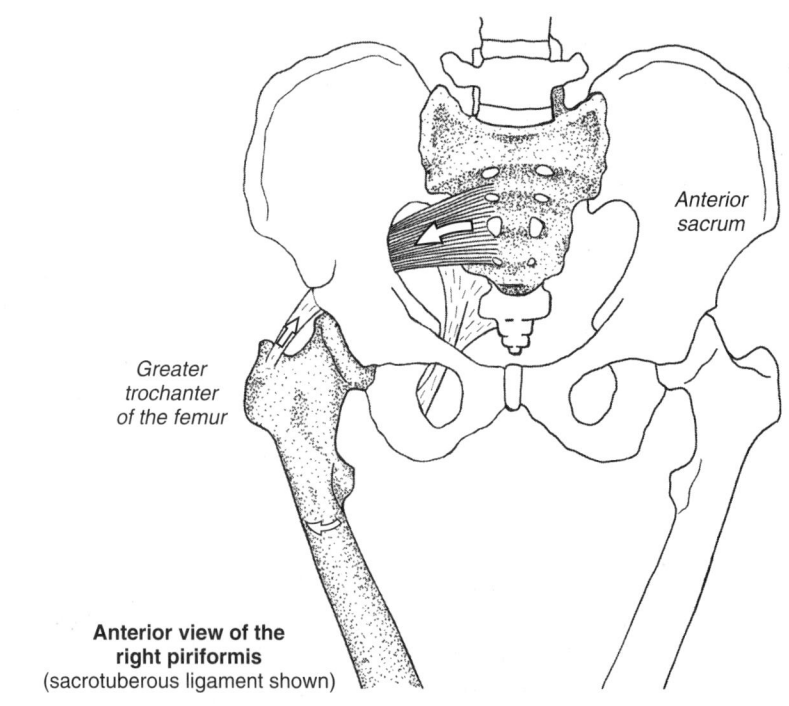

Anterior view of the
right piriformis
(sacrotuberous ligament shown)

Actions
Lateral rotation of the thigh at the hip joint
Horizontal extension (horizontal abduction) of the thigh at the hip joint (if the thigh is flexed)
Medial rotation of the thigh at the hip joint (if the thigh is flexed)
Contralateral rotation of the pelvis at the hip joint

Innervation
The lumbosacral plexus

Arterial Supply
The superior and inferior gluteal arteries

THE MUSCULAR SYSTEM Muscles of the Pelvis

> **DID YOU KNOW?**
> A tight piriformis can compress the sciatic nerve causing symptoms of sciatica. This condition is called piriformis syndrome.

SUPERIOR GEMELLUS
(OF THE DEEP LATERAL ROTATORS OF THE THIGH)

su-**pee**-ree-or jee-**mel**-us

Actions
Lateral rotation of the thigh at the hip joint
Horizontal extension (horizontal abduction) of the thigh at the hip joint (if the thigh is flexed)
Contralateral rotation of the pelvis at the hip joint

Innervation
The lumbosacral plexus

Arterial Supply
The inferior gluteal artery

Posterior view of the right superior gemellus
Ischial spine
Greater trochanter of the femur

OBTURATOR INTERNUS
(OF THE DEEP LATERAL ROTATORS OF THE THIGH)

ob-too-**ray**-tor in-**ter**-nus

Actions
Lateral rotation of the thigh at the hip joint
Horizontal extension (horizontal abduction) of the thigh at the hip joint (if the thigh is flexed)
Contralateral rotation of the pelvis at the hip joint

Innervation
The lumbosacral plexus

Arterial Supply
The superior and inferior gluteal arteries

Posterior view of the right obturator internus
Internal surface of the pelvic bone surrounding the obturator foramen
Greater trochanter of the femur

THE MUSCULAR SYSTEM Muscles of the Pelvis   189

Superior
gemellus

Obturator
internus

DID YOU KNOW?

The distal tendons of the superior gemellus, obturator internus, and inferior gemellus usually blend together.

INFERIOR GEMELLUS
(OF THE DEEP LATERAL ROTATORS OF THE THIGH)
in-**fee**-ree-or jee-**mel**-us

Posterior view of the right inferior gemellus

Actions
Lateral rotation of the thigh at the hip joint
Horizontal extension (horizontal abduction) of the thigh at the hip joint (if the thigh is flexed)
Contralateral rotation of the pelvis at the hip joint

Innervation
The lumbosacral plexus

Arterial Supply
The inferior gluteal artery

THE MUSCULAR SYSTEM Muscles of the Pelvis

DID YOU KNOW?
The distal tendons of the superior gemellus, obturator internus, and inferior gemellus usually blend together.

Inferior gemellus

OBTURATOR EXTERNUS
(OF THE DEEP LATERAL ROTATORS OF THE THIGH)
ob-too-**ray**-tor ex-**ter**-nus

Actions
Lateral rotation of the thigh at the hip joint
Contralateral rotation of the pelvis at the hip joint

Innervation
The obturator nerve

Arterial Supply
The obturator artery

THE MUSCULAR SYSTEM: Muscles of the Pelvis

 DID YOU KNOW? The obturator externus is located deeper and has a different innervation than the other deep lateral rotators of the thigh.

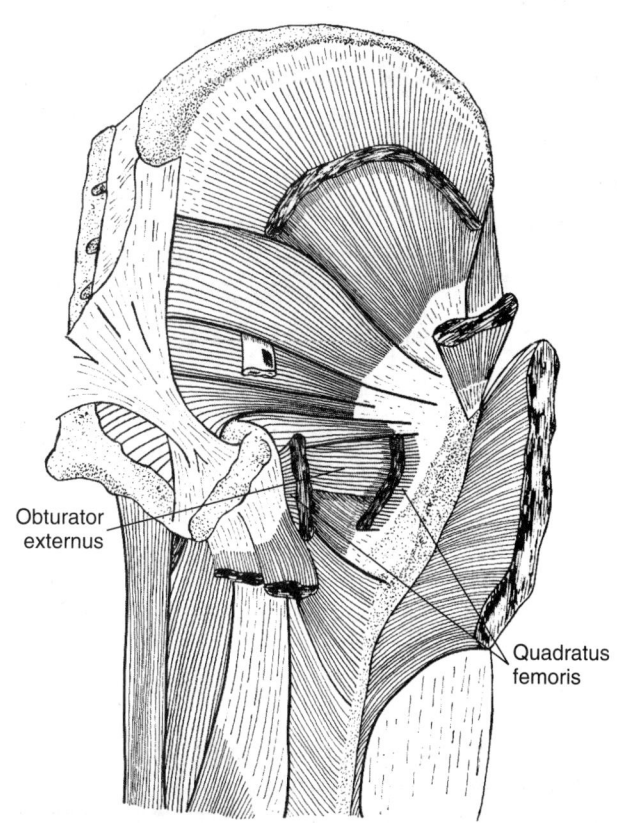

THE MUSCULAR SYSTEM Muscles of the Pelvis

QUADRATUS FEMORIS
(OF THE DEEP LATERAL ROTATORS OF THE THIGH)
kwod-**rate**-us **fem**-o-ris

Posterior view of the right quadratus femoris

Actions
Lateral rotation of the thigh at the hip joint
Adduction of the thigh at the hip joint
Contralateral rotation of the pelvis at the hip joint

Innervation
The lumbosacral plexus

Arterial Supply
The inferior gluteal artery

THE MUSCULAR SYSTEM Muscles of the Pelvis

Quadratus femoris

DID YOU KNOW?

The quadratus femoris attaches sufficiently distal on the femur to be able to do adduction of the thigh at the hip joint.

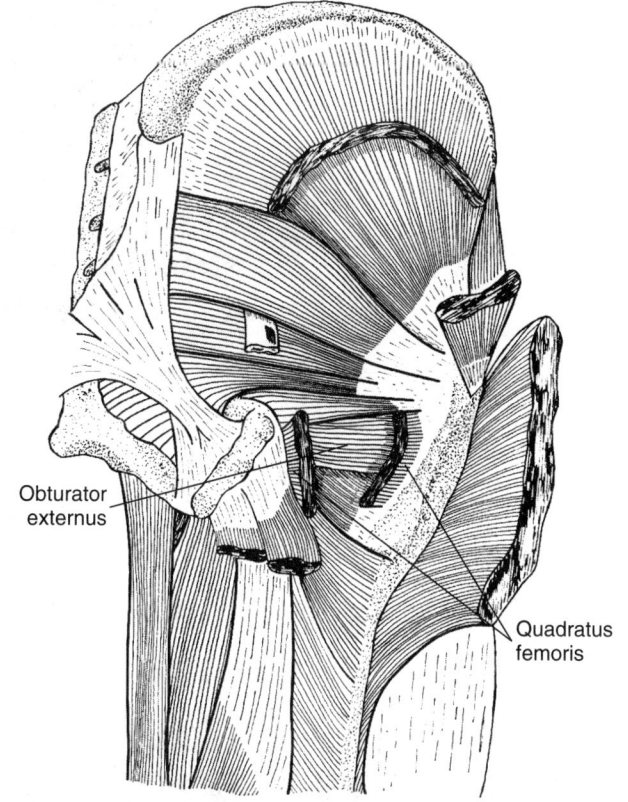

Obturator externus

Quadratus femoris

THE MUSCULAR SYSTEM Muscles of the Pelvis

ANTERIOR VIEW OF THE RIGHT PELVIS

Answers to labeling exercises are on p. 465.

THE MUSCULAR SYSTEM Muscles of the Pelvis

LATERAL VIEW OF THE RIGHT PELVIS

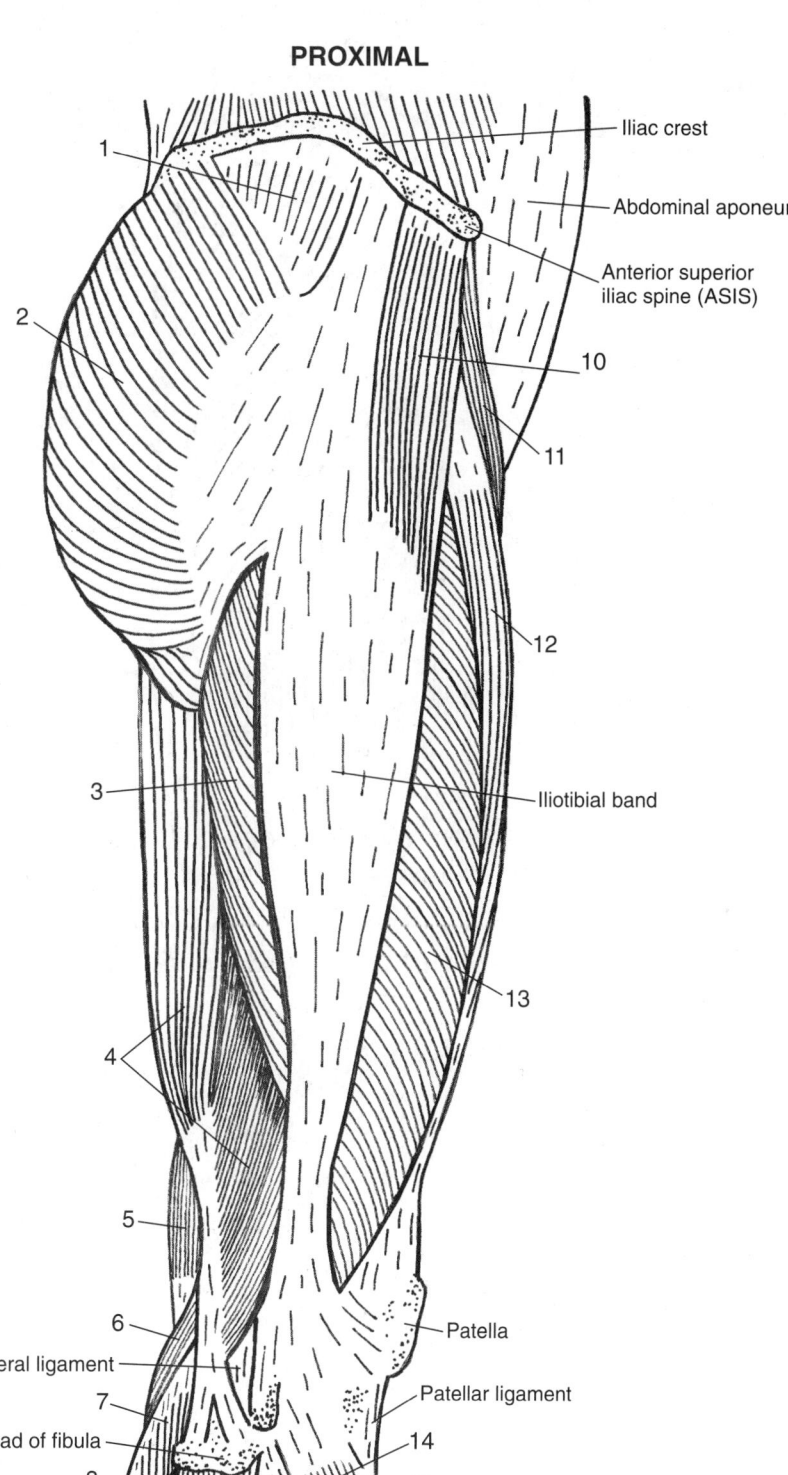

198 THE MUSCULAR SYSTEM Muscles of the Pelvis

POSTERIOR VIEW OF THE RIGHT PELVIS (SUPERFICIAL)

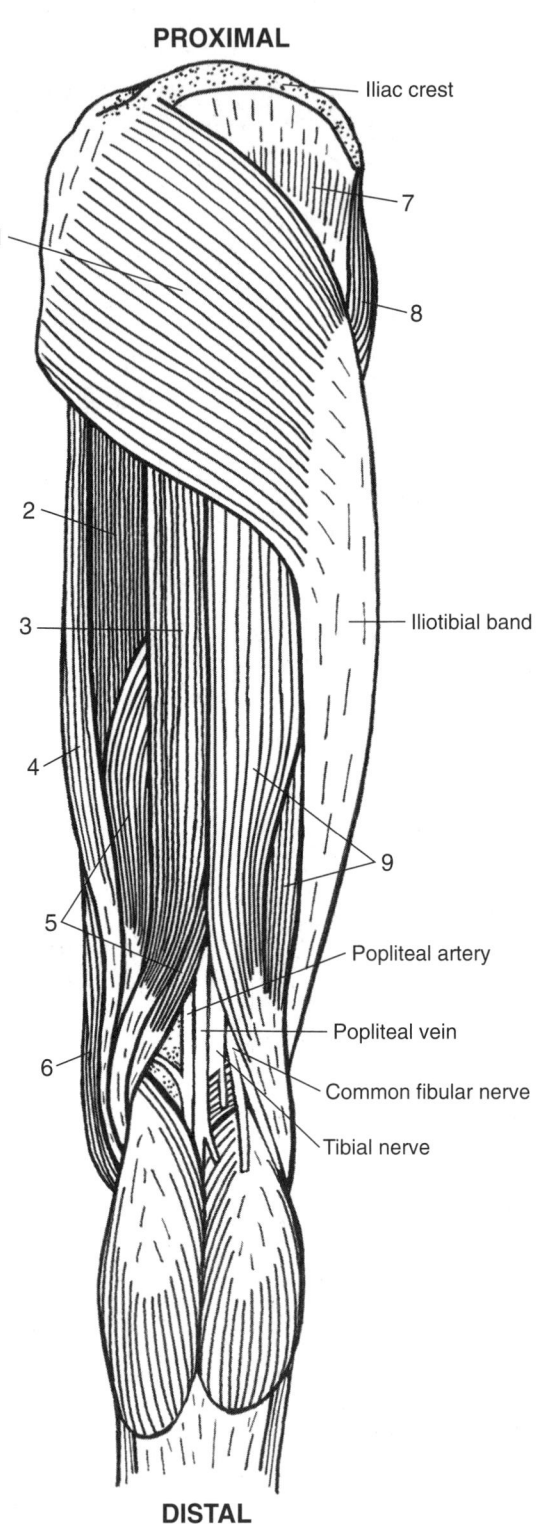

THE MUSCULAR SYSTEM Muscles of the Pelvis

POSTERIOR VIEW OF THE RIGHT PELVIS (DEEP)

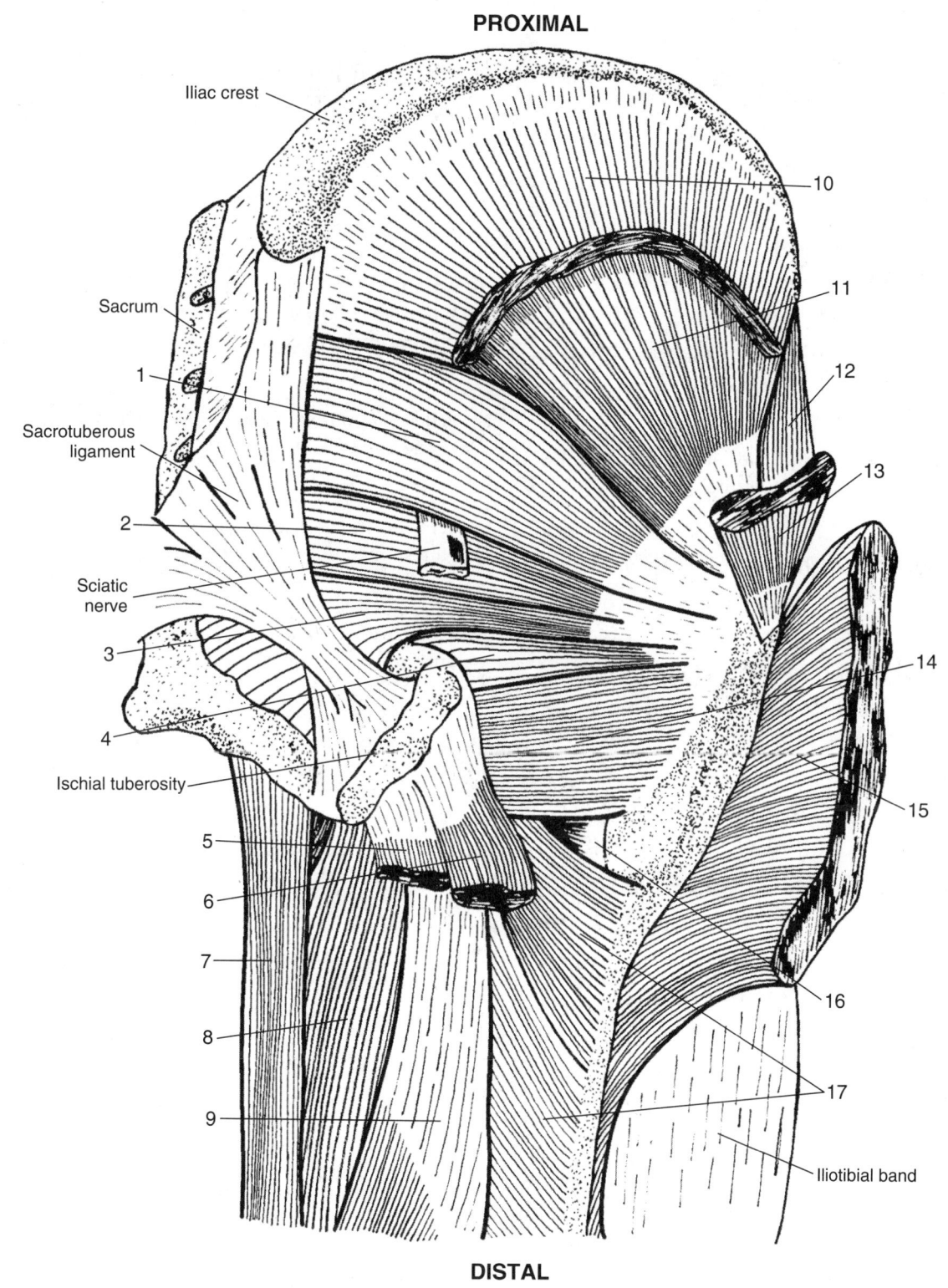

Review Questions

Muscles of the Pelvis
Answers to these questions are found on page 466.

1. What muscle is immediately superior to the inferior gemellus?

2. What muscle is immediately superior to the superior gemellus?

3. If the quadratus femoris is being lengthened, what joint action of the thigh is occurring?

4. What are the most superior and inferior muscles of the deep lateral rotators of the thigh group?

5. What two muscles attach to the periphery of the obturator foramen?

6. What effect would passive flexion of the thigh at the hip joint have upon the length of the gluteus maximus?

7. What three muscles comprise the gluteal group?

8. What is the largest muscle in the human body?

9. The distal tendons of what two muscles usually blend with the distal tendon of the obturator internus?

10. Name an antagonist to the obturator externus' action upon the thigh.

11. Are the superior gemellus and obturator internus synergistic with or antagonistic to each other?

12. What muscle is immediately deep to the psoas minor?

13. Passive extension of the trunk at the spinal joints results in what change in length to the psoas minor?

14. What rotation of the pelvis at the hip joint does the right piriformis create?

15. Besides the gluteus maximus, what other muscle attaches into the iliotibial band?

16. Are the upper fibers of the gluteus maximus synergistic with or antagonistic to the lower fibers of the gluteus maximus?

17. What two muscles attach onto the lesser trochanter of the femur?

18. What is the most important joint action of the gluteus medius?

19. What frontal plane action of the thigh can the quadratus femoris do?

20. Relative to the gluteus maximus, where is the piriformis located?

21. The superior gemellus and obturator internus are members of what group?

22. Where does the sciatic nerve usually exit the pelvis relative to the piriformis?

23. Are the gluteus medius and minimus synergistic with or antagonistic to each other?

24. If the thigh is passively laterally rotated at the hip joint, what happens to the length of the obturator externus?

25. What joint action of the thigh is occurring if there is a concentric contraction of the superior gemellus?

More review activities on Evolve at http://evolve.elsevier.com/Muscolino/muscular/

26. What muscle is superficial to the inferior gemellus?

27. What muscle is directly inferior to the piriformis?

28. How are the psoas major and psoas minor synergistic with each other?

29. How is the gluteus medius antagonistic to itself?

30. How can the two quadratus femoris muscles be antagonistic to each other?

31. What muscle is superficial to the piriformis?

32. If the right psoas major is eccentrically contracting, what sagittal plane joint motion of the thigh is occurring?

33. If the thigh is first flexed, what joint actions of the thigh could be done to stretch the piriformis?

34. Are the psoas major and iliacus synergistic with or antagonistic to the sartorius? Why?

35. What two muscles are superficial to the gluteus medius?

36. Would passive medial rotation of the thigh at the hip joint shorten or lengthen the psoas major and iliacus?

37. What joint action of the thigh occurs when the superior gemellus eccentrically contracts?

38. What other muscles share the quadratus femoris' proximal attachment?

39. If the thigh is medially rotated at the hip joint, what happens to the length of the inferior gemellus?

40. What effect would active flexion of the thigh at the hip joint have upon the length of the gluteus maximus?

41. What joint action is occurring if the left psoas minor is concentrically contracting?

42. What muscle is immediately superficial to the obturator externus?

43. What two muscles of the lower extremity attach to the anterolateral lumbar spine?

44. If the thigh is actively extended and laterally rotated, what happens to the length of the piriformis?

45. What muscle is immediately superior to the obturator externus?

46. What six muscles comprise the deep lateral rotators of the thigh group?

47. What muscle is immediately inferior to the obturator internus?

48. What muscle of the abdomen and pelvis is absent in approximately 40% of individuals?

49. What pelvic action is created by the right inferior gemellus?

50. Old-fashioned straight-leg sit-ups are no longer recommended because they overly strengthen what muscle?

51. What muscle's tendon is located directly lateral to the distal tendon of the iliacus?

52. Which muscle is deeper, the gluteus medius or the gluteus minimus?

53. If the thigh is moving and the obturator externus is eccentrically contracting, what joint action is occurring?

54. What muscle is immediately deep to the quadratus femoris?

THE MUSCULAR SYSTEM Muscles of the Thigh

ANTERIOR VIEW OF THE RIGHT THIGH (SUPERFICIAL)

Relationship of femoral vessels to anterior thigh

THE MUSCULAR SYSTEM Muscles of the Thigh

ANTERIOR VIEW OF THE RIGHT THIGH (DEEP)

THE MUSCULAR SYSTEM Muscles of the Thigh

POSTERIOR VIEW OF THE RIGHT THIGH (SUPERFICIAL)

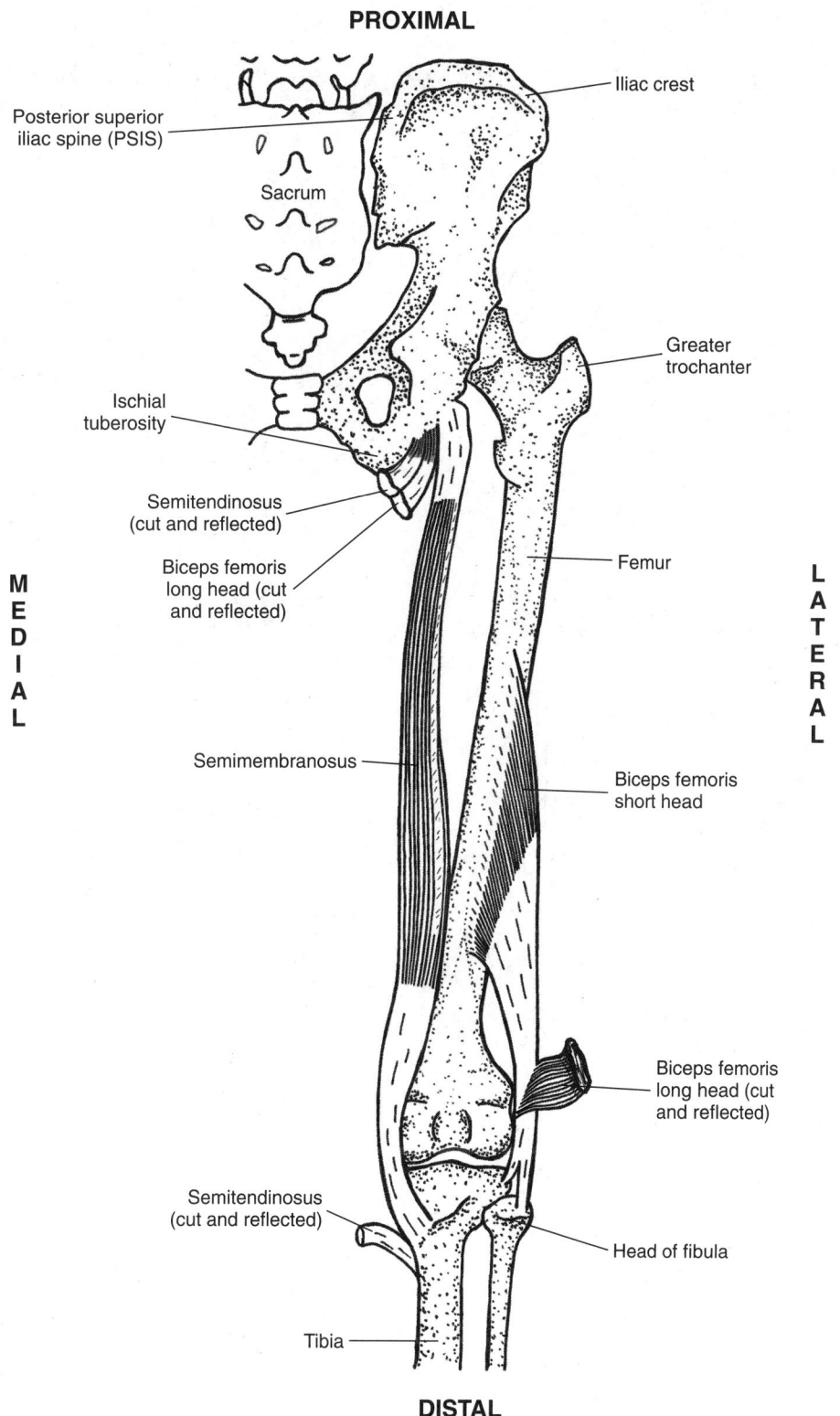

THE MUSCULAR SYSTEM — Muscles of the Thigh

LATERAL VIEW OF THE RIGHT THIGH

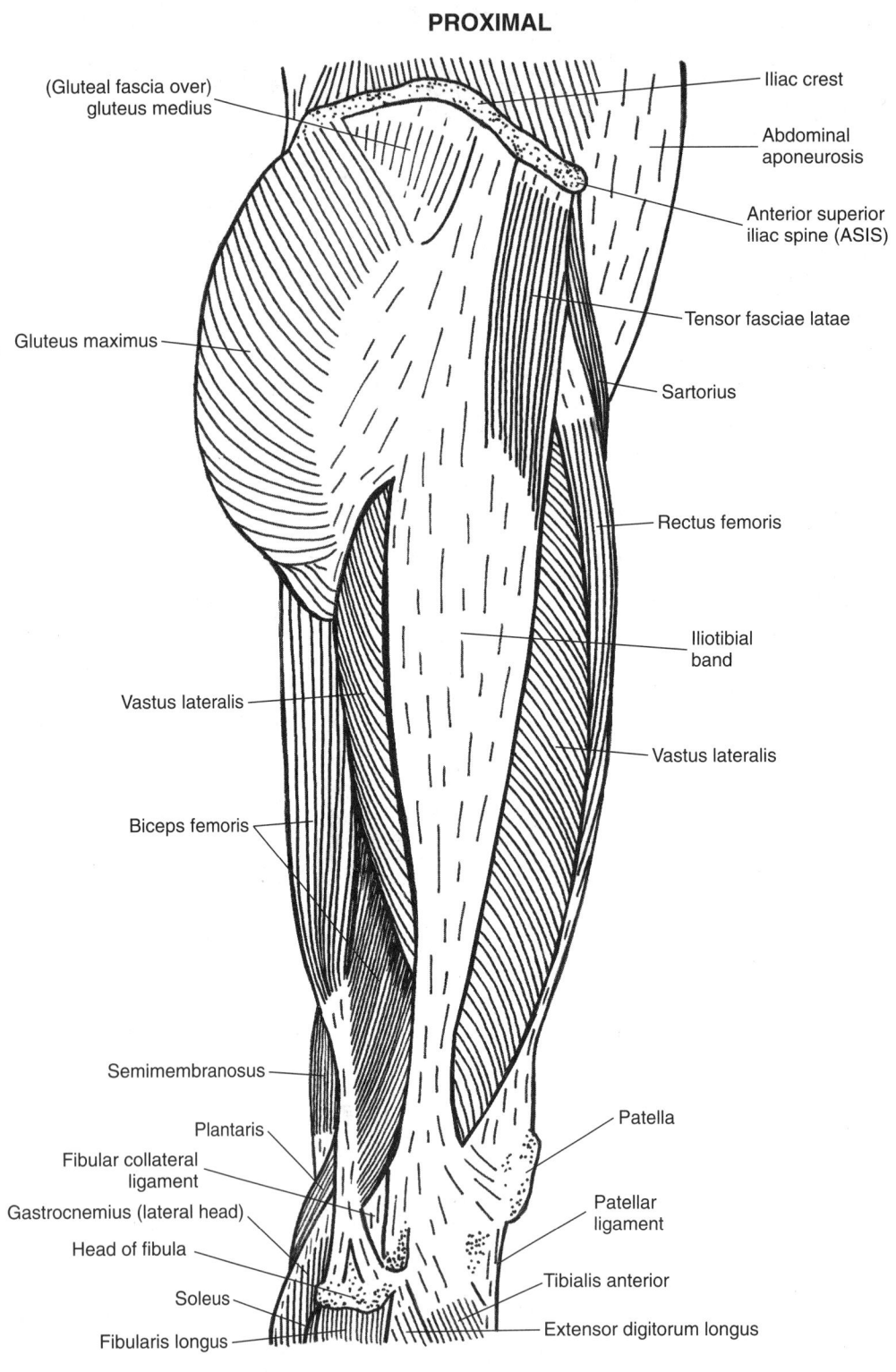

THE MUSCULAR SYSTEM Muscles of the Thigh

MEDIAL VIEW OF THE RIGHT THIGH

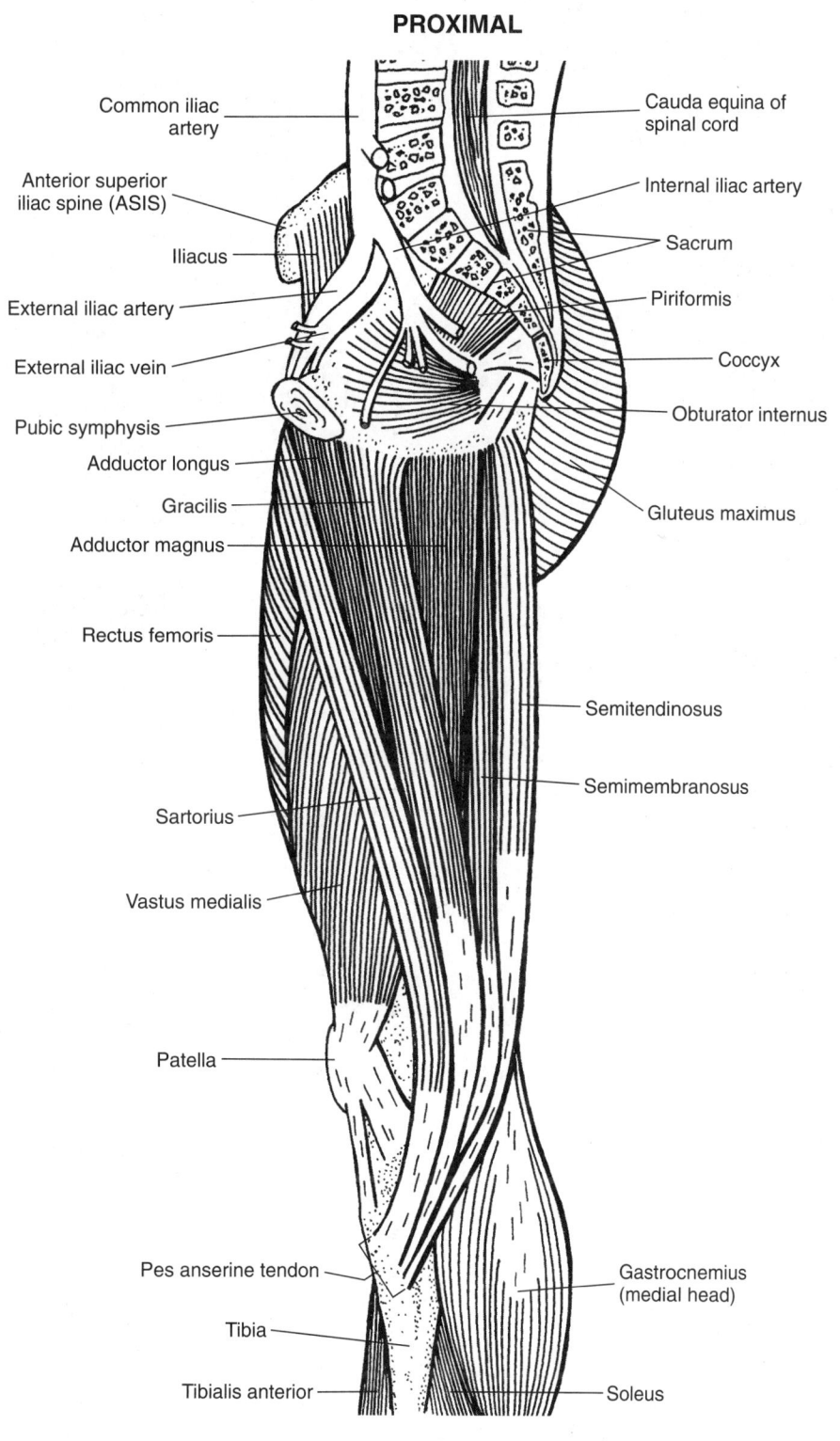

TENSOR FASCIAE LATAE ("TFL")
ten-sor fash-ee-a la-tee

Actions
Flexion of the thigh at the hip joint
Abduction of the thigh at the hip joint
Medial rotation of the thigh at the hip joint
Anterior tilt of the pelvis at the hip joint
Depression (lateral tilt) of the pelvis at the hip joint
Ipsilateral rotation of the pelvis at the hip joint
Extension of the leg at the knee joint

Innervation
The superior gluteal nerve

Arterial Supply
The superior gluteal artery

Lateral view of the right tensor fasciae latae

THE MUSCULAR SYSTEM Muscles of the Thigh   209

The tensor fasciae latae is one of two muscles that attach into the iliotibial band.

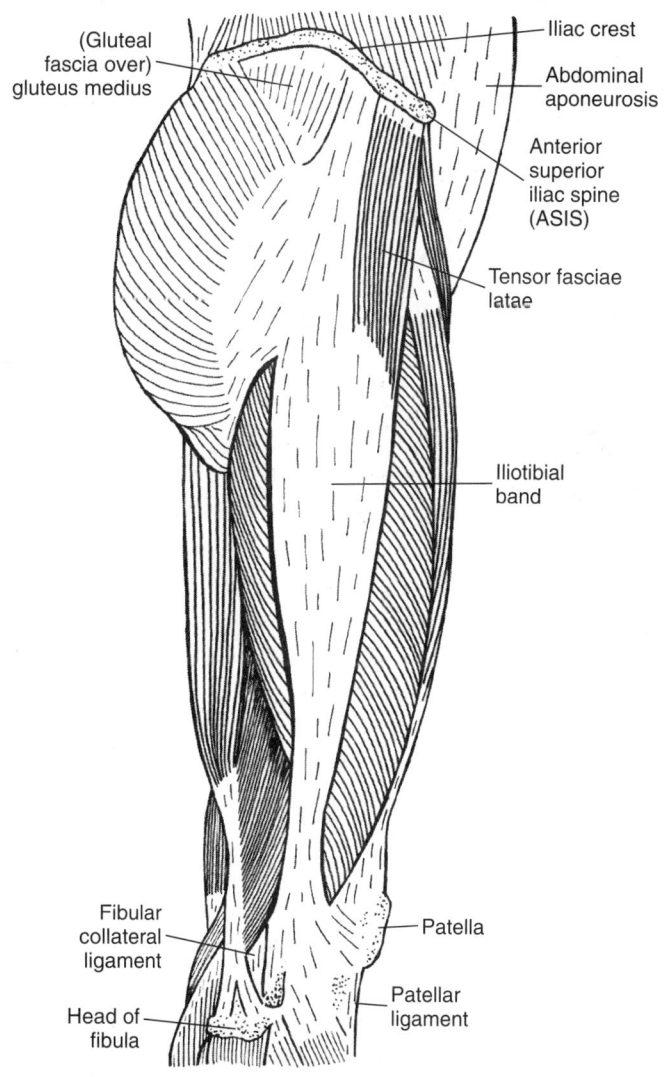

SARTORIUS
sar-**tor**-ee-us

Actions
Flexion of the thigh at the hip joint
Abduction of the thigh at the hip joint
Lateral rotation of the thigh at the hip joint
Flexion of the leg at the knee joint
Anterior tilt of the pelvis at the hip joint
Medial rotation of the leg at the knee joint
Depression (lateral tilt) of the pelvis at the hip joint
Contralateral rotation of the pelvis at the hip joint

Innervation
The femoral nerve

Arterial Supply
The femoral artery

Anterior superior iliac spine (ASIS)

Anterior view of the right sartorius

Pes anserine tendon

THE MUSCULAR SYSTEM Muscles of the Thigh

The sartorius is the longest muscle in the human body. It is also one of three muscles that attach into the pes anserine tendon.

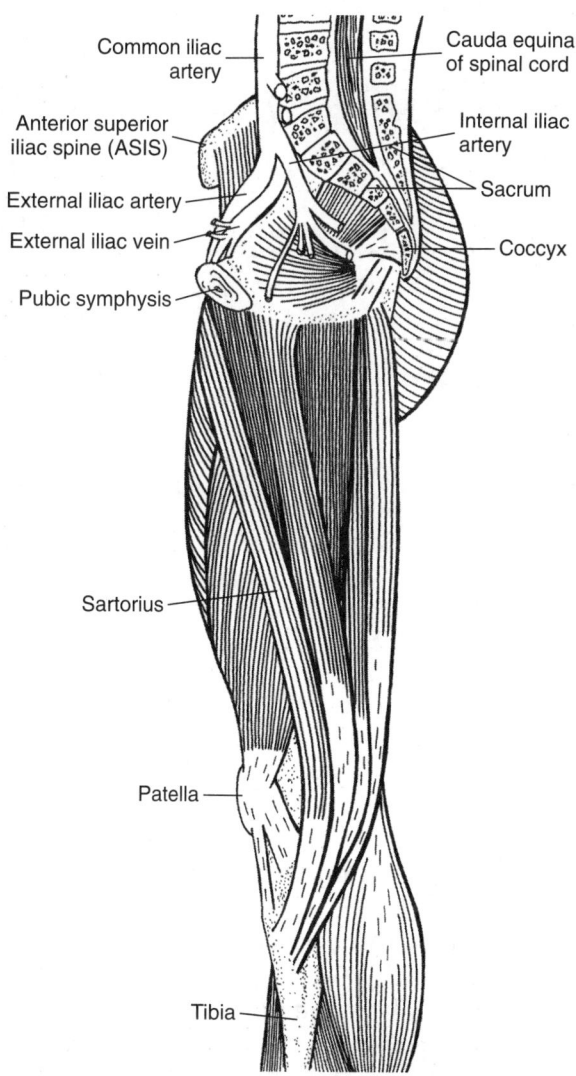

THE MUSCULAR SYSTEM — Muscles of the Thigh

RECTUS FEMORIS
(OF THE QUADRICEPS FEMORIS GROUP)

rek-tus **fem**-o-ris

Anterior inferior iliac spine (AIIS)

Tibial tuberosity

Anterior view of the right rectus femoris

Actions
Extension of the leg at the knee joint
Flexion of the thigh at the hip joint
Anterior tilt of the pelvis at the hip joint

Innervation
The femoral nerve

Arterial Supply
The femoral artery and the deep femoral artery

THE MUSCULAR SYSTEM Muscles of the Thigh

Rectus femoris

DID YOU KNOW?

The rectus femoris is the only quadriceps femoris muscle that can create movement of the thigh or pelvis at the hip joint, because it is the only one that crosses the hip joint.

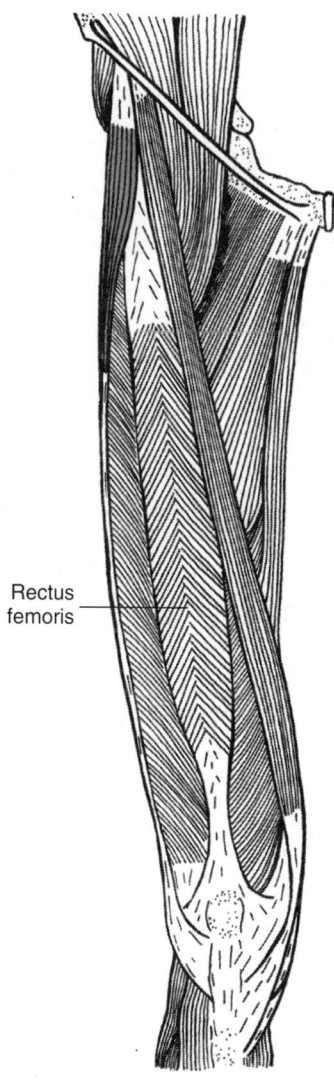

Rectus femoris

VASTUS LATERALIS
(OF THE QUADRICEPS FEMORIS GROUP)

vas-tus lat-er-**a**-lis

> **Action**
> Extension of the leg at the knee joint
>
> **Innervation**
> The femoral nerve
>
> **Arterial Supply**
> The femoral artery and the deep femoral artery

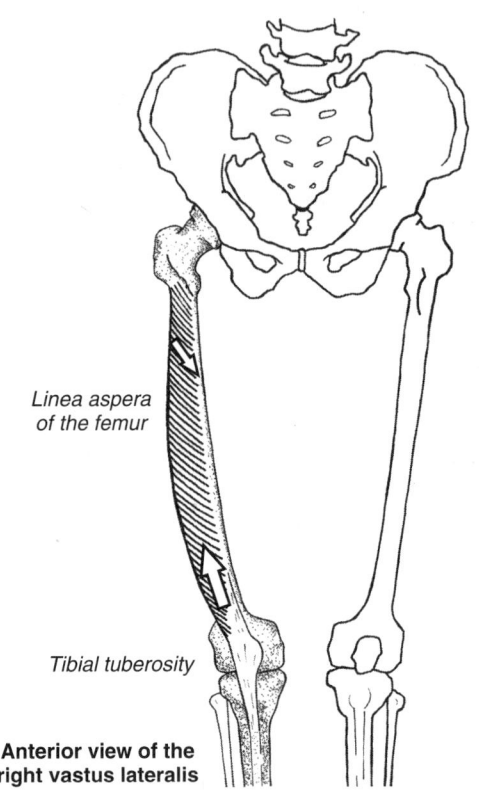

Anterior view of the right vastus lateralis

VASTUS MEDIALIS
(OF THE QUADRICEPS FEMORIS GROUP)

vas-tus mee-dee-**a**-lis

> **Action**
> Extension of the leg at the knee joint
>
> **Innervation**
> The femoral nerve
>
> **Arterial Supply**
> The femoral artery

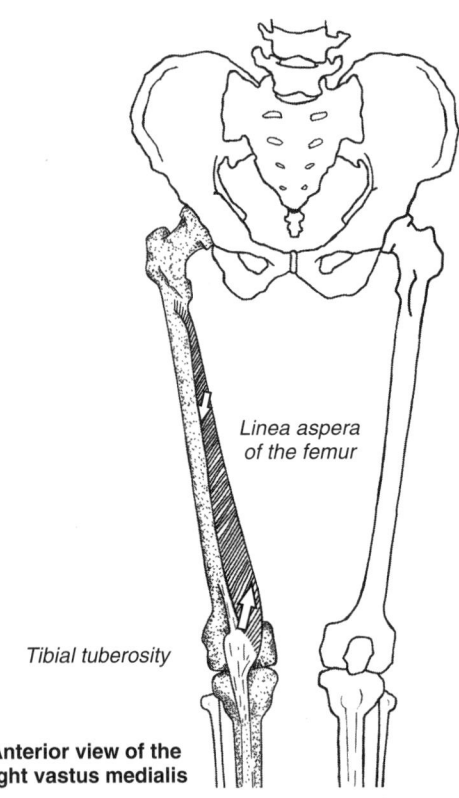

Anterior view of the right vastus medialis

THE MUSCULAR SYSTEM Muscles of the Thigh 215

Vastus lateralis — Vastus medialis

DID YOU KNOW?

The vastus lateralis is the largest of the four quadriceps femoris muscles. Pain attributed to the iliotibial band is often due to this large muscle that lies deep to it.

Vastus lateralis — Vastus medialis

DID YOU KNOW?

The most distal aspect of the vastus medialis is bulky and may form a bulge in well-toned individuals.

VASTUS INTERMEDIUS
(OF THE QUADRICEPS FEMORIS GROUP)

vas-tus in-ter-**mee**-dee-us

Action
Extension of the leg at the knee joint

Innervation
The femoral nerve

Arterial Supply
The deep femoral artery

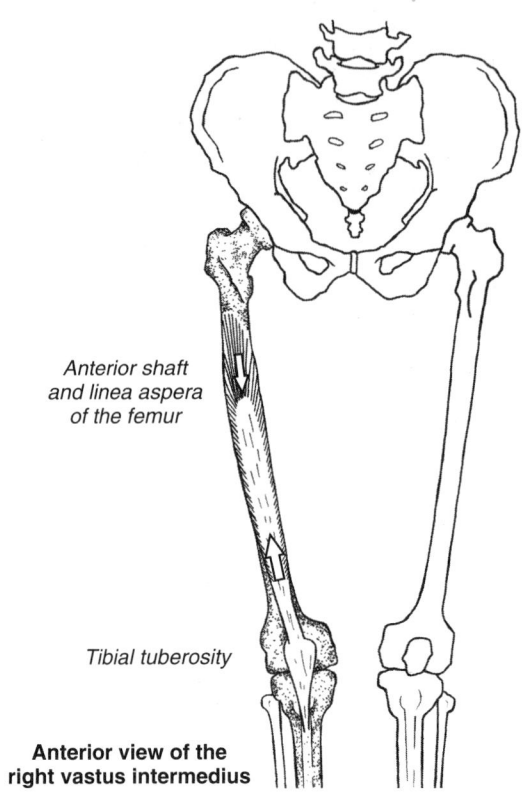

Anterior shaft and linea aspera of the femur

Tibial tuberosity

Anterior view of the right vastus intermedius

ARTICULARIS GENUS

ar-**tik**-you-**la**-ris **je**-new

Action
Tenses and pulls the joint capsule of the knee joint proximally

Innervation
The femoral nerve

Arterial Supply
The deep femoral artery

Anterior distal femoral shaft

Joint capsule of the knee joint

Anterior view of the right articularis genus

THE MUSCULAR SYSTEM Muscles of the Thigh 217

Vastus intermedius

From most perspectives, the vastus intermedius is the deepest of the four quadriceps femoris muscles.

Vastus intermedius

The articularis genus has no skeletal function to move bones. It acts to move the joint capsule of the knee so that it doesn't get pinched between the femur and tibia when the knee joint moves.

PECTINEUS
(OF THE ADDUCTOR GROUP)

pek-**tin**-ee-us

Actions
Adduction of the thigh at the hip joint
Flexion of the thigh at the hip joint
Anterior tilt of the pelvis at the hip joint
Elevation of the pelvis at the hip joint

Innervation
The femoral nerve

Arterial Supply
The femoral artery and the deep femoral artery

Pectineal line of the pubis

Pectineal line of the femur

Anterior view of the right pectineus

GRACILIS
(OF THE ADDUCTOR GROUP)

gra-**sil**-is

Actions
Adduction of the thigh at the hip joint
Flexion of the thigh at the hip joint
Flexion of the leg at the knee joint
Anterior tilt of the pelvis at the hip joint
Medial rotation of the leg at the knee joint
Elevation of the pelvis at the hip joint

Innervation
The obturator nerve

Arterial Supply
The deep femoral artery

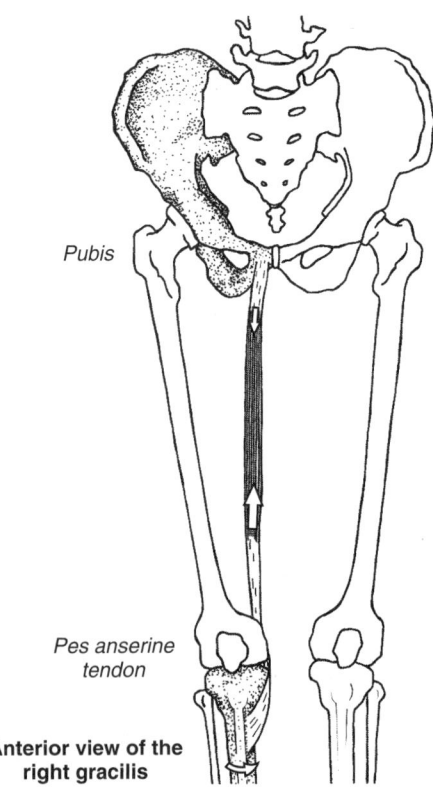

Pubis

Pes anserine tendon

Anterior view of the right gracilis

THE MUSCULAR SYSTEM Muscles of the Thigh   219

The pectineus attaches from the pectineal line of the pubis to the pectineal line of the femur.

The gracilis muscle is the second longest muscle in the human body. It is also one of three muscles that attach into the pes anserine tendon.

ADDUCTOR LONGUS
(OF THE ADDUCTOR GROUP)
ad-**duk**-tor **long**-us

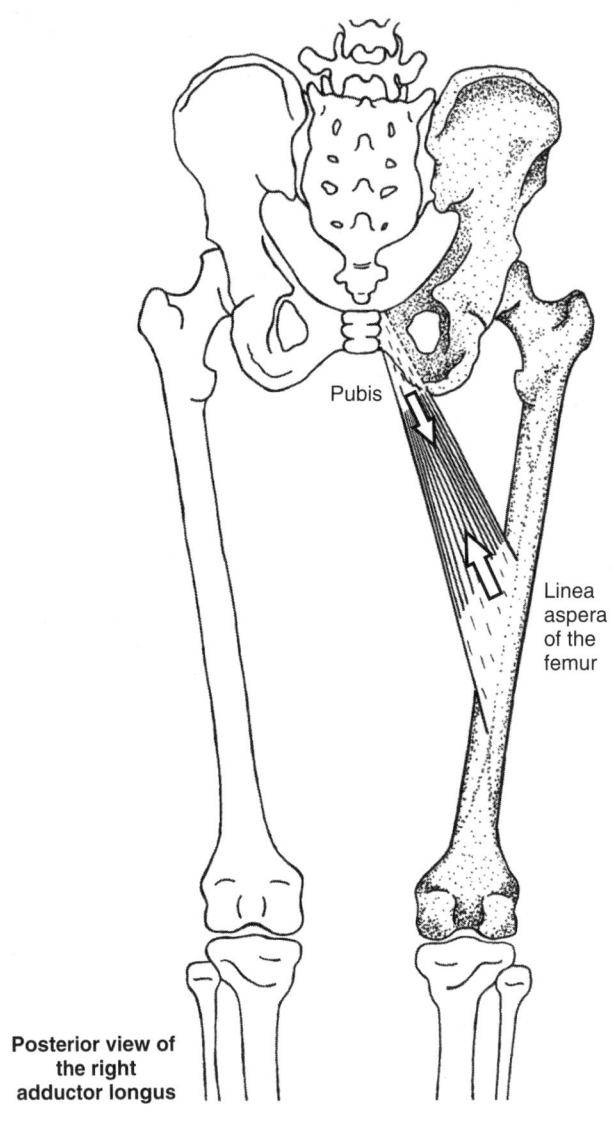

Posterior view of the right adductor longus

Actions
Adduction of the thigh at the hip joint
Flexion of the thigh at the hip joint
Anterior tilt of the pelvis at the hip joint
Elevation of the pelvis at the hip joint

Innervation
The obturator nerve

Arterial Supply
The femoral artery and the deep femoral artery

THE MUSCULAR SYSTEM Muscles of the Thigh 221

DID YOU KNOW?

The adductor longus is easy to locate because it has the most prominent tendon in the groin region. Its proximal tendon can also be useful as a landmark for palpating other muscles of the region.

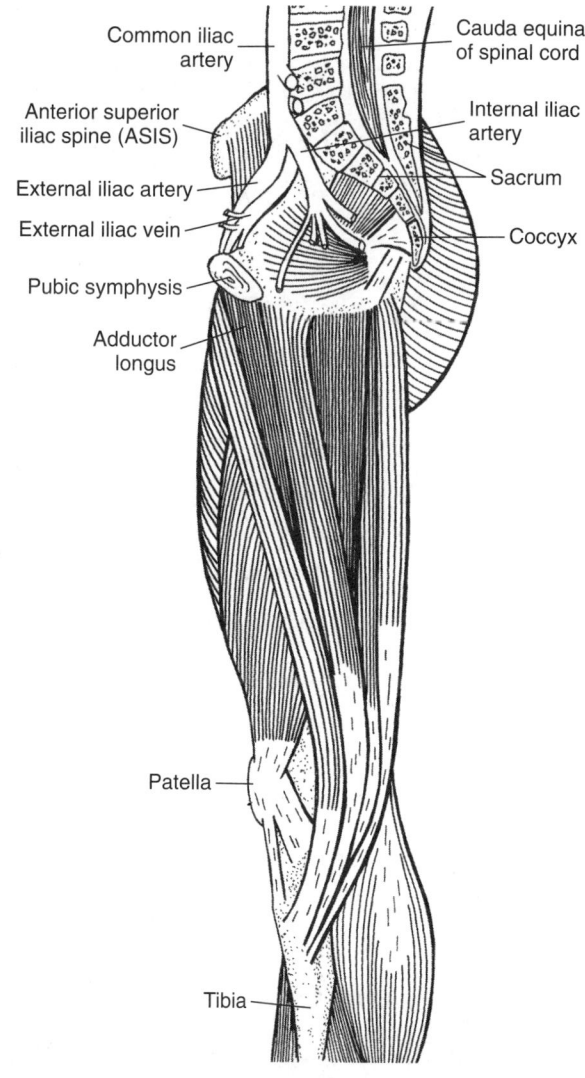

ADDUCTOR BREVIS
(OF THE ADDUCTOR GROUP)
ad-**duk**-tor **bre**-vis

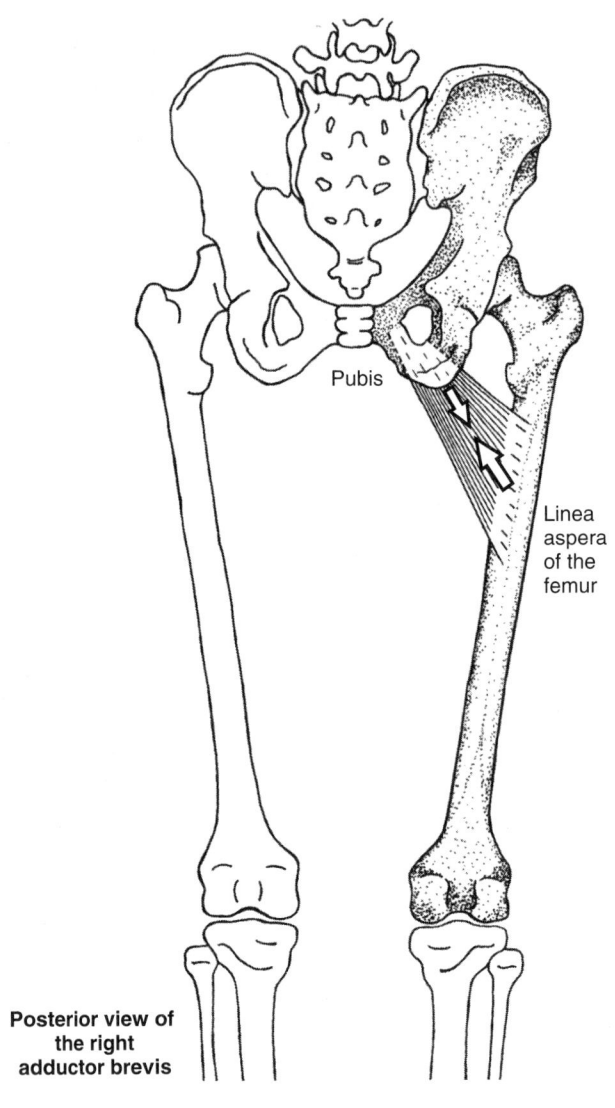

Posterior view of the right adductor brevis

Actions	Innervation	Arterial Supply
Adduction of the thigh at the hip joint Flexion of the thigh at the hip joint Anterior tilt of the pelvis at the hip joint Elevation of the pelvis at the hip joint	The obturator nerve	The femoral artery and the deep femoral artery

THE MUSCULAR SYSTEM Muscles of the Thigh

Adductor brevis

DID YOU KNOW

The adductor brevis is located between the adductor longus and adductor magnus.

ADDUCTOR MAGNUS
(OF THE ADDUCTOR GROUP)
ad-**duk**-tor **mag**-nus

Actions
Adduction of the thigh at the hip joint
Extension of the thigh at the hip joint
Posterior tilt of the pelvis at the hip joint
Elevation of the pelvis at the hip joint

Innervation
The obturator nerve and the sciatic nerve

Arterial Supply
Anterior head: the femoral artery and the deep femoral artery
Posterior head: the deep femoral artery and the inferior gluteal artery

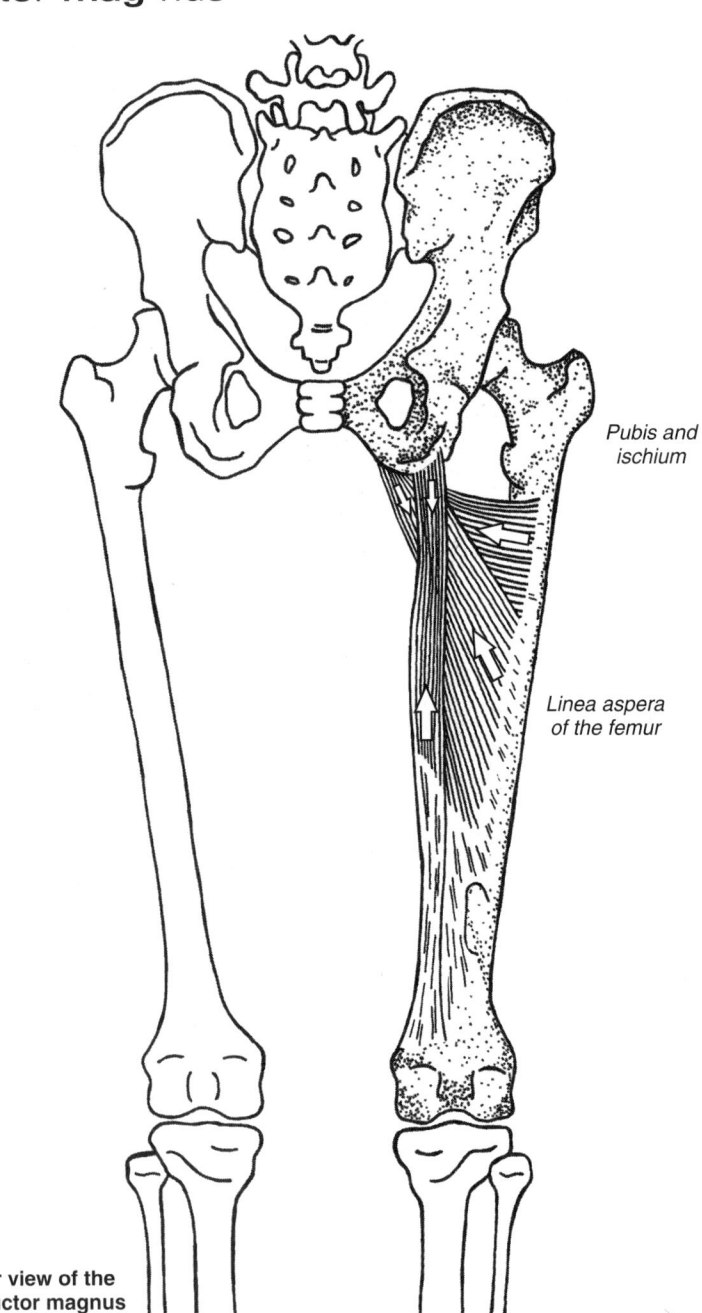

Pubis and ischium

Linea aspera of the femur

Posterior view of the right adductor magnus

THE MUSCULAR SYSTEM Muscles of the Thigh   225

DID YOU KNOW

Because the adductor magnus is so far posterior, attaches to the ischial tuberosity, and can extend the thigh at the hip joint, it is sometimes called the 4th hamstring.

BICEPS FEMORIS
(OF THE HAMSTRING GROUP)
by-seps **fem**-o-ris

Actions
Flexion of the leg at the knee joint (entire muscle)
Extension of the thigh at the hip joint (long head)
Posterior tilt of the pelvis at the hip joint (long head)
Lateral rotation of the leg at the knee joint (entire muscle)
Adduction of the thigh at the hip joint (long head)
Lateral rotation of the thigh at the hip joint (long head)

Innervation
The sciatic nerve

Arterial Supply
Long head: the inferior gluteal artery and perforating branches of the deep femoral artery
Short head: perforating branches of the deep femoral artery

Ischial tuberosity and the linea aspera of the femur

Head of the fibula and the tibia

Posterior view of the right biceps femoris

THE MUSCULAR SYSTEM Muscles of the Thigh

 DID YOU KNOW

The biceps femoris is a lateral hamstring muscle. Its short head is the only part of the hamstring group that does not cross the hip joint.

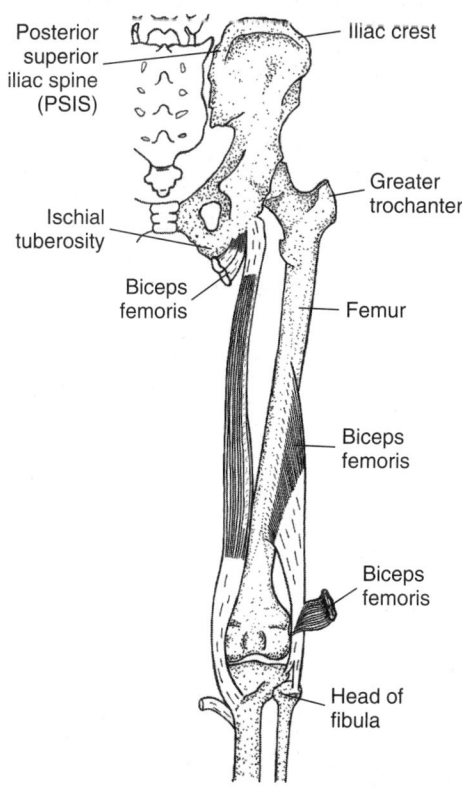

SEMITENDINOSUS
(OF THE HAMSTRING GROUP)
sem-i-**ten**-di-**no**-sus

Actions
Flexion of the leg at the knee joint
Extension of the thigh at the hip joint
Posterior tilt of the pelvis at the hip joint
Medial rotation of the leg at the knee joint
Medial rotation of the thigh at the hip joint

Innervation
The sciatic nerve

Arterial Supply
The inferior gluteal artery and perforating branches of the deep femoral artery

Posterior view of the right semitendinosus

SEMIMEMBRANOSUS
(OF THE HAMSTRING GROUP)
sem-i-**mem**-bra-**no**-sus

Actions
Flexion of the leg at the knee joint
Extension of the thigh at the hip joint
Posterior tilt of the pelvis at the hip joint
Medial rotation of the leg at the knee joint
Medial rotation of the thigh at the hip joint

Innervation
The sciatic nerve

Arterial Supply
The inferior gluteal artery and perforating branches of the deep femoral artery

Posterior view of the right semimembranosus

THE MUSCULAR SYSTEM Muscles of the Thigh

DID YOU KNOW

The semitendinosus is named for its long distal tendon. It is also one of three muscles that attach into the pes anserine tendon.

DID YOU KNOW

The semimembranosus is named for its long membranous proximal tendon.

THE MUSCULAR SYSTEM   Muscles of the Thigh

ANTERIOR VIEW OF THE RIGHT THIGH (SUPERFICIAL)

Relationship of femoral vessels to anterior thigh

Answers to labeling exercises are on p. 466.

THE MUSCULAR SYSTEM Muscles of the Thigh 231

ANTERIOR VIEW OF THE RIGHT THIGH (DEEP)

232 THE MUSCULAR SYSTEM Muscles of the Thigh

POSTERIOR VIEW OF THE RIGHT THIGH (SUPERFICIAL)

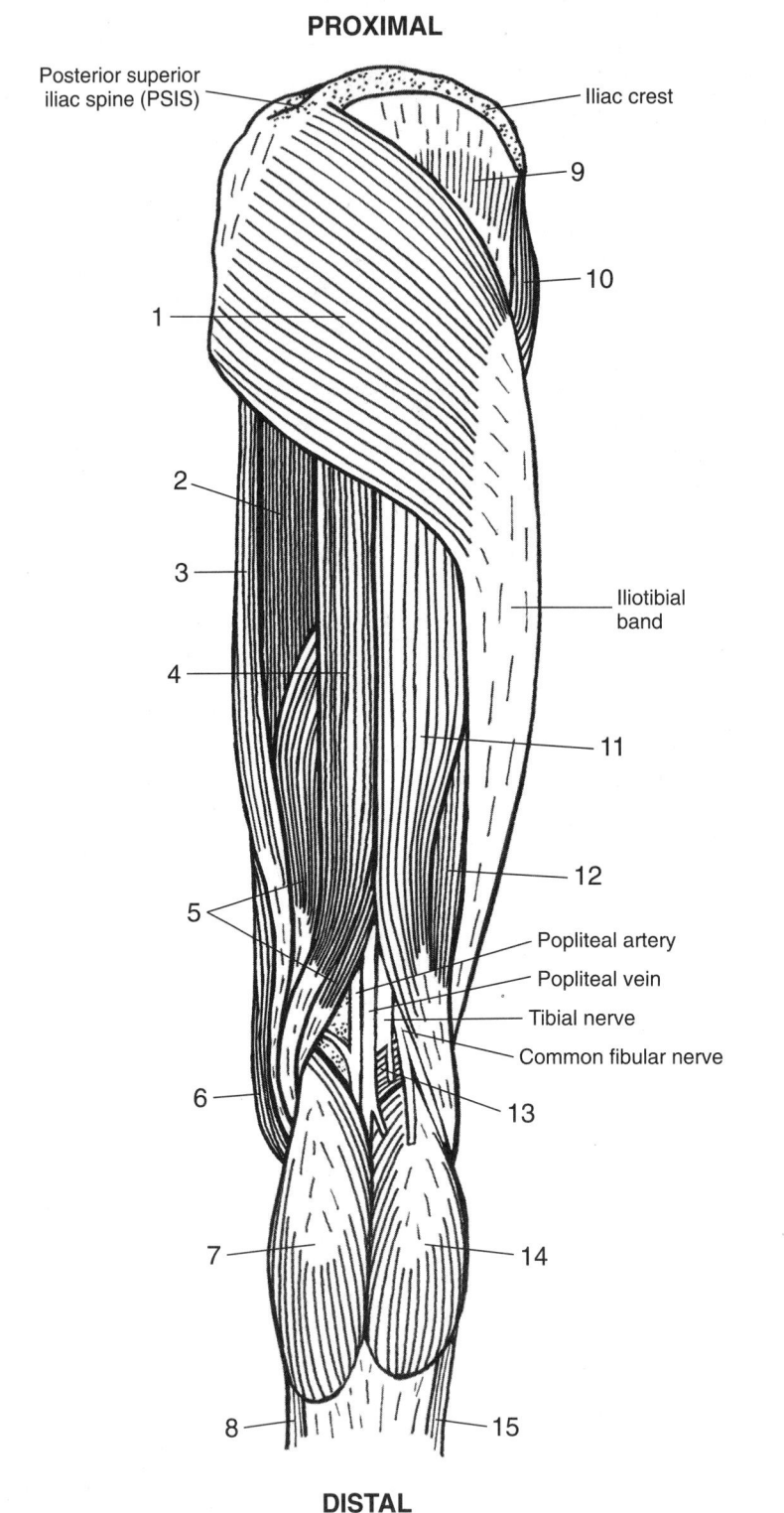

THE MUSCULAR SYSTEM Muscles of the Thigh

POSTERIOR VIEW OF THE RIGHT THIGH (DEEP)

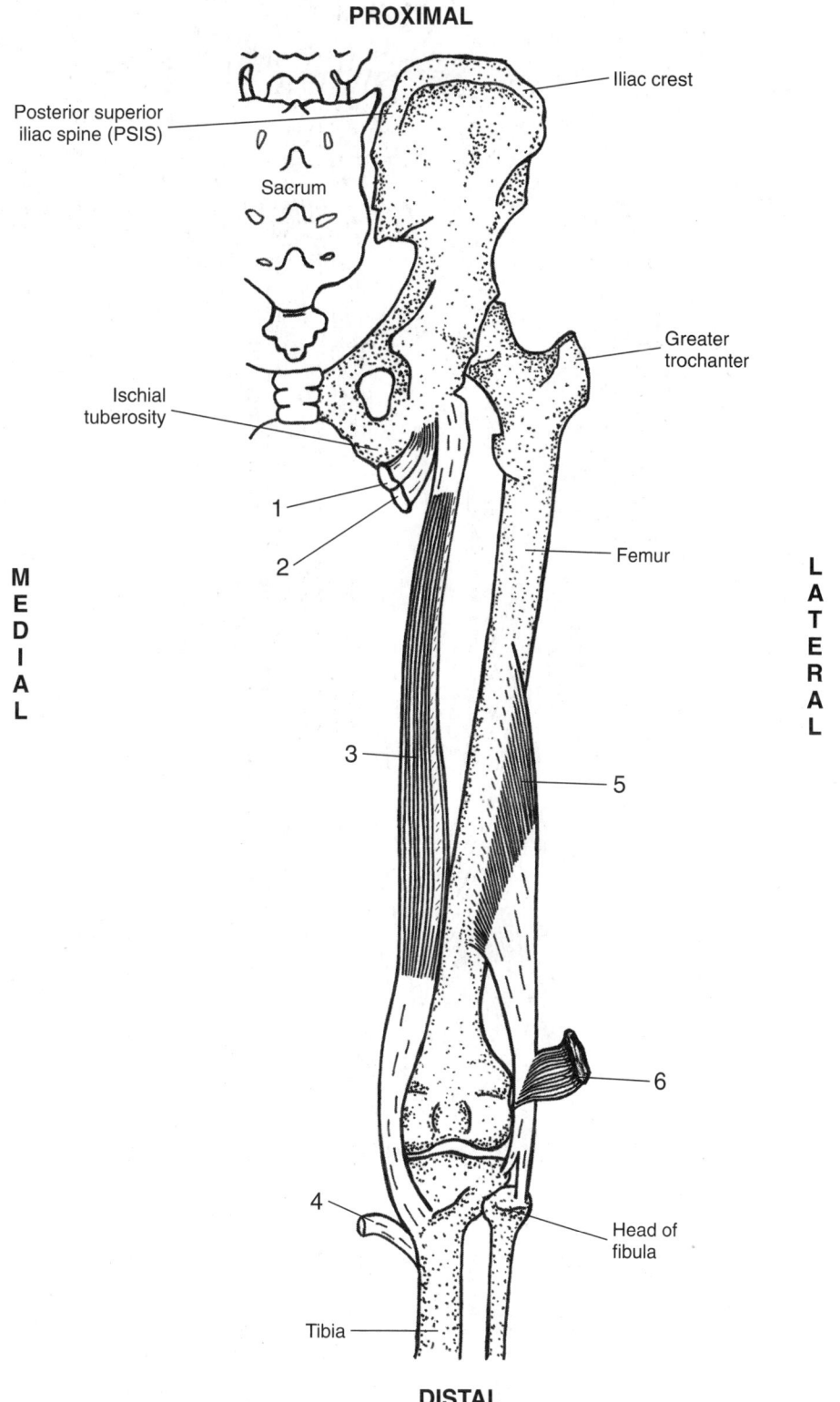

THE MUSCULAR SYSTEM — Muscles of the Thigh

LATERAL VIEW OF THE RIGHT THIGH

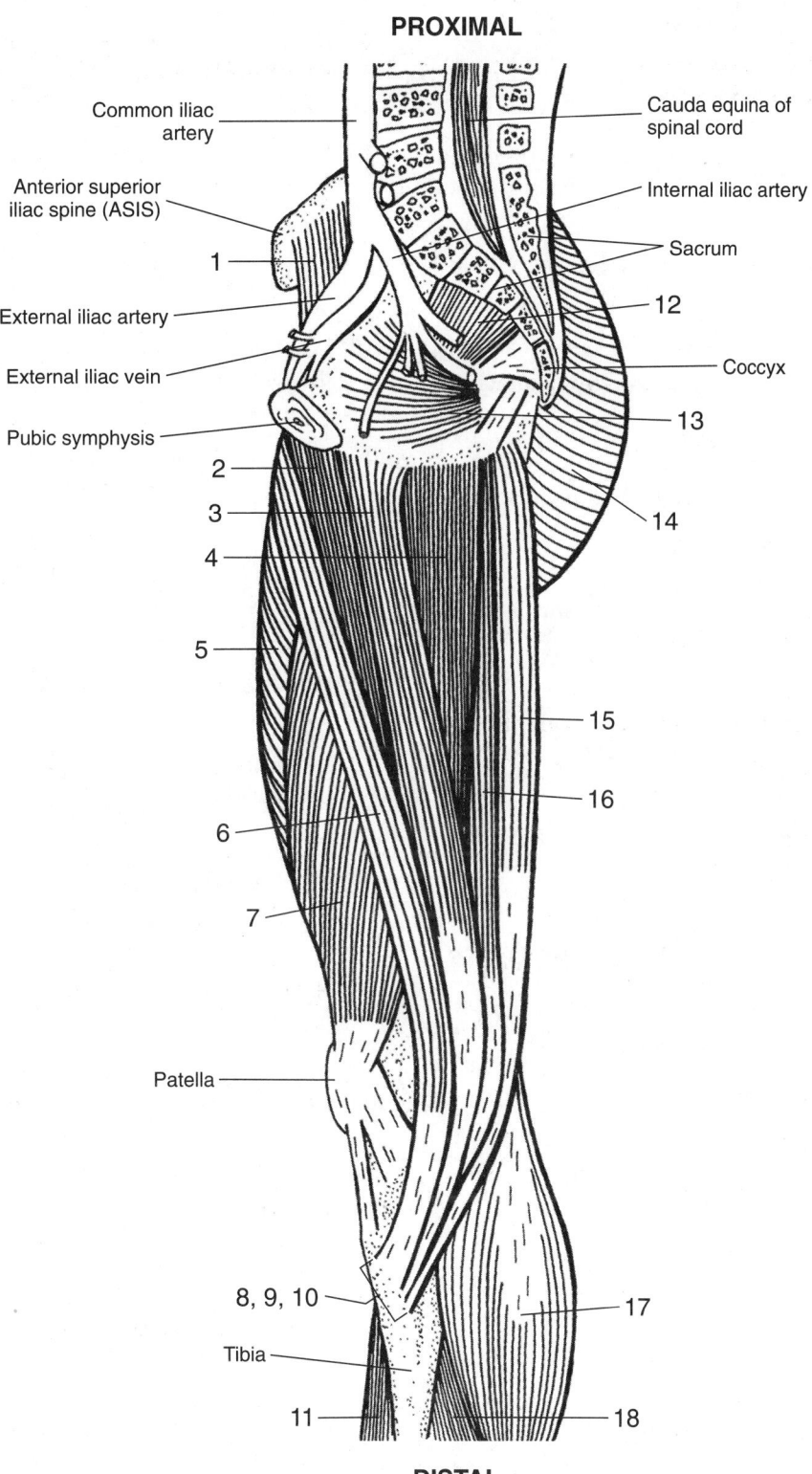

Review Questions

Muscles of the Thigh
Answers to these questions are found on page 466.

1. Proximally, the rectus femoris is located between what two muscles?

2. What muscle is superficial to the proximal attachment of the biceps femoris?

3. How many muscles of the adductor group attach to the linea aspera?

4. Which thigh muscle is named for its long distal tendon?

5. What joint action is occurring if the vastus lateralis is eccentrically contracting?

6. Name a muscle that is antagonistic to both of the pectineus' joint actions of the thigh?

7. What muscle is located immediately medial to the medial hamstrings?

8. What happens to the length of the semitendinosus if the pelvis is anteriorly tilted?

9. What is the only part of the hamstring group that cannot extend the thigh at the hip joint?

10. Besides the TFL, what muscle attaches to the anterior superior iliac spine of the pelvis?

11. What muscle acts to move the joint capsule of the knee?

12. Which of the following joint actions of the pelvis at the hip joint is occurring if the semimembranosus concentrically contracts? anterior tilt / posterior tilt

13. Name three synergists to the rectus femoris at the knee joint.

14. How many of the muscles of the adductor group can flex the thigh at the hip joint?

15. How are the biceps femoris and the semitendinosus antagonistic to each other?

16. How are all four quadriceps femoris muscles synergistic with each other?

17. Why are the hamstrings antagonistic to the TFL?

18. What is the only part of the hamstring group that does not cross the hip joint?

19. What is the common distal attachment of all four quadriceps femoris muscles?

20. What two muscles attach into the iliotibial band?

21. What three muscles attach into the pes anserine tendon?

22. What happens to the length of the sartorius when the knee joint extends?

23. What muscle's tendon is located directly medial to the distal tendon of the sartorius?

24. How is the pectineus synergistic with the rectus femoris?

25. During what joint actions of the pelvis does the adductor longus lengthen?

26. What joint action of the knee lengthens the biceps femoris?

27. What joint actions are antagonistic to the pelvic actions of the adductor longus?

28. What three muscles attach into the pes anserine tendon?

29. What muscle is sometimes known as the 4th hamstring?

More review activities on Evolve at http://evolve.elsevier.com/Muscolino/muscular/

30. What muscle is deep to the vastus intermedius?

31. Which muscle of the adductor group is the most posterior?

32. What three muscles comprise the hamstring group?

33. What happens to the length of the adductor magnus if the thigh is actively extended at the hip joint?

34. Which of the following joint actions of the thigh at the hip joint occurs if the adductor magnus eccentrically contracts? extension / flexion

35. Which quadriceps femoris muscle is the largest?

36. If the thigh is passively flexed at the hip joint, what happens to the length of the TFL?

37. What is the only muscle of the adductor group that crosses the knee joint?

38. Which hamstring muscle is located the most laterally?

39. What happens to the length of the vastus intermedius if the leg is passively extended at the knee joint?

40. Why is the semitendinosus antagonistic to the sartorius?

41. What muscle is immediately deep to the TFL?

42. If the sartorius is eccentrically contracting, what action is occurring at the hip joint?

43. What muscle is immediately medial to the pectineus?

44. What muscle is deep to the iliotibial band for most of its length?

45. What muscle is immediately lateral to the pectineus?

46. What muscle is immediately deep to the adductor longus?

47. How can the rectus abdominis be considered to be synergistic with the adductor magnus?

48. How many of the quadriceps femoris muscles attach to the linea aspera of the femur?

49. What is the longest muscle in the human body?

50. Which muscle of the adductor group has the most prominent proximal tendon?

51. What muscle is located directly deep to the rectus femoris?

52. If the thigh is passively laterally rotated at the hip joint, what happens to the length of the TFL?

53. What seven muscles attach to the linea aspera of the femur?

54. What happens to the length of the rectus femoris if the hip joint flexes?

55. What five muscles comprise the adductors of the thigh group?

56. What happens to the length of the gracilis if the pelvis is posteriorly tilted at the hip joint?

57. What is the only quadriceps femoris muscle that crosses the hip joint?

58. What four muscles comprise the quadriceps femoris group?

59. Name a synergist to the vastus intermedius.

ANTERIOR VIEW OF THE RIGHT LEG

THE MUSCULAR SYSTEM Muscles of the Leg

POSTERIOR VIEW OF THE RIGHT LEG (SUPERFICIAL)

THE MUSCULAR SYSTEM Muscles of the Leg

POSTERIOR VIEW OF THE RIGHT LEG (INTERMEDIATE)

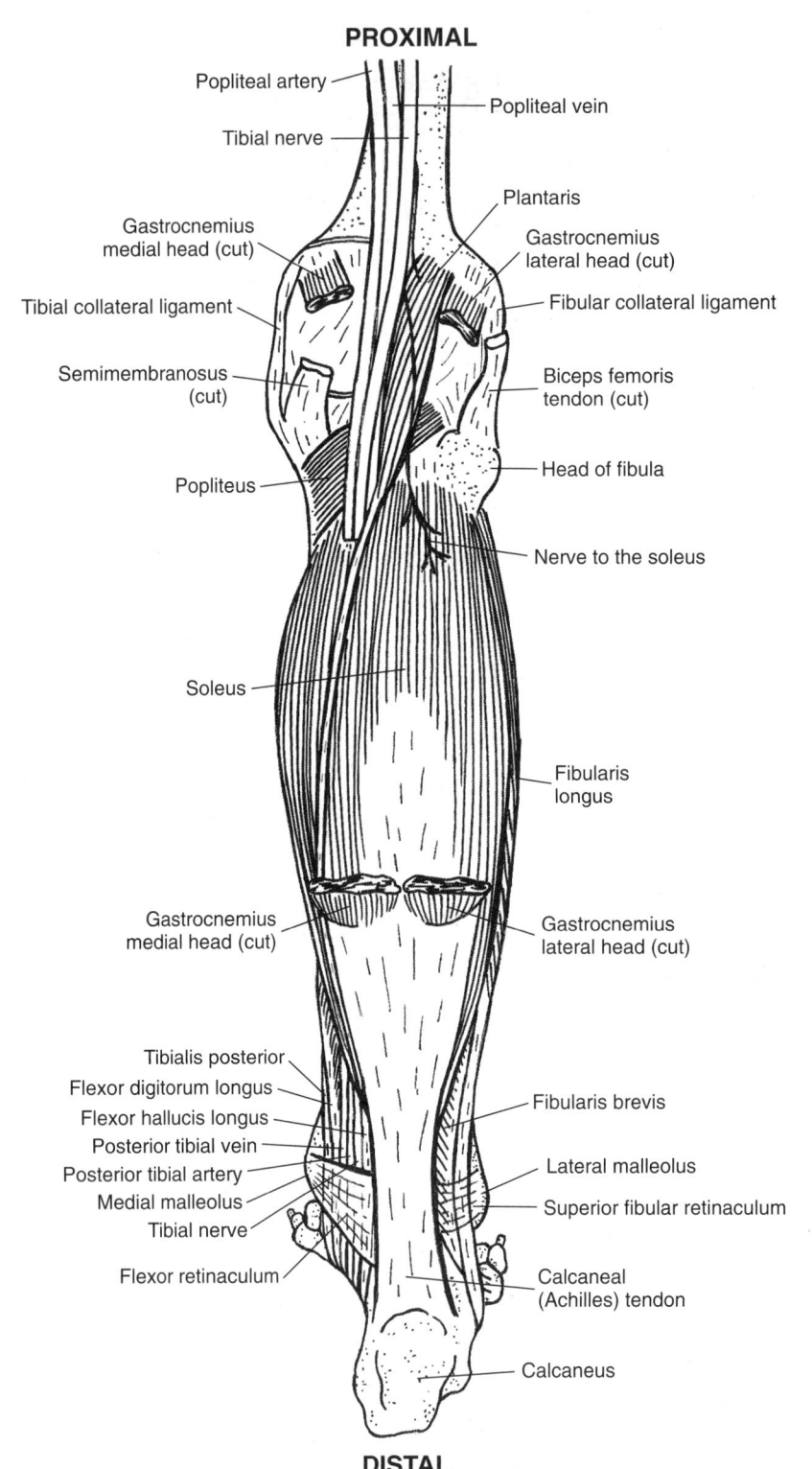

THE MUSCULAR SYSTEM Muscles of the Leg

POSTERIOR VIEW OF THE RIGHT LEG (DEEP)

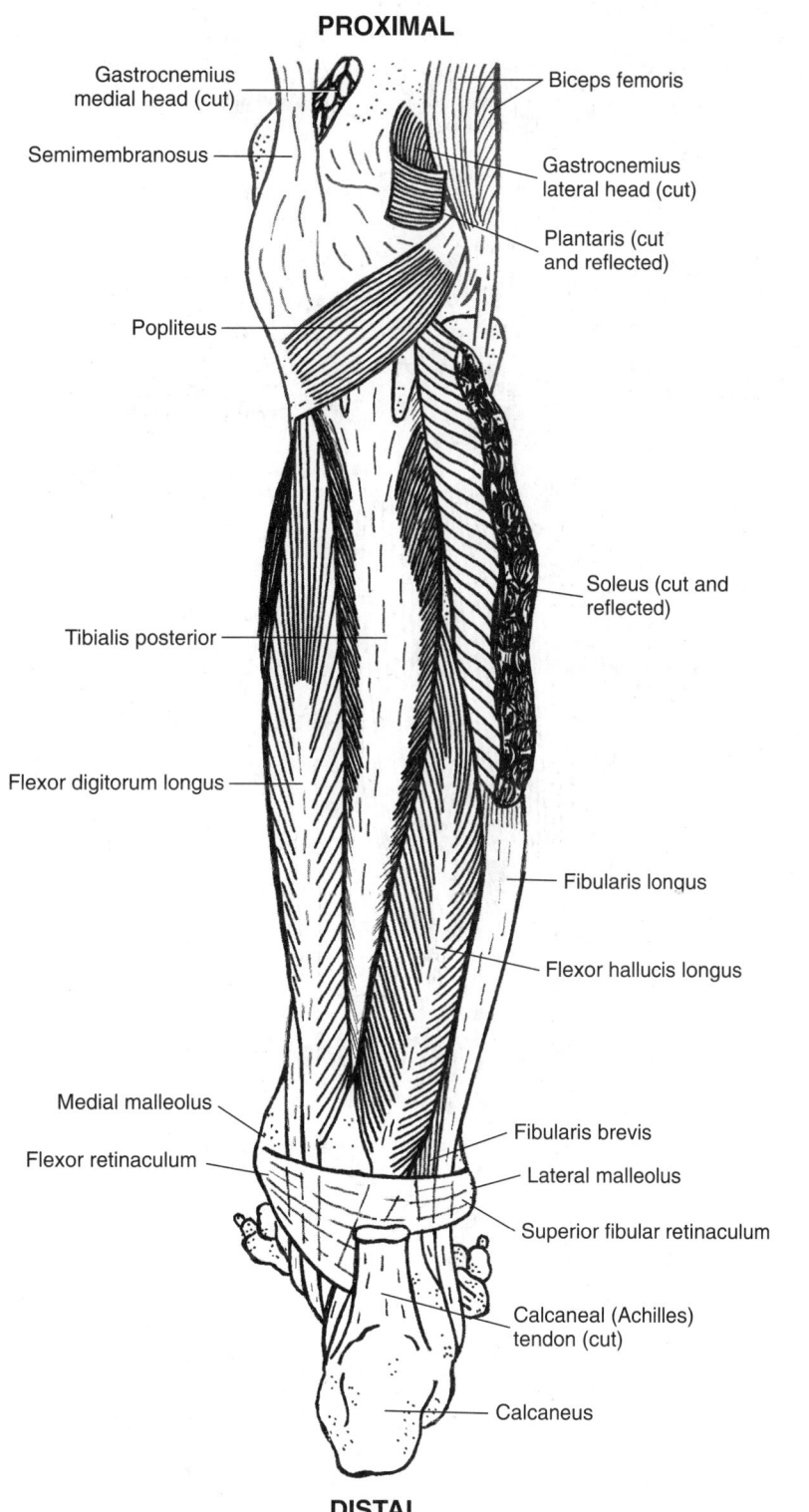

THE MUSCULAR SYSTEM Muscles of the Leg

LATERAL VIEW OF THE RIGHT LEG

THE MUSCULAR SYSTEM Muscles of the Leg

TIBIALIS ANTERIOR
(IN THE ANTERIOR COMPARTMENT)
tib-ee-**a**-lis an-**tee**-ri-or

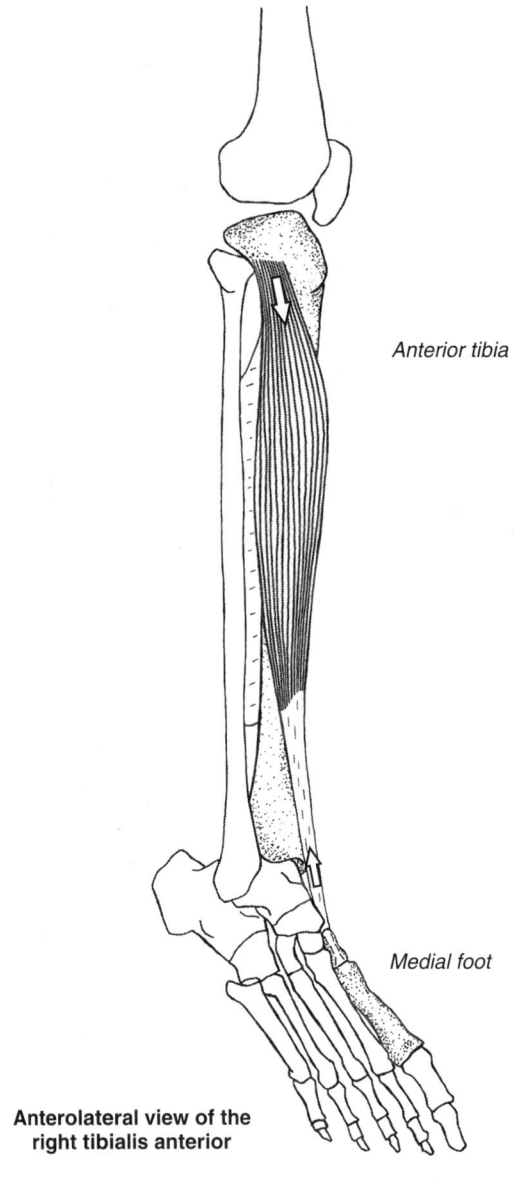

Anterior tibia

Medial foot

Anterolateral view of the right tibialis anterior

Actions
Dorsiflexion of the foot at the ankle joint
Inversion of the foot at the subtalar joint

Innervation
The deep fibular nerve

Arterial Supply
The anterior tibial artery

THE MUSCULAR SYSTEM Muscles of the Leg

Tibialis anterior

DID YOU KNOW?

The tibialis anterior is the most commonly affected muscle when a person has shin splints. The tibialis anterior is also one of the two "stirrup muscles."

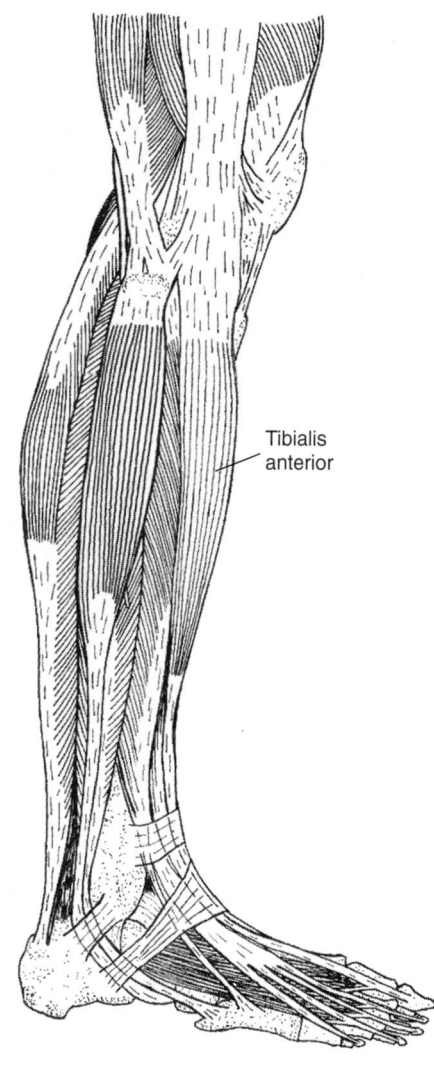

Tibialis anterior

EXTENSOR HALLUCIS LONGUS
(IN THE ANTERIOR COMPARTMENT)
eks-**ten**-sor hal-**oo**-sis **long**-us

Actions
Extension of the big toe (toe #1) at the metatarsophalangeal joint and the interphalangeal joint
Dorsiflexion of the foot at the ankle joint
Inversion of the foot at the subtalar joint

Innervation
The deep fibular nerve

Arterial Supply
The anterior tibial artery

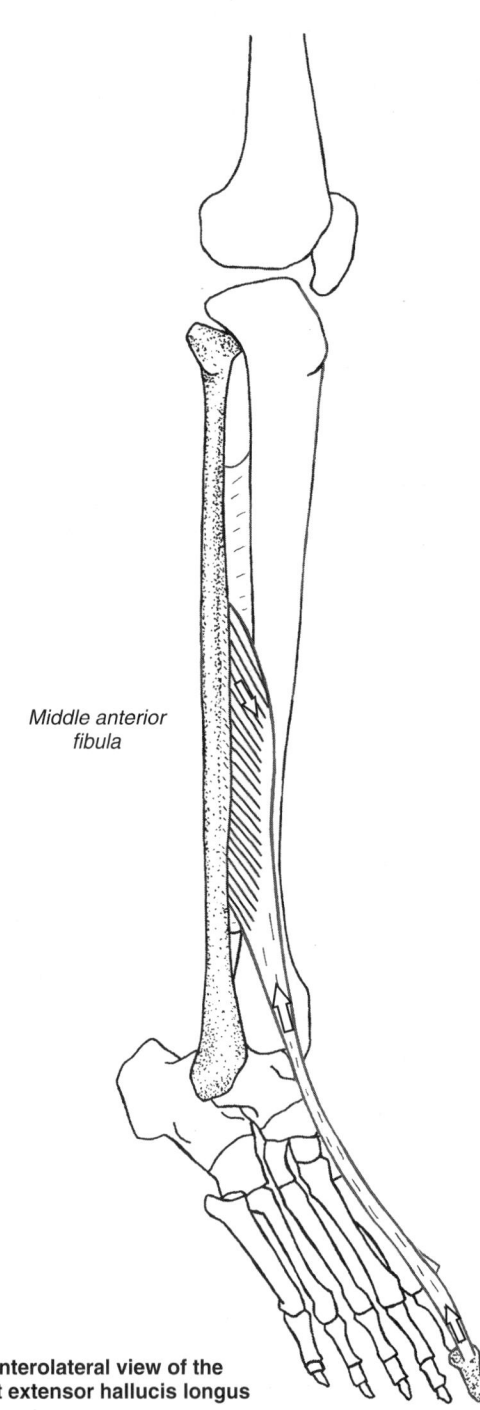

Middle anterior fibula

Anterolateral view of the right extensor hallucis longus

Dorsal surface of the big toe (toe #1)

THE MUSCULAR SYSTEM: Muscles of the Leg

DID YOU KNOW? The extensor hallucis longus is the only muscle that can extend the distal phalanx of the big toe.

Extensor hallucis longus

EXTENSOR DIGITORUM LONGUS
(IN THE ANTERIOR COMPARTMENT)

eks-**ten**-sor dij-i-**toe**-rum **long**-us

Actions
Extension of toes #2-5 at the metatarsophalangeal joint and the proximal and distal interphalangeal joints
Dorsiflexion of the foot at the ankle joint
Eversion of the foot at the subtalar joint

Innervation
The deep fibular nerve

Arterial Supply
The anterior tibial artery

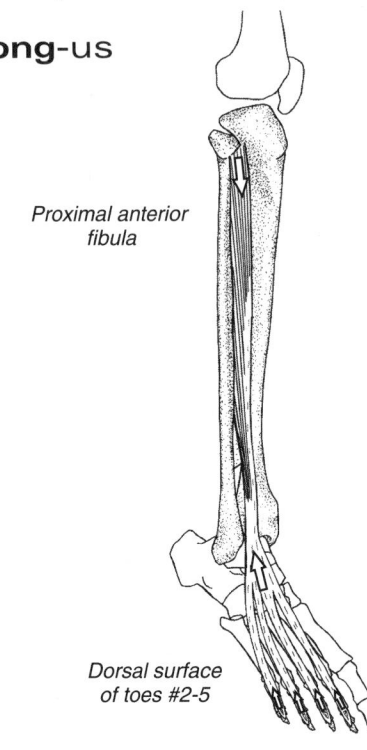

Anterolateral view of the right extensor digitorum longus

FIBULARIS TERTIUS
(IN THE ANTERIOR COMPARTMENT)

fib-you **la**-ris **ter**-she-us

Actions
Dorsiflexion of the foot at the ankle joint
Eversion of the foot at the subtalar joint

Innervation
The deep fibular nerve

Arterial Supply
The anterior tibial artery

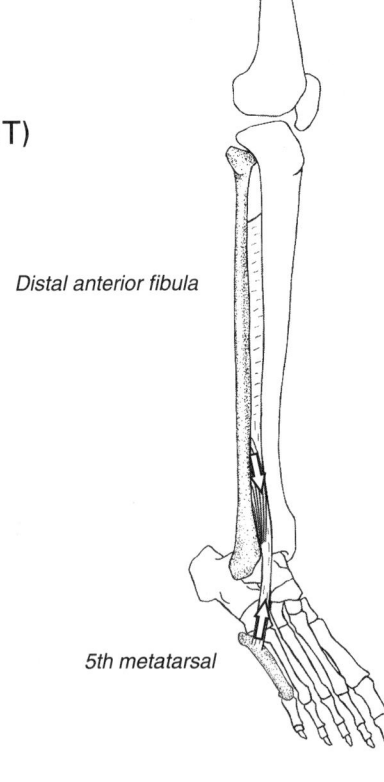

Anterolateral view of the right fibularis tertius

THE MUSCULAR SYSTEM Muscles of the Leg 249

DID YOU KNOW

The most distal and lateral part of the extensor digitorum longus does not attach onto "digits", therefore it is given another name, the fibularis tertius. Therefore, the fibularis tertius is actually the most distal and lateral part of the extensor digitorum longus. It is given a separate name because it does not attach onto "digits."

FIBULARIS LONGUS
(IN THE LATERAL COMPARTMENT)

fib-you-la-ris **long**-us

Actions
Eversion of the foot at the subtalar joint
Plantarflexion of the foot at the ankle joint

Innervation
The superficial fibular nerve

Arterial Supply
The fibular artery

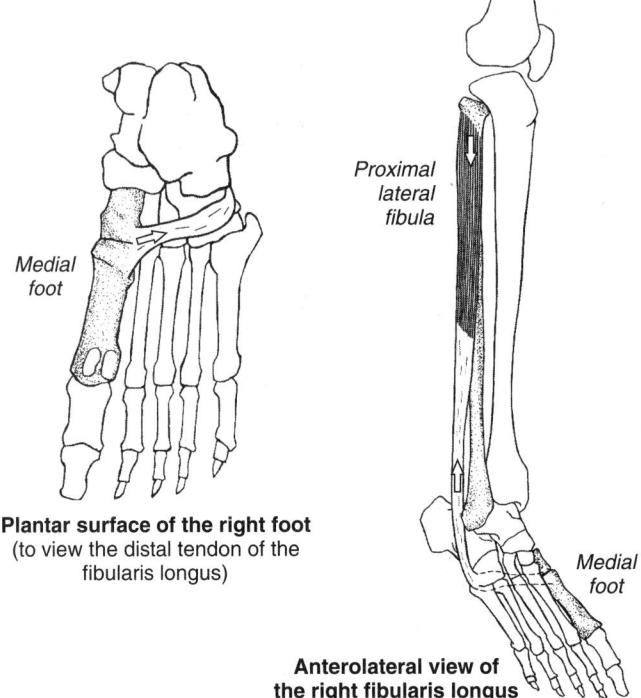

Plantar surface of the right foot
(to view the distal tendon of the fibularis longus)

Anterolateral view of the right fibularis longus

FIBULARIS BREVIS
(IN THE LATERAL COMPARTMENT)

fib-you-la-ris **bre**-vis

Actions
Eversion of the foot at the subtalar joint
Plantarflexion of the foot at the ankle joint

Innervation
The superficial fibular nerve

Arterial Supply
The fibular artery

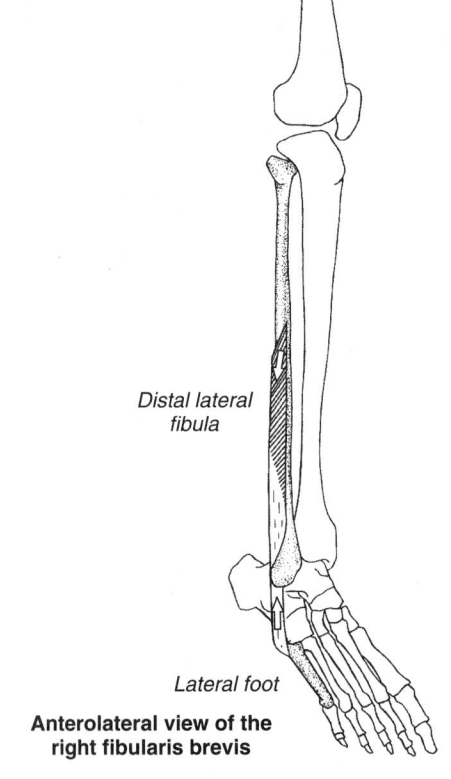

Anterolateral view of the right fibularis brevis

THE MUSCULAR SYSTEM Muscles of the Leg 251

DID YOU KNOW

The fibularis longus, along with the tibialis anterior, are often called the "stirrup muscles" because their distal tendons form a stirrup around the foot.

DID YOU KNOW

The fibularis brevis is located deep to the fibularis longus and has the same actions as the fibularis longus.

GASTROCNEMIUS ("GASTROC")
(OF THE TRICEPS SURAE AND IN THE SUPERFICIAL POSTERIOR COMPARTMENT)

gas-trok-**nee**-me-us

Actions
Plantarflexion of the foot at the ankle joint
Flexion of the leg at the knee joint
Inversion of the foot at the subtalar joint

Innervation
The tibial nerve

Arterial Supply
Sural branches of the popliteal artery

Medial and lateral femoral condyles

Calcaneus via the calcaneal (Achilles) tendon

Posterior view of the right gastrocnemius
(with the foot plantarflexed)

SOLEUS
(OF THE TRICEPS SURAE AND IN THE SUPERFICIAL POSTERIOR COMPARTMENT)

so-lee-us

Actions
Plantarflexion of the foot at the ankle joint
Inversion of the foot at the subtalar joint

Innervation
The tibial nerve

Arterial Supply
Sural branches of the popliteal artery

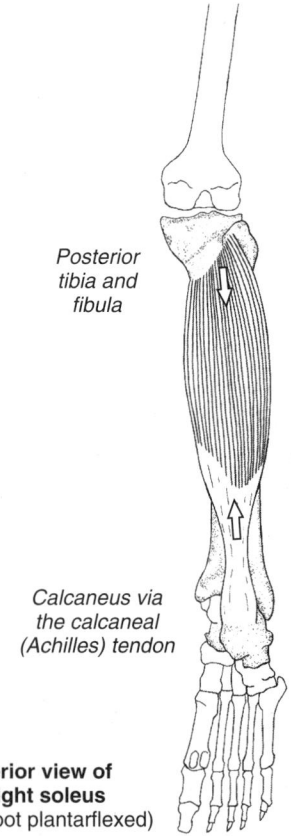

Posterior tibia and fibula

Calcaneus via the calcaneal (Achilles) tendon

Posterior view of the right soleus
(with the foot plantarflexed)

THE MUSCULAR SYSTEM Muscles of the Leg

The gastrocnemius (and soleus) attaches into the calcaneus via the calcaneal tendon, which is more well known as the Achilles tendon.

The soleus is actually quite large and massive, accounting for the contours of the gastrocnemius being so visible. "Behind every great gastrocnemius is a great soleus ☺."

PLANTARIS
(IN THE SUPERFICIAL POSTERIOR COMPARTMENT)

plan-**ta**-ris

Actions
Plantarflexion of the foot at the ankle joint
Flexion of the leg at the knee joint

Innervation
The tibial nerve

Arterial Supply
Sural branches of the popliteal artery

Posterior view of the right plantaris
(with the foot plantarflexed)

POPLITEUS
(IN THE DEEP POSTERIOR COMPARTMENT)

pop-**lit**-ee-us

Actions
Medial rotation of the leg at the knee joint
Flexion of the leg at the knee joint
Lateral rotation of the thigh at the knee joint

Innervation
The tibial nerve

Arterial Supply
Branches of the popliteal artery

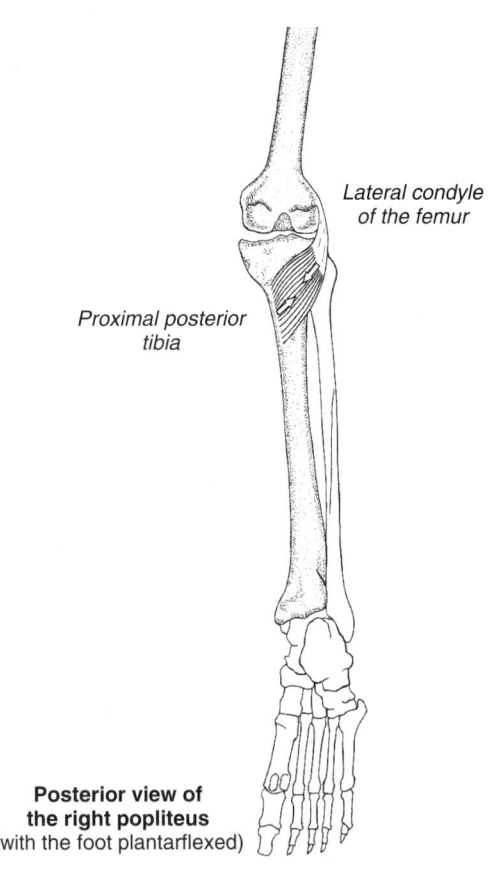

Posterior view of the right popliteus
(with the foot plantarflexed)

THE MUSCULAR SYSTEM Muscles of the Leg

DID YOU KNOW

The vast majority of the length of the plantaris is its long, slender, distal tendon.

DID YOU KNOW

The popliteus is considered important for its rotation action at the knee joint, which is said to "unlock" the extended knee.

TIBIALIS POSTERIOR
(IN THE DEEP POSTERIOR COMPARTMENT)
tib-ee-**a**-lis pos-**tee**-ri-or

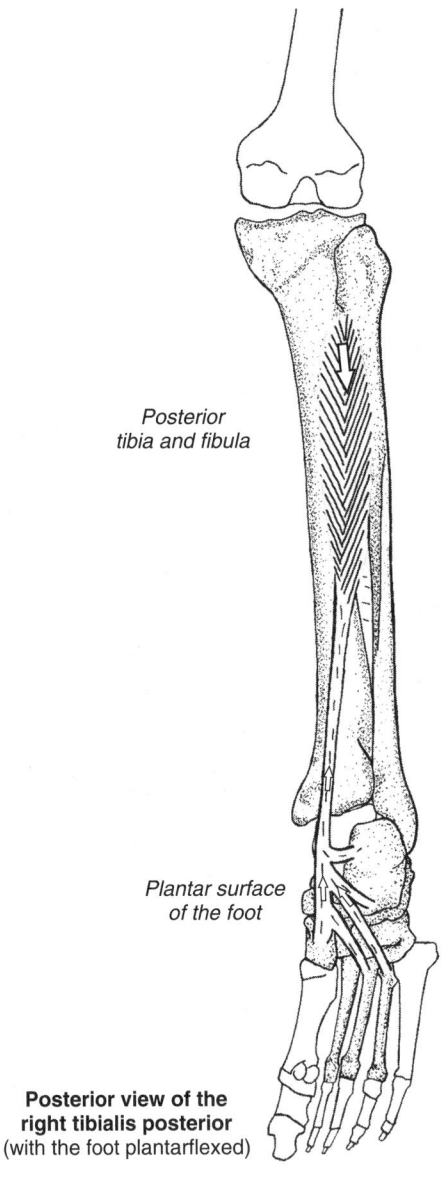

Posterior tibia and fibula

Plantar surface of the foot

Posterior view of the right tibialis posterior (with the foot plantarflexed)

Actions
Plantarflexion of the foot at the ankle joint
Inversion of the foot at the subtalar joint

Innervation
The tibial nerve

Arterial Supply
The posterior tibial artery

THE MUSCULAR SYSTEM Muscles of the Leg

Tibialis posterior

DID YOU KNOW?

The tibialis posterior is "Tom" of the "Tom, Dick, and Harry muscles." "Tom, Dick, and Harry muscles" are grouped together because their distal tendons all cross posterior to the medial malleolus of the tibia.

Tibialis posterior

FLEXOR DIGITORUM LONGUS
(IN THE DEEP POSTERIOR COMPARTMENT)
fleks-or dij-i-toe-rum long-us

Actions
Flexion of toes #2-5 at the metatarsophalangeal joint and the proximal and distal interphalangeal joints
Plantarflexion of the foot at the ankle joint
Inversion of the foot at the subtalar joint

Innervation
The tibial nerve

Arterial Supply
The posterior tibial artery

Middle posterior tibia

Posterior view of the right flexor digitorum longus
(with the foot plantarflexed)

Plantar surface of toes #2-5

THE MUSCULAR SYSTEM: Muscles of the Leg

Flexor digitorum longus

 DID YOU KNOW

The flexor digitorum longus is "Dick" of the "Tom, Dick, and Harry muscles." "Tom, Dick, and Harry muscles" are grouped together because their distal tendons all cross posterior to the medial malleolus of the tibia.

Flexor digitorum longus

FLEXOR HALLUCIS LONGUS
(IN THE DEEP POSTERIOR COMPARTMENT)
fleks-or hal-oo-sis long-us

Actions
Flexion of the big toe (toe #1) at the metatarsophalangeal joint and the interphalangeal joint
Plantarflexion of the foot at the ankle joint
Inversion of the foot at the subtalar joint

Innervation
The tibial nerve

Arterial Supply
The posterior tibial artery

Distal posterior fibula

Plantar surface of the big toe (toe #1)

Posterior view of the right flexor hallucis longus (with the foot plantarflexed)

THE MUSCULAR SYSTEM Muscles of the Leg

Flexor hallucis longus

DID YOU KNOW

The flexor hallucis longus is "Harry" of the "Tom, Dick, and Harry muscles." "Tom, Dick, and Harry muscles" are grouped together because their distal tendons all cross posterior to the medial malleolus of the tibia.

Flexor hallucis longus

THE MUSCULAR SYSTEM Muscles of the Leg

ANTERIOR VIEW OF THE RIGHT LEG

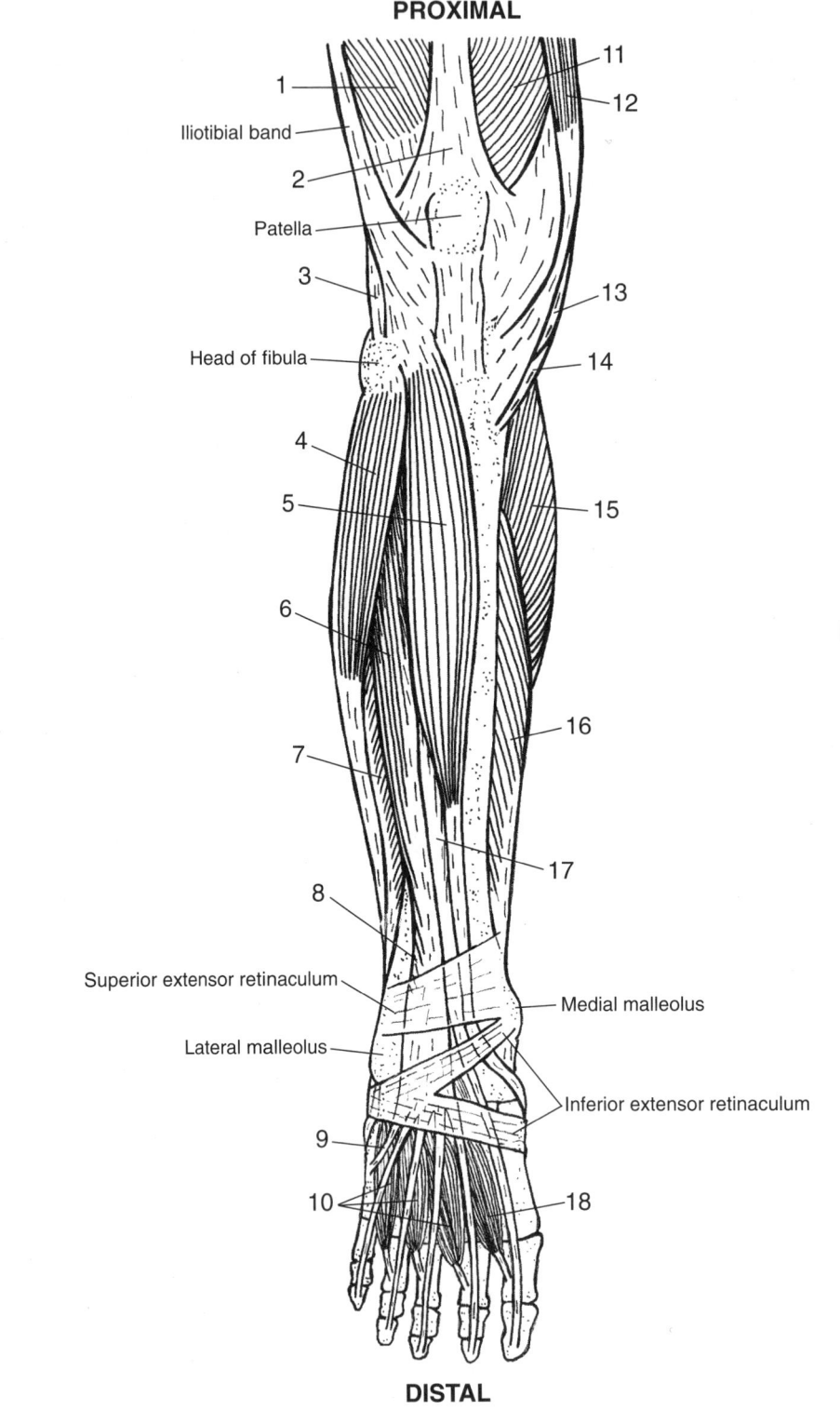

Answers to labeling exercises are on p. 467.

THE MUSCULAR SYSTEM Muscles of the Leg 263

POSTERIOR VIEW OF THE RIGHT LEG (SUPERFICIAL)

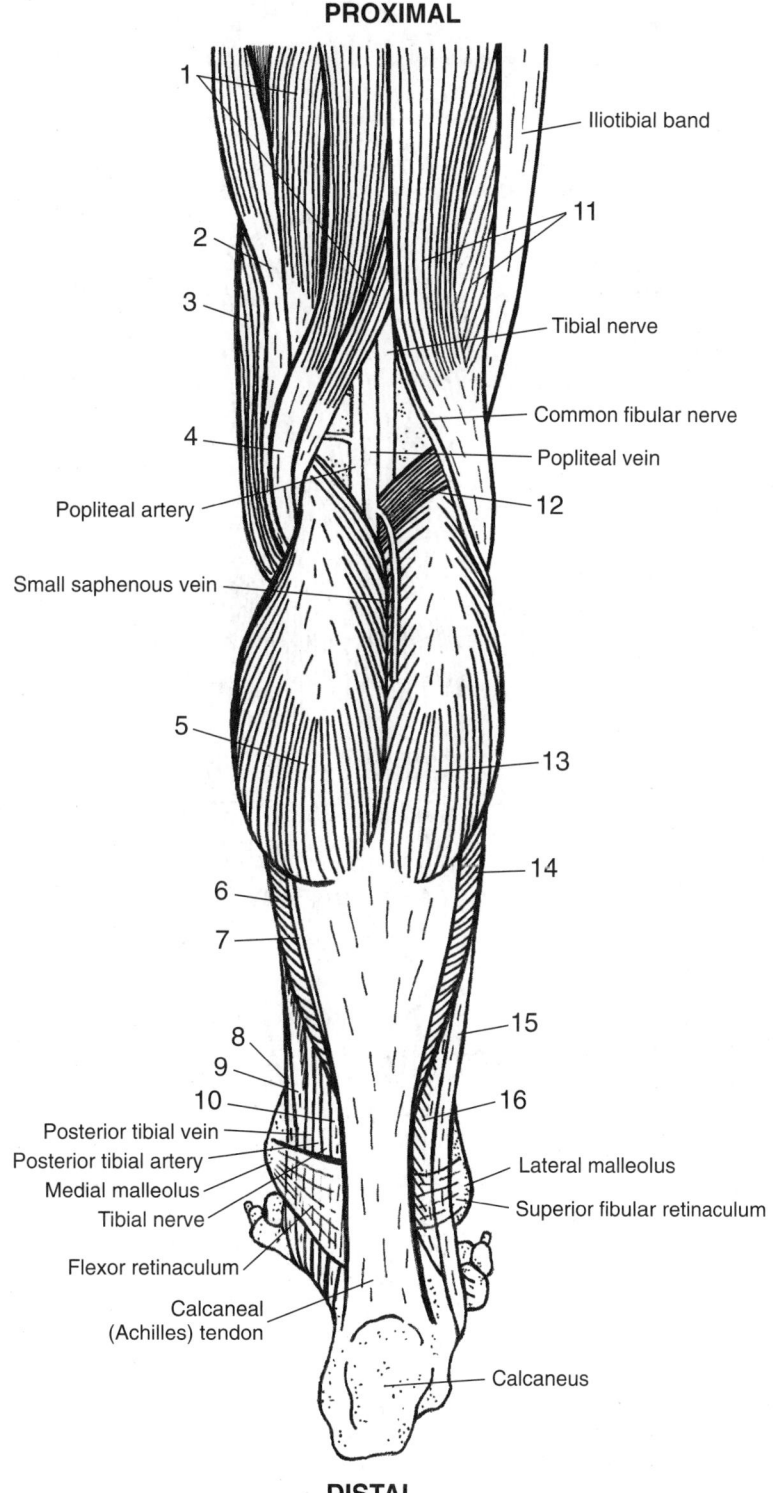

THE MUSCULAR SYSTEM Muscles of the Leg

POSTERIOR VIEW OF THE RIGHT LEG (INTERMEDIATE)

THE MUSCULAR SYSTEM Muscles of the Leg   265

POSTERIOR VIEW OF THE RIGHT LEG (DEEP)

PROXIMAL

1
2
3
4
5
6
7
8
9
10
11
12

MEDIAL

LATERAL

Medial malleolus
Flexor retinaculum
Lateral malleolus
Superior fibular retinaculum
Calcaneal (Achilles) tendon (cut)
Calcaneus

DISTAL

THE MUSCULAR SYSTEM Muscles of the Leg

LATERAL VIEW OF THE RIGHT LEG

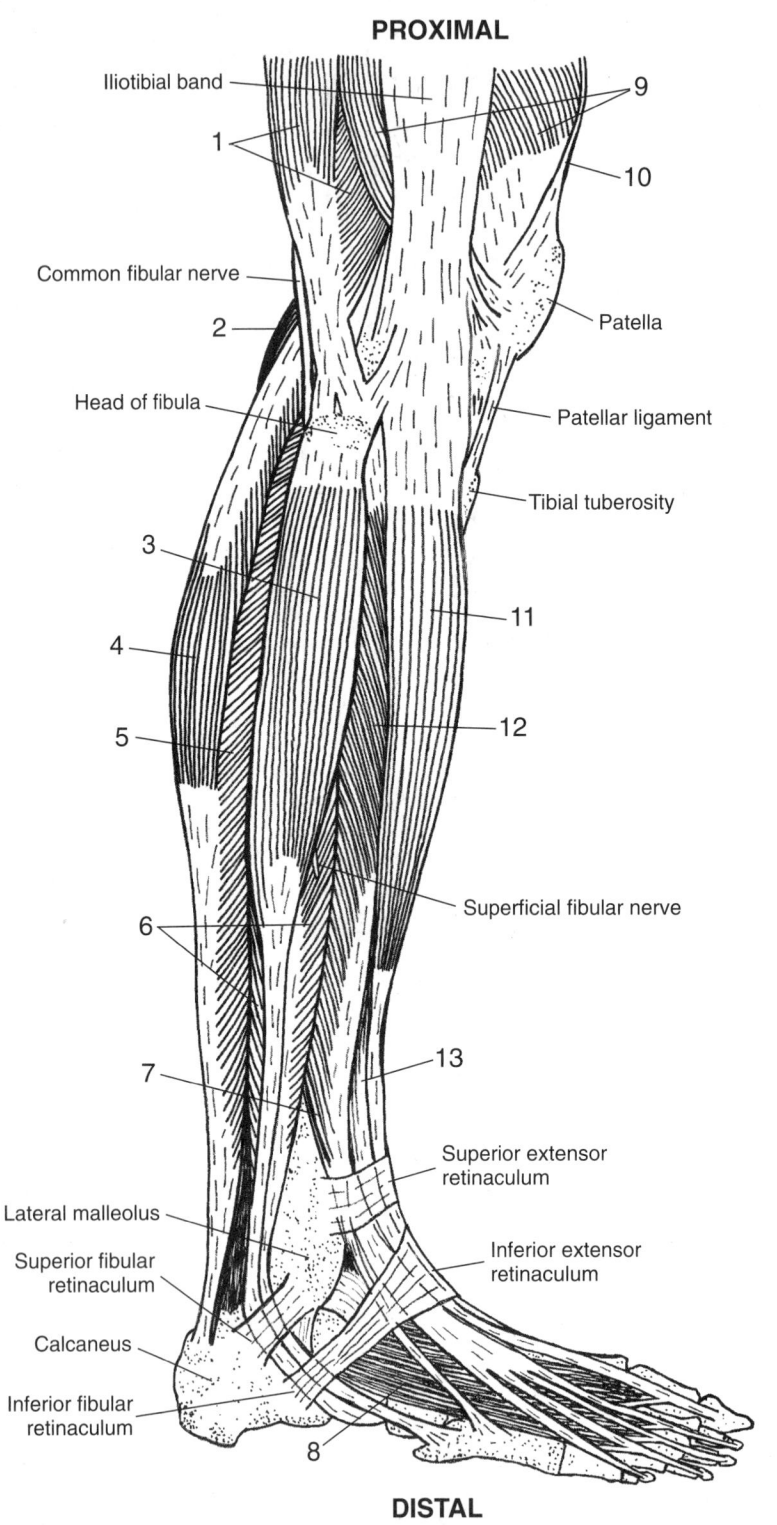

THE MUSCULAR SYSTEM Muscles of the Leg   267

MEDIAL VIEW OF THE RIGHT LEG

Review Questions

Muscles of the Leg
Answers to these questions are found on page 467.

1. How are the fibularis tertius and brevis synergistic with each other?

2. Where are the Tom, Dick, and Harry muscles most superficial?

3. What muscle is considered to be important for its rotation action at the knee joint?

4. All three fibularis muscles attach proximally to what bone?

5. How are the fibularis tertius and brevis antagonistic to each other?

6. The fibularis tertius is actually the most distal part of what muscle?

7. What action(s) would an antagonist to the fibularis longus have?

8. Which fibularis muscle travels in the deep plantar foot?

9. How are the tibialis anterior and extensor digitorum longus synergistic with each other?

10. What three muscles are located in the superficial posterior compartment of the leg?

11. What two muscles attach to the 5th metatarsal?

12. What happens to the length of the flexor digitorum longus when the knee joint is passively flexed?

13. What muscles make up the triceps surae group?

14. To which phalanx/phalanges do the flexor digitorum and flexor hallucis longus muscles attach?

15. The distal tendon of what two muscles is known as the Achilles tendon?

16. Who are the Tom, Dick, and Harry muscles?

17. Which muscle is deeper, the extensor digitorum longus or the extensor hallucis longus?

18. What muscle is immediately superficial to the plantaris?

19. What muscle is located superficially immediately posterior to the fibularis longus?

20. What four muscles are located in the anterior compartment of the leg?

21. If the tibialis anterior is concentrically contracting, what joint action(s) is/are occurring?

22. What two muscles attach to the lateral condyle of the femur?

23. If the big toe is flexed at the metatarsophalangeal and interphalangeal joints, what happens to the length of the extensor hallucis longus?

24. Which Tom, Dick, and Harry muscle lies closest to the medial malleolus of the tibia?

25. Which Tom, Dick, and Harry muscle has the most superficial exposure in the distal medial leg?

26. What muscle is immediately posterior to the fibularis longus?

27. What are the two stirrup muscles?

28. Is the tibialis anterior synergistic with or antagonistic to the gastrocnemius?

29. Which muscle is deeper, the fibularis longus or brevis?

30. What is the only muscle of the posterior compartments of the leg that does not cross the ankle joint?

31. How can the popliteus both medially and laterally rotate the knee joint?

32. What joint actions are shared by all three Tom, Dick, and Harry muscles?

33. What two muscles attach to the first metatarsal and first cuneiform?

34. What two muscles are located in the lateral compartment of the leg?

35. What muscle is immediately superficial to the Tom, Dick, and Harry muscles?

36. What muscle is antagonistic to both actions of the foot of the flexor hallucis longus?

37. What is the only tarsal bone to which the tibialis posterior does not attach?

38. What muscle lies immediately medial to the belly of the tibialis posterior?

39. If the fibularis longus and brevis are eccentrically contracting, what joint motion(s) is/are occurring?

40. From a posterior perspective, what muscle is immediately deep to the gastrocnemius?

41. What happens to the length of the tibialis posterior if the ankle joint is passively or actively plantarflexed?

42. What four muscles are located in the deep posterior compartment of the leg?

THE MUSCULAR SYSTEM Intrinsic Muscles of the Foot

DORSAL VIEW OF THE RIGHT FOOT

PROXIMAL

Fibularis longus
Fibularis brevis
Extensor digitorum longus
Lateral malleolus
Fibularis brevis tendon
5th metatarsal
Fibularis tertius tendon
Extensor digitorum brevis
Abductor digiti minimi pedis
3rd and 4th dorsal interossei pedis

Extensor hallucis longus
Tibialis anterior
Soleus
Superior extensor retinaculum
Medial malleolus
Inferior extensor retinaculum
Extensor hallucis brevis
Abductor hallucis
1st and 2nd dorsal interossei pedis

LATERAL

MEDIAL

DISTAL

EXTENSOR DIGITORUM BREVIS
(DORSAL SURFACE)

eks-**ten**-sor dij-i-**toe**-rum **bre**-vis

Action
Extension of toes #2-4 at the metatarsophalangeal and proximal and distal interphalangeal joints

Innervation
The deep fibular nerve

Arterial Supply
The dorsalis pedis artery

Dorsolateral view of the right extensor digitorum brevis

EXTENSOR HALLUCIS BREVIS
(DORSAL SURFACE)

eks-**ten**-sor hal-**oo**-sis **bre**-vis

Action
Extension of the big toe (toe #1) at the metatarsophalangeal joint

Innervation
The deep fibular nerve

Arterial Supply
The dorsalis pedis artery

Dorsolateral view of the right extensor hallucis brevis

THE MUSCULAR SYSTEM Intrinsic Muscles of the Foot 275

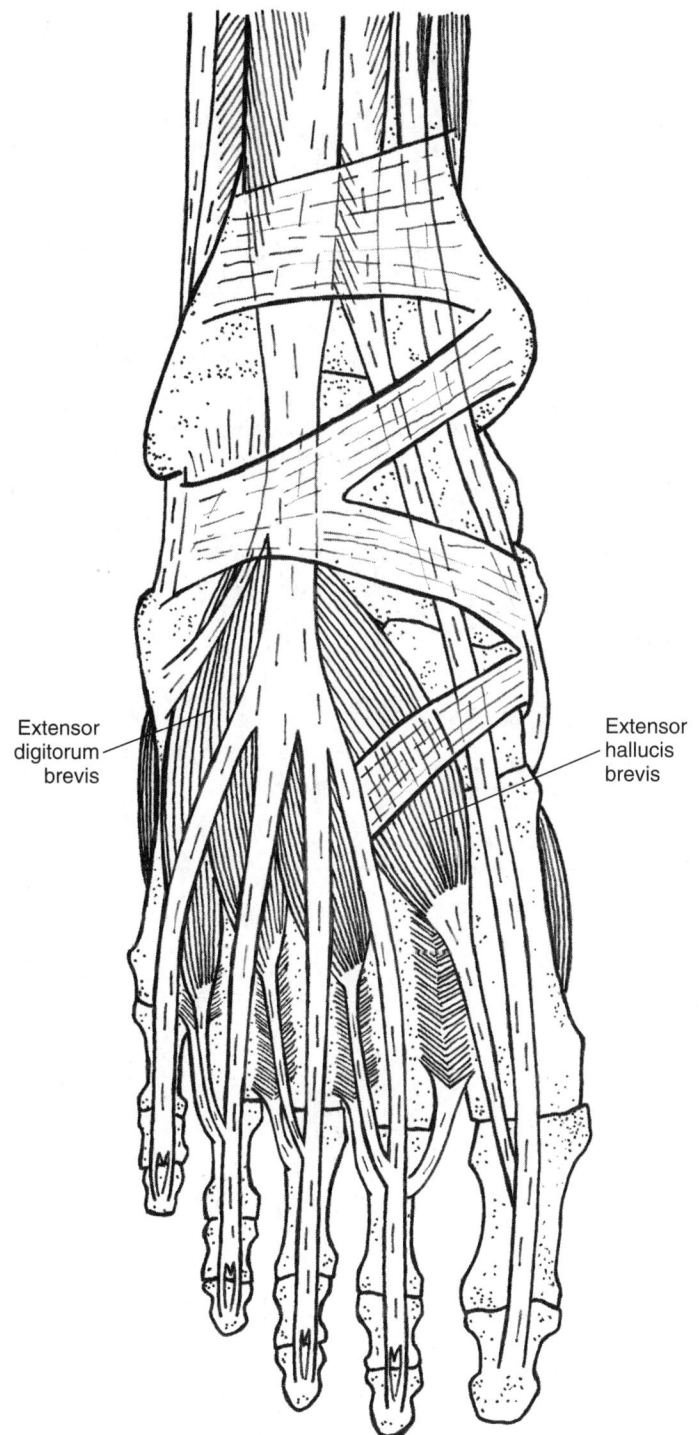

Extensor digitorum brevis

Extensor hallucis brevis

DID YOU KNOW

The extensor digitorum brevis and extensor hallucis brevis are actually parts of the same muscle and are the only intrinsic foot muscles located on the dorsal side.

ABDUCTOR HALLUCIS
(PLANTAR SURFACE—LAYER I)

ab-**duk**-tor hal-**oo**-sis

Actions
Abduction of the big toe (toe #1) at the metatarsophalangeal joint
Flexion of the big toe (toe #1) at the metatarsophalangeal joint

Innervation
The medial plantar nerve

Arterial Supply
The medial plantar artery

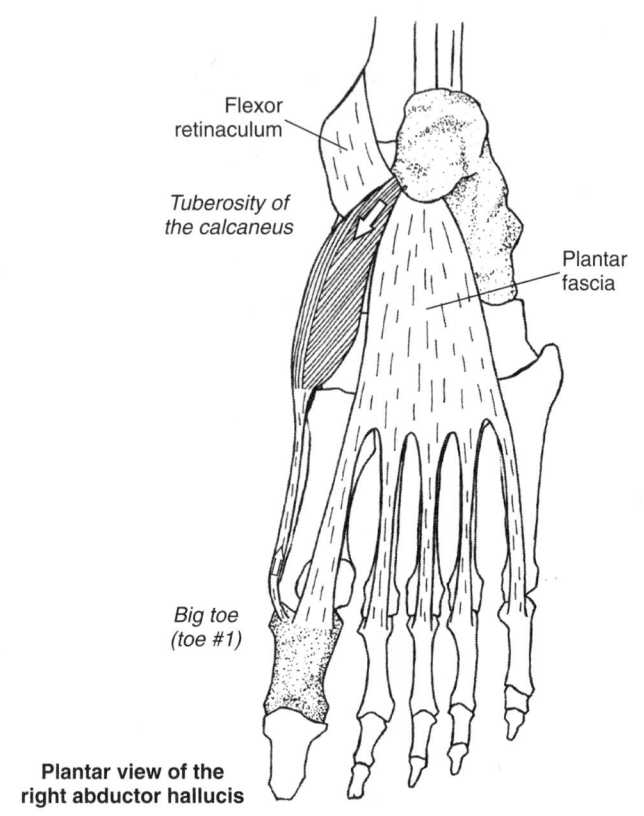

Plantar view of the right abductor hallucis

ABDUCTOR DIGITI MINIMI PEDIS
(PLANTAR SURFACE—LAYER I)

ab-**duk**-tor **dij**-i-tee **min**-i-mee **peed**-us

Actions
Abduction of the little toe (toe #5) at the metatarsophalangeal joint
Flexion of the little toe (toe #5) at the metatarsophalangeal joint

Innervation
The lateral plantar nerve

Arterial Supply
The lateral plantar artery

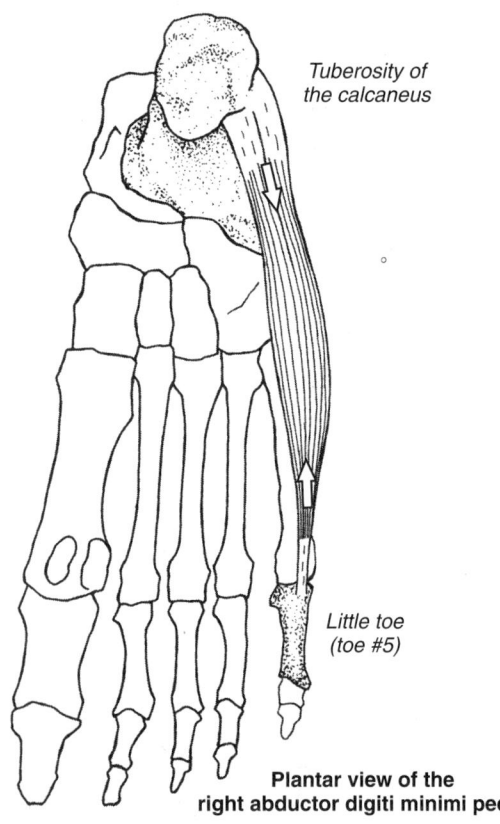

Plantar view of the right abductor digiti minimi pedis

THE MUSCULAR SYSTEM Intrinsic Muscles of the Foot

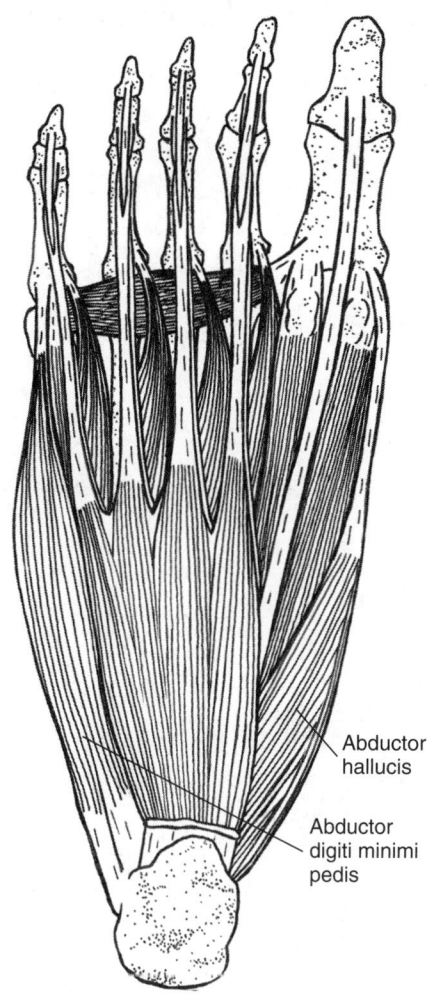

Abductor hallucis
Abductor digiti minimi pedis

DID YOU KNOW?
The abductor hallucis is easily palpable on the medial side of the plantar surface of the foot.

DID YOU KNOW?
The abductor digiti minimi pedis is often known simply as the abductor digiti minimi. But there is an abductor digiti minimi (manus) of the hand as well and confusion can result.

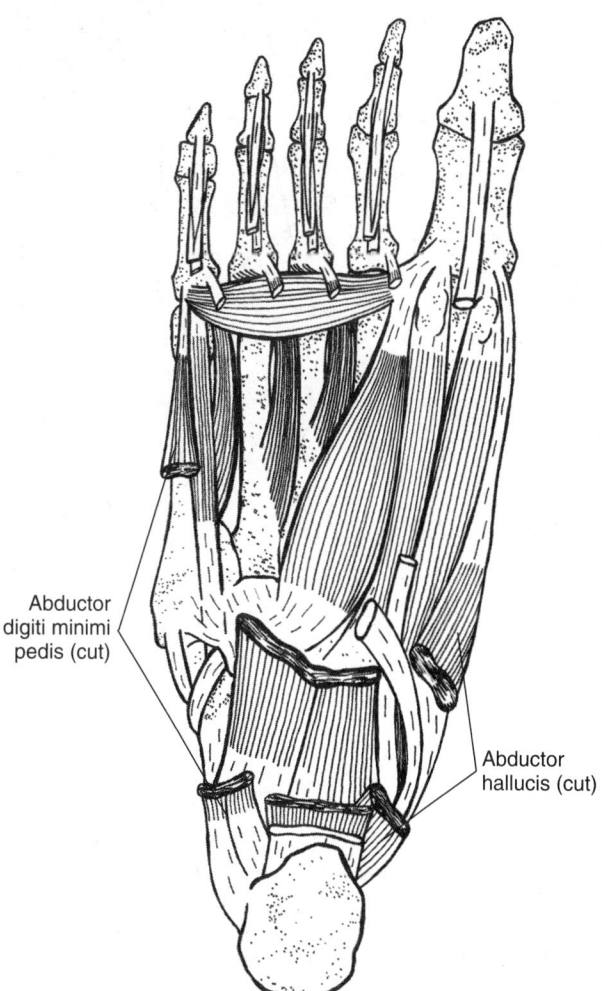

Abductor digiti minimi pedis (cut)
Abductor hallucis (cut)

FLEXOR DIGITORUM BREVIS
(PLANTAR SURFACE—LAYER I)
fleks-or dij-i-toe-rum bre-vis

Plantar view of the right flexor digitorum brevis

Toes #2-5

Action	Innervation	Arterial Supply
Flexion of toes #2-5 at the metatarsophalangeal and the proximal interphalangeal joints	The medial plantar nerve	The medial and lateral plantar arteries

THE MUSCULAR SYSTEM Intrinsic Muscles of the Foot 279

Flexor digitorum brevis

DID YOU KNOW?

The distal tendons of the flexor digitorum brevis split to allow passage of the distal tendons of the flexor digitorum longus to the distal phalanges of toes #2-5.

QUADRATUS PLANTAE
(PLANTAR SURFACE—LAYER II)

kwod-**ray**-tus **plan**-tee

Action
Flexion of toes #2-5 at the metatarsophalangeal and the proximal and distal interphalangeal joints

Innervation
The lateral plantar nerve

Arterial Supply
The medial and lateral plantar arteries

Plantar view of the right quadratus plantae

LUMBRICALS PEDIS
(PLANTAR SURFACE—LAYER II)

(There are four lumbrical pedis muscles, named #1, #2, #3, and #4.)

lum-bri-kuls **peed**-us

Actions
Extension of toes #2-5 at the proximal and distal interphalangeal joints
Flexion of toes #2-5 at the metatarsophalangeal joint

Innervation
The medial and lateral plantar nerves

Arterial Supply
The medial and lateral plantar arteries

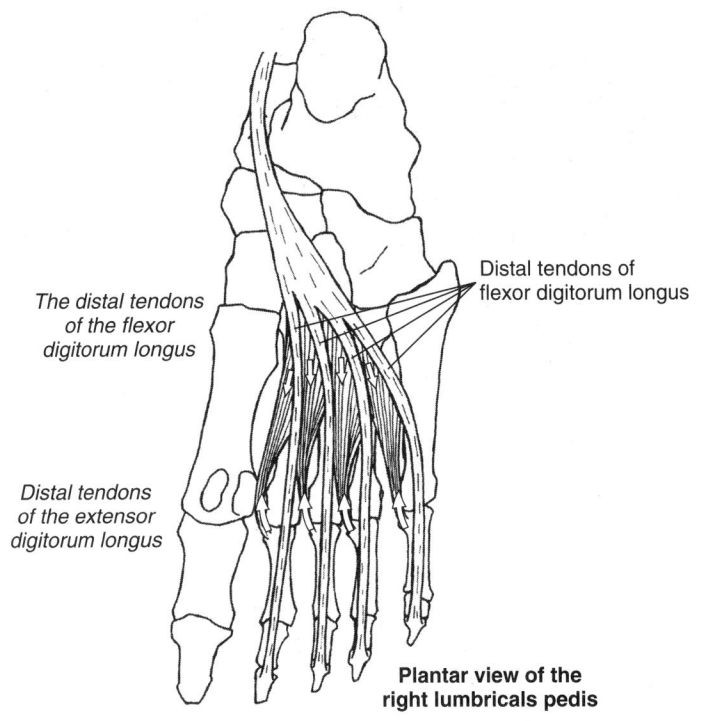

Plantar view of the right lumbricals pedis

THE MUSCULAR SYSTEM Intrinsic Muscles of the Foot

The quadratus plantae assists the flexor digitorum longus by straightening out the line of pull of this muscle upon the toes. For this reason, the quadratus plantae is also known as the flexor digitorum accessorius.

The lumbricals pedis are named for looking like earthworms; "lumbrical" is Latin for earthworm. There are four lumbricals pedis muscles in each foot.

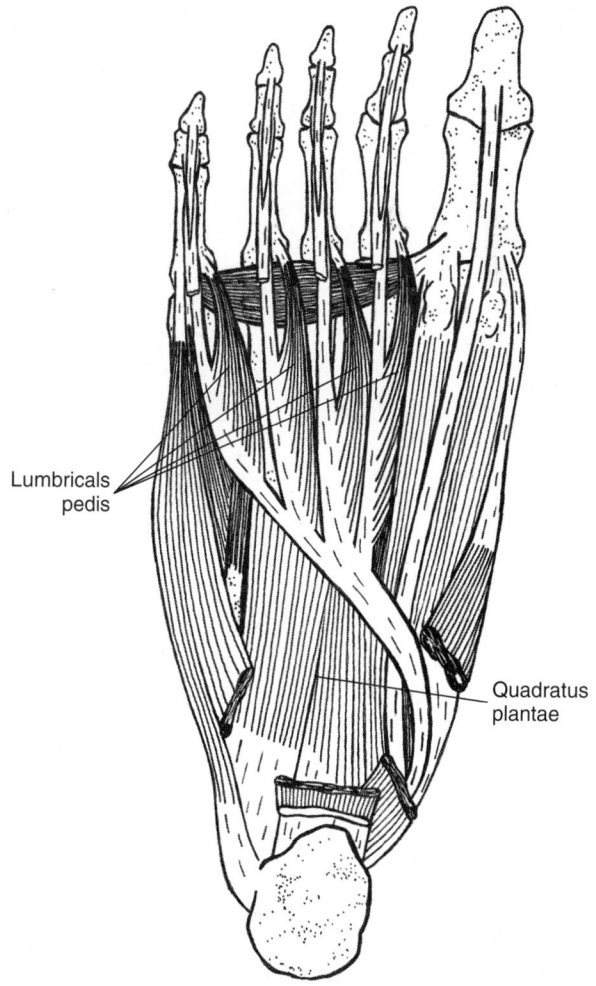

FLEXOR HALLUCIS BREVIS
(PLANTAR SURFACE—LAYER III)

fleks-or hal-**oo**-sis **bre**-vis

Action
Flexion of the big toe (toe #1) at the metatarsophalangeal joint

Innervation
The medial plantar nerve

Arterial Supply
The medial plantar artery

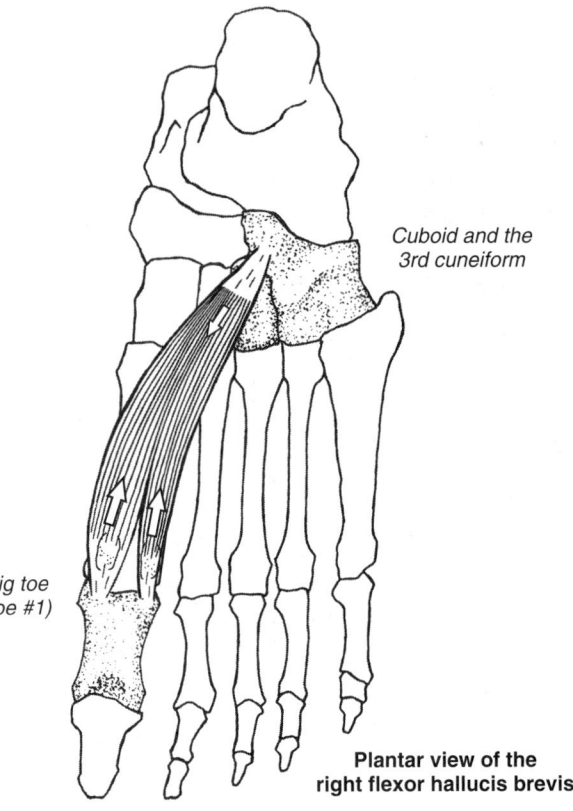

Plantar view of the right flexor hallucis brevis

FLEXOR DIGITI MINIMI PEDIS
(PLANTAR SURFACE—LAYER III)

fleks-or **dij**-i-tee **min**-i-mee **peed**-us

Action
Flexion of the little toe (toe #5) at the metatarsophalangeal joint

Innervation
The lateral plantar nerve

Arterial Supply
The lateral plantar artery

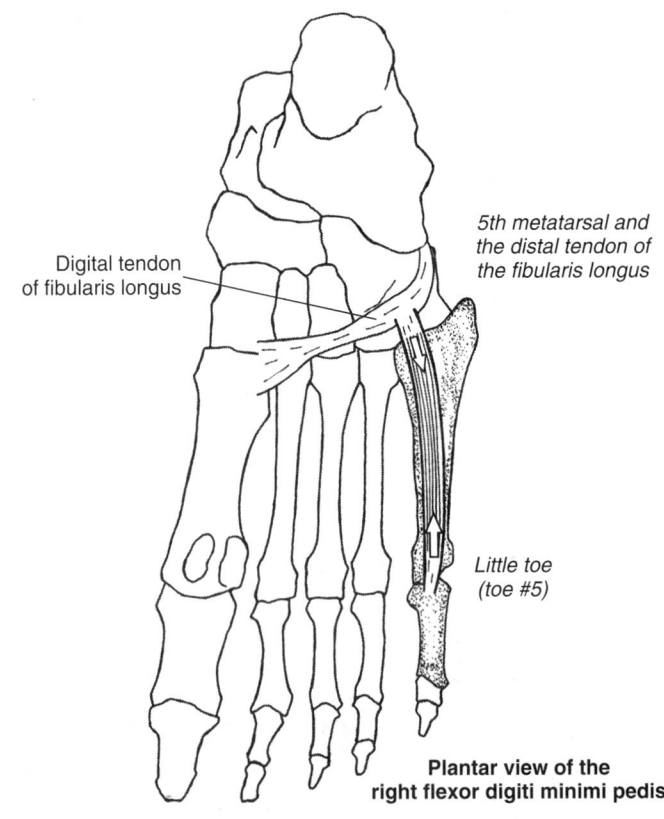

Plantar view of the right flexor digiti minimi pedis

THE MUSCULAR SYSTEM Intrinsic Muscles of the Foot

Distally, there is a sesamoid bone in the medial and lateral tendons of the flexor hallucis brevis.

The flexor digiti minimi pedis is often known as simply the flexor digiti minimi or the flexor digiti minimi brevis. However, there is a flexor digiti minimi (manus) of the hand, and confusion can result.

ADDUCTOR HALLUCIS
(PLANTAR SURFACE—LAYER III)
ad-**duk**-tor hal-**oo**-sis

Plantar view of the right adductor hallucis

Actions
Adduction of the big toe (toe #1) at the metatarsophalangeal joint
Flexion of the big toe (toe #1) at the metatarsophalangeal joint

Innervation
The lateral plantar nerve

Arterial Supply
Branches of the plantar arch

THE MUSCULAR SYSTEM Intrinsic Muscles of the Foot

DID YOU KNOW

The adductor hallucis occasionally has attachments onto the 1st metatarsal that can create opposition of the big toe toward the other toes. When this occurs, this muscle is called the opponens hallucis. This arrangement is common in apes, whose feet are more "handy" than ours ☺.

PLANTAR INTEROSSEI
(PLANTAR SURFACE—LAYER IV)

(There are three plantar interossei muscles, named #1, #2, and #3.)

plan-tar in-ter-**oss**-ee-eye

Actions
Adduction of toes #3-5 at the metatarsophalangeal joint
Flexion of toes #3-5 at the metatarsophalangeal joint
Extension of toes #3-5 at the proximal and distal interphalangeal joints

Innervation
The lateral plantar nerve

Arterial Supply
Branches of the plantar arch

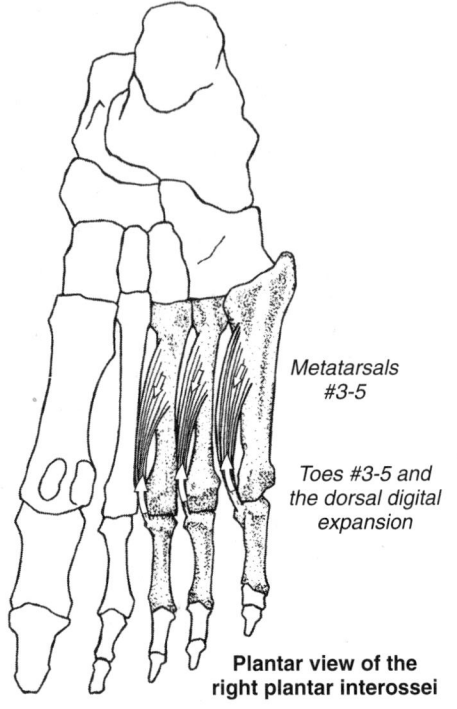

Metatarsals #3-5

Toes #3-5 and the dorsal digital expansion

Plantar view of the right plantar interossei

DORSAL INTEROSSEI PEDIS
(PLANTAR SURFACE—LAYER IV)

(There are four dorsal interossei pedis muscles, named #1, #2, #3, and #4.)

plan-tar in-ter-**oss**-ee-eye **peed**-us

Actions
Abduction of toes #2-4 at the metatarsophalangeal joint
Flexion of toes #2-4 at the metatarsophalangeal joint at the metatarsophalangeal joint
Extension of toes #2-4 at the proximal and distal interphalangeal joints

Innervation
The lateral plantar nerve

Arterial Supply
Branches of the plantar arch

Metatarsals

Dorsolateral view of the right dorsal interossei pedis

Toes #2-4 and the dorsal digital expansion

THE MUSCULAR SYSTEM Intrinsic Muscles of the Foot   287

DID YOU KNOW?

*The main action of the dorsal interossei pedis is abduction of the toes at the metatarsophalangeal joints. The main action of the plantar interossei is adduction of the toes at the metatarsophalangeal joints. The mnemonic to remember these actions is **DAB PAD**; **D**orsals **AB**duct, **P**lantars **AD**duct.*

288 THE MUSCULAR SYSTEM Intrinsic Muscles of the Foot

DORSAL VIEW OF THE RIGHT FOOT

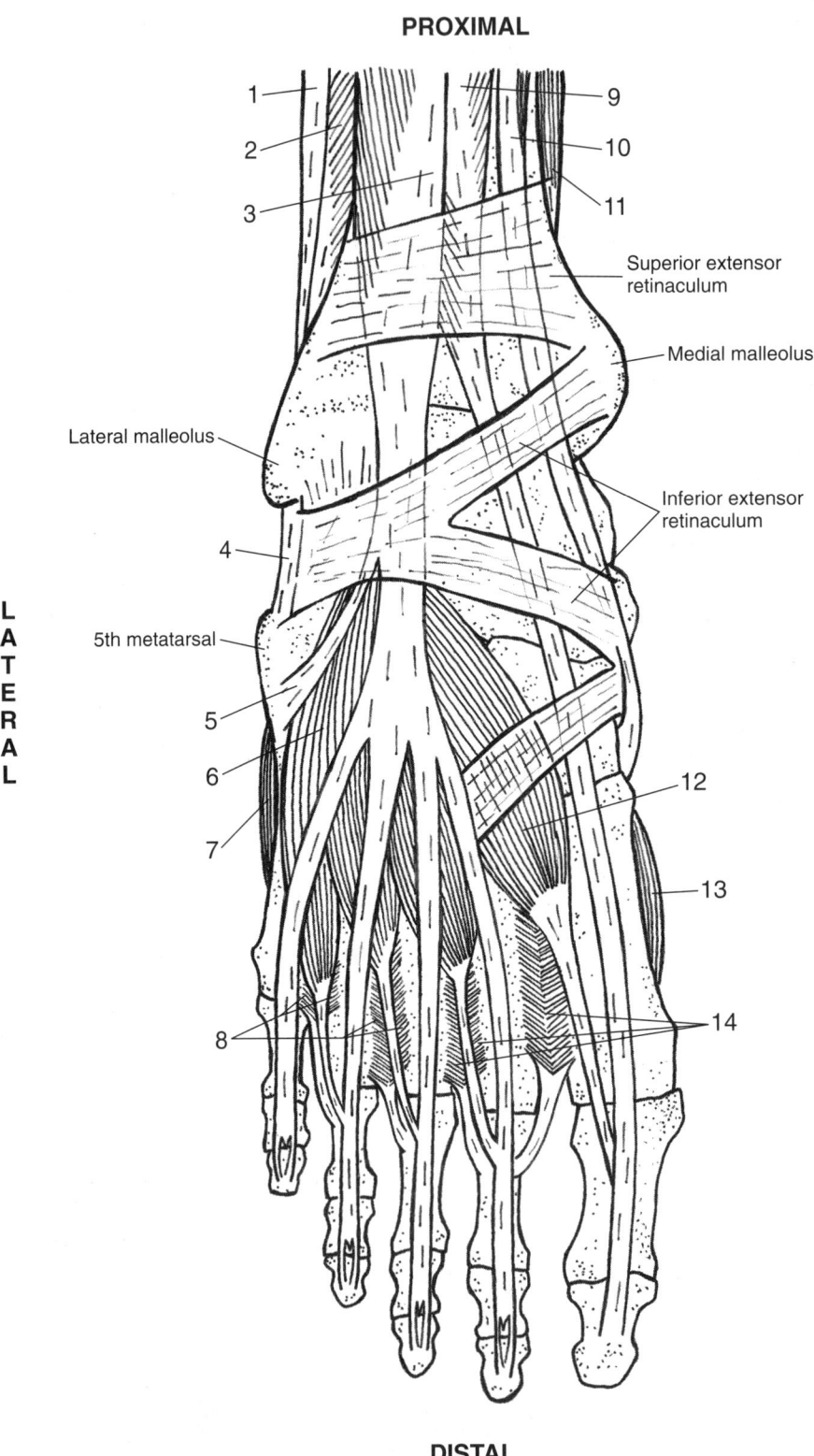

Answers to labeling exercises are on p. 467.

THE MUSCULAR SYSTEM — Intrinsic Muscles of the Foot

PLANTAR VIEW OF THE RIGHT FOOT (SUPERFICIAL MUSCULAR LAYER)

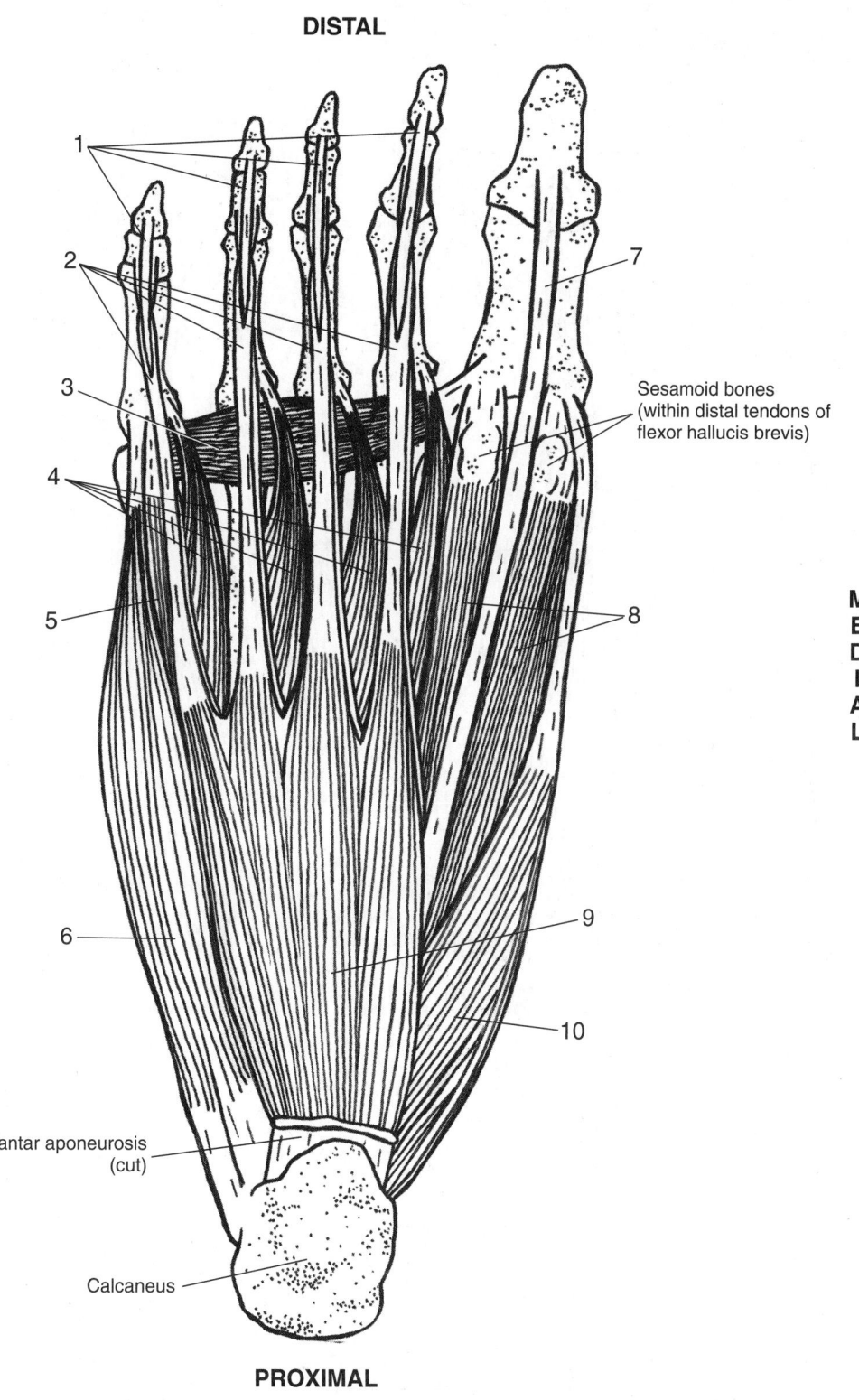

290 THE MUSCULAR SYSTEM Intrinsic Muscles of the Foot

PLANTAR VIEW OF THE RIGHT FOOT
(INTERMEDIATE MUSCULAR LAYER)

THE MUSCULAR SYSTEM | Intrinsic Muscles of the Foot

PLANTAR VIEW OF THE RIGHT FOOT
(DEEP MUSCULAR LAYER)

Review Questions

Intrinsic Muscles of the Foot
Answers to these questions are found on page 468.

1. What is another name for the quadratus plantae?

2. What muscle is synergistic with the extensor digitorum brevis?

3. What joint actions are occurring when the flexor digitorum brevis is concentrically contracting?

4. What two muscles are antagonistic to the flexor hallucis brevis?

5. What joint action occurs when the adductor hallucis concentrically contracts?

6. What muscle is antagonistic to the adductor hallucis?

7. If the big toe is passively extended at the metatarsophalangeal joint, what happens to the length of the extensor hallucis brevis?

8. Which interosseus muscle is lengthened if the 2nd toe tibially abducts?

9. What are the three muscles located in Layer III of the plantar foot?

10. What intrinsic muscle of the foot has sesamoid bones within its distal tendons?

11. What muscle is immediately medial to the oblique head of the adductor hallucis?

12. How many intrinsic muscles of the foot are located on the dorsal side?

13. What muscle is immediately deep to the transverse head of the adductor hallucis?

14. What three muscles are located in Layer I of the plantar foot?

15. What is the relationship of the lumbricals pedis to the transverse head of the adductor hallucis?

16. What is the mnemonic for the actions of the dorsal interossei pedis and plantar interossei?

17. In the proximal foot, what muscle is immediately deep to the flexor digitorum brevis?

18. What is the common proximal attachment of the extensors hallucis and digitorum brevis?

19. What muscle is antagonistic to the abductor digiti minimi pedis?

20. The tendons of what muscles are superficial to the extensor digitorum brevis?

21. What two muscles are located in Layer II of the plantar foot?

22. From the plantar perspective, which muscle group is deeper, the plantar interossei or the dorsal interossei pedis?

23. When the distal tendons of the flexor digitorum brevis split, what muscle's tendons pass through?

24. What is the common proximal attachment of the abductor hallucis and abductor digiti minimi pedis?

25. What are the names of the two heads of the adductor hallucis?

26. Which two dorsal interosseus pedis (DIP) muscles are antagonistic to each other?

27. What muscle is immediately medial to the abductor digiti minimi pedis?

28. In the proximal foot, what muscle is immediately lateral to the flexor digitorum brevis?

29. What three muscles attach to the tuberosity of the calcaneus?

30. What distal tendon of the foot serves as a proximal attachment of the flexor digiti minimi pedis?

31. What muscle is synergistic with the extensor hallucis brevis?

32. What muscle is superficial to the quadratus plantae?

33. What joint action(s) is/are occurring when the flexor digitorum brevis is lengthened?

34. What muscle is antagonistic to the adduction action of the plantar interosseus muscle of the little (5th) toe?

35. What muscle is antagonistic to the abductor hallucis?

36. What joint action occurs when the abductor hallucis eccentrically contracts?

37. What muscle is synergistic with the quadratus plantae's actions of flexion of toes #2-5 at the distal interphalangeal joint?

38. What is the proximal attachment of the lumbricals pedis?

39. What two muscles are located in Layer IV of the plantar foot?

40. What intrinsic muscle of the foot contains sesamoid bones?

41. What happens to the length of the flexor digiti minimi pedis when the little toe extends at the metatarsophalangeal joint?

42. Do the lumbricals flex and/or extend the toes (#2-5)?

THE MUSCULAR SYSTEM — Muscles of the Scapula/Arm

ANTERIOR VIEW OF THE RIGHT SHOULDER

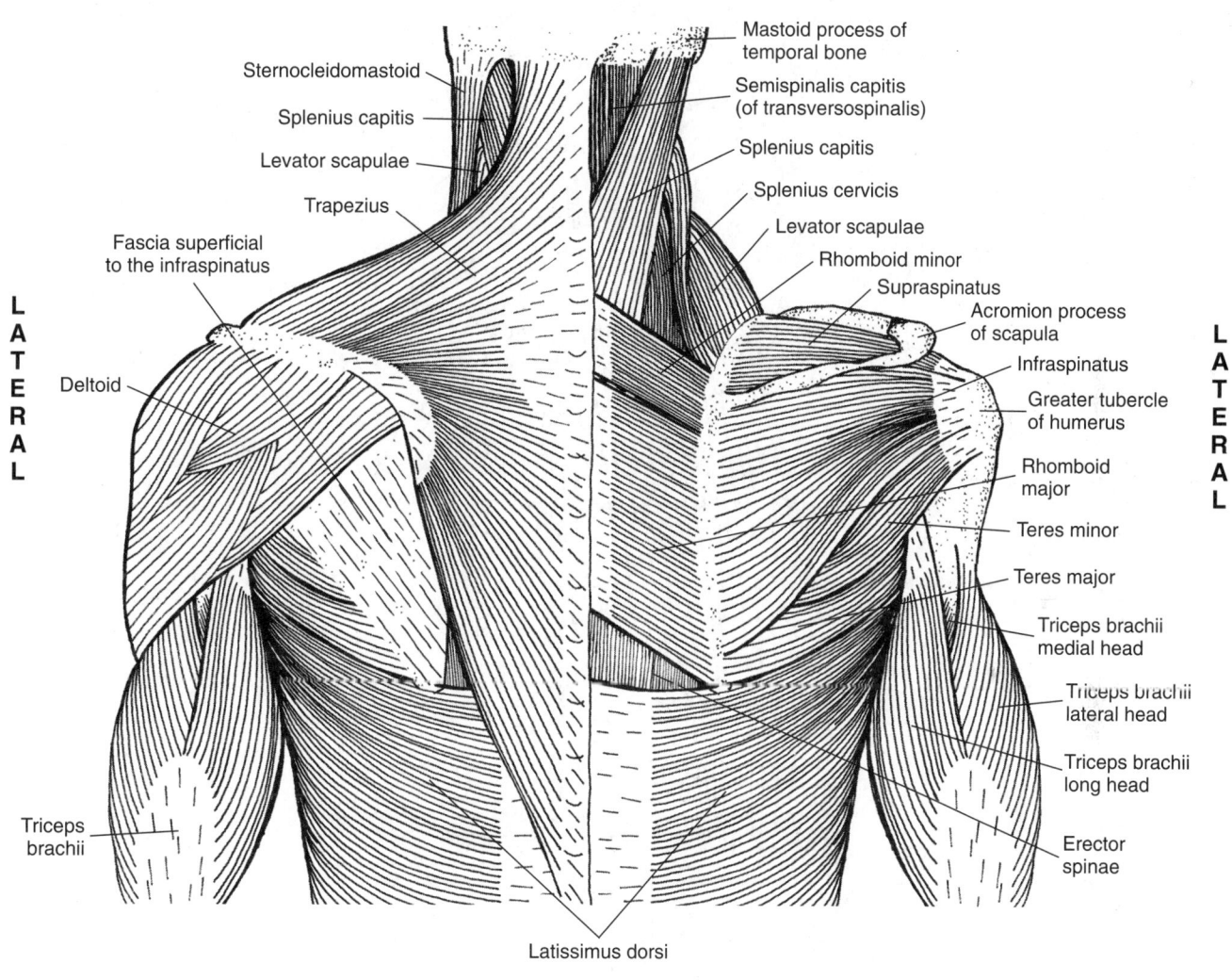

THE MUSCULAR SYSTEM: Muscles of the Scapula/Arm

ANTERIOR VIEW OF THE RIGHT ARM (SUPERFICIAL)

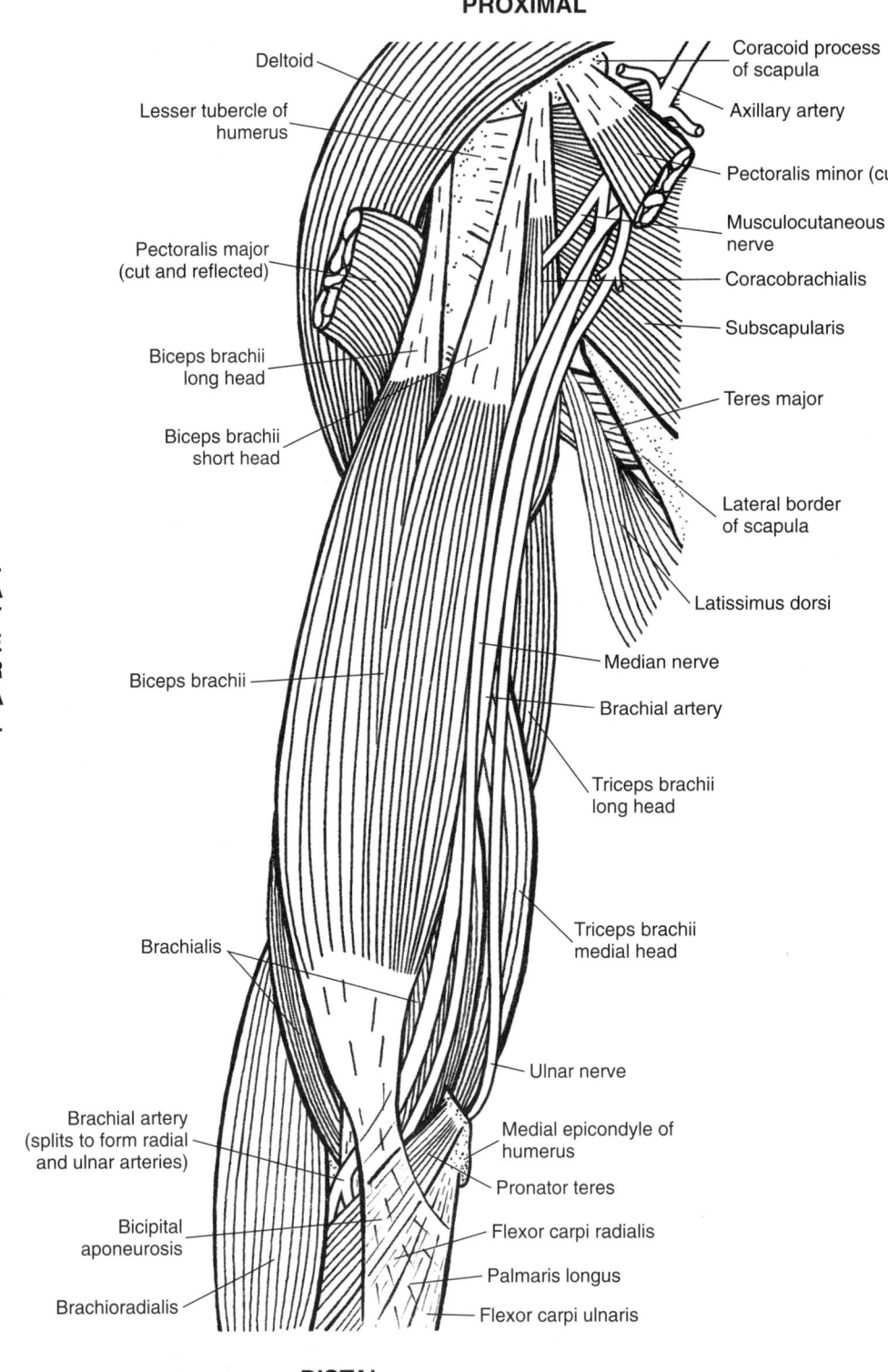

THE MUSCULAR SYSTEM Muscles of the Scapula/Arm

ANTERIOR VIEW OF THE RIGHT ARM (DEEP)

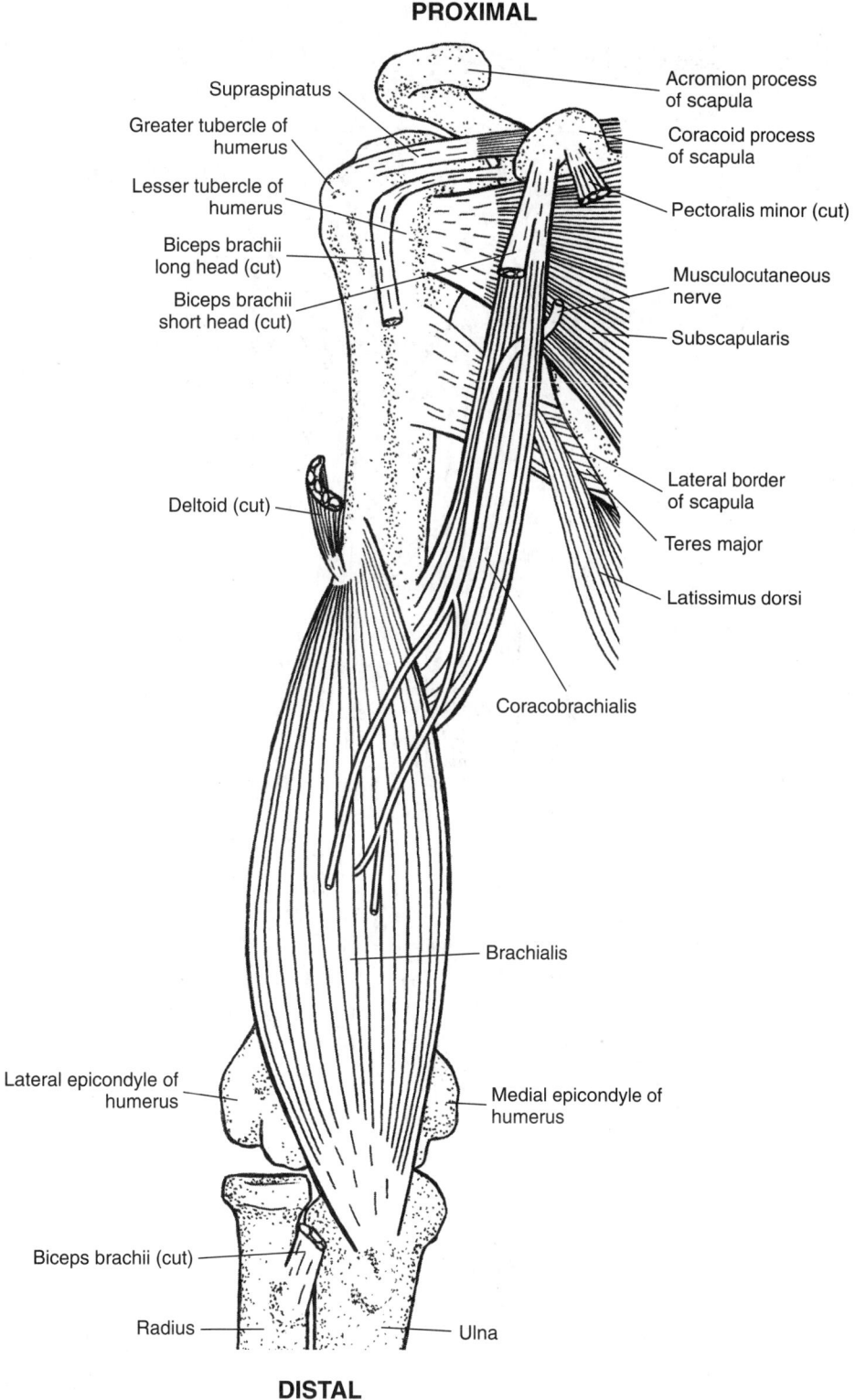

THE MUSCULAR SYSTEM — Muscles of the Scapula/Arm

MEDIAL VIEW OF THE RIGHT ARM

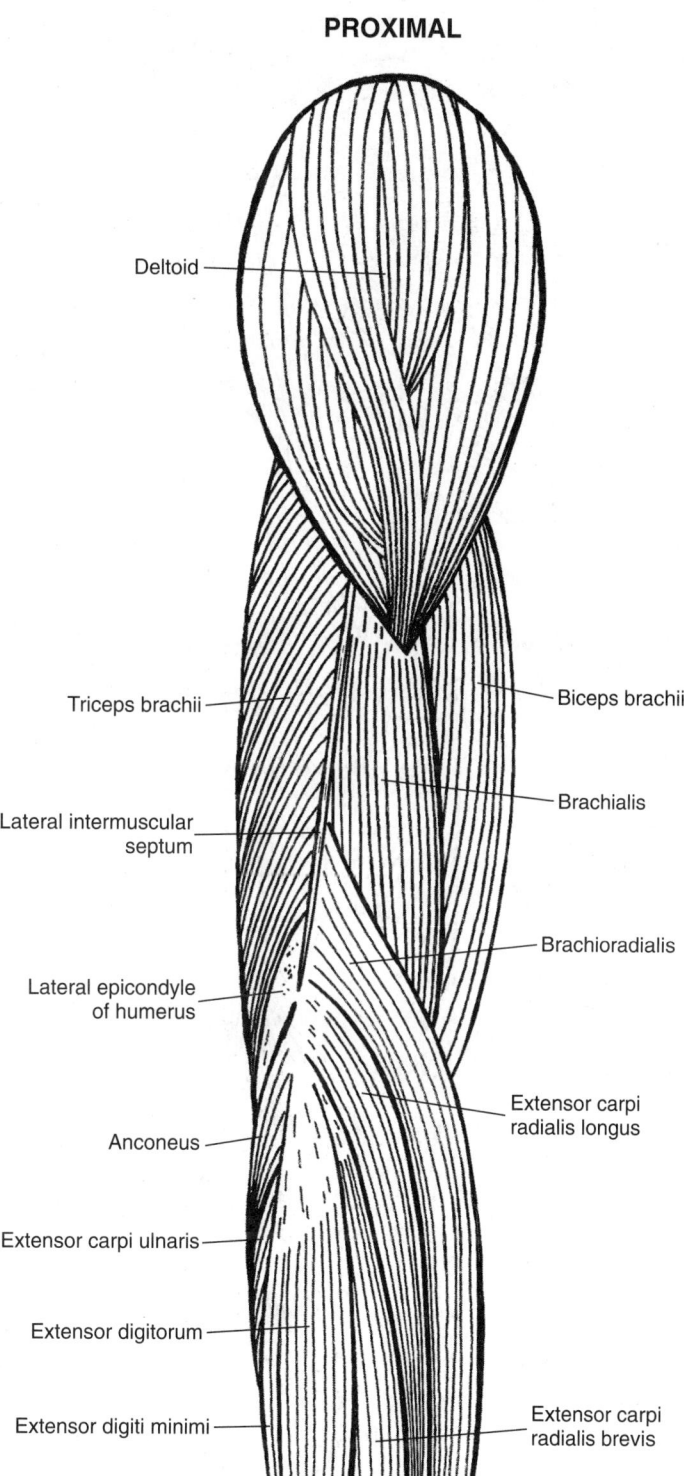

POSTERIOR VIEW OF THE RIGHT ARM

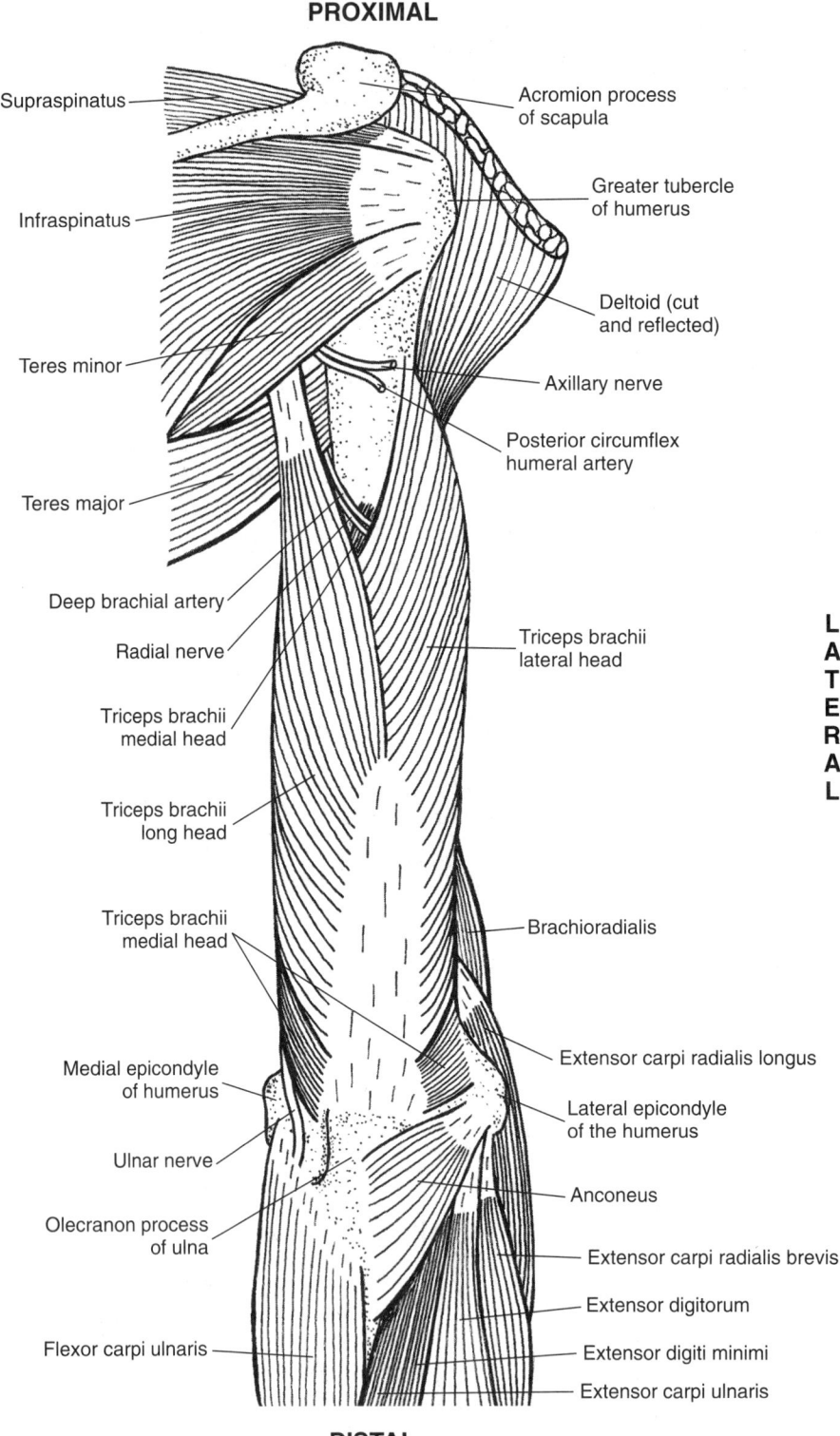

THE MUSCULAR SYSTEM Muscles of the Scapula/Arm

ANTERIOR VIEW OF THE RIGHT GLENOHUMERAL JOINT

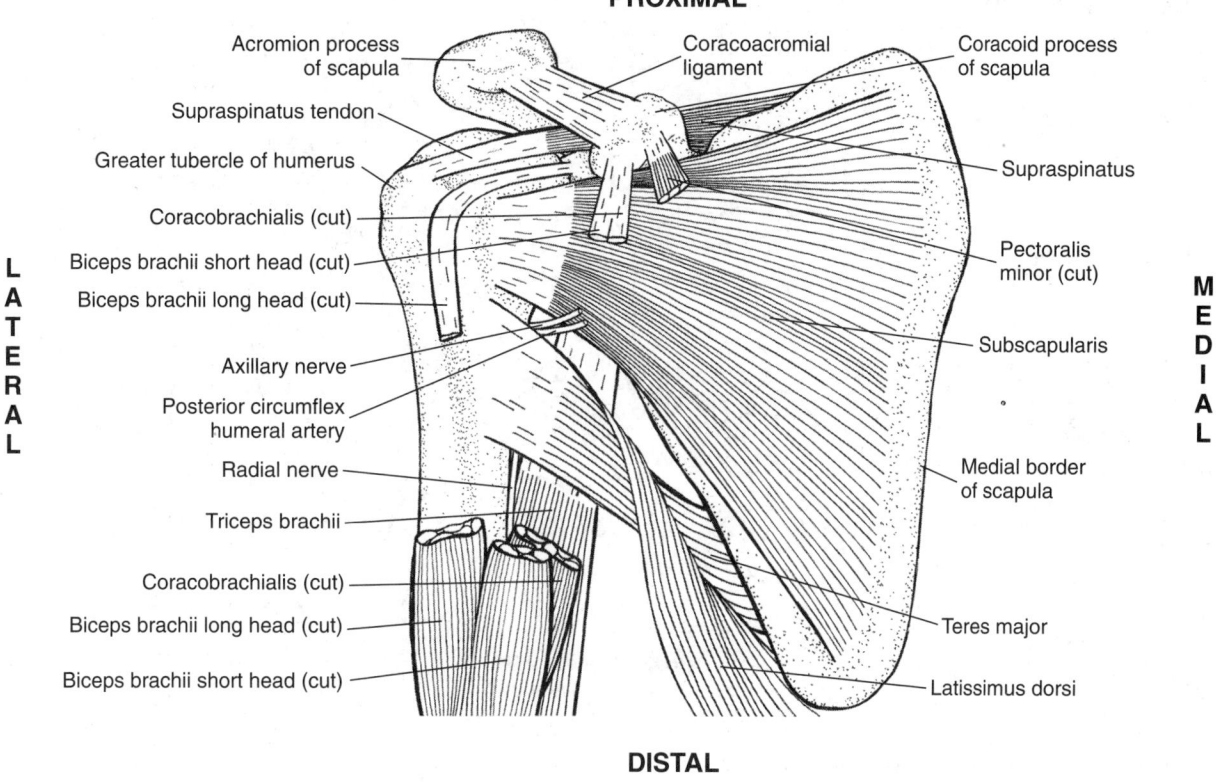

POSTERIOR VIEW OF THE RIGHT GLENOHUMERAL JOINT

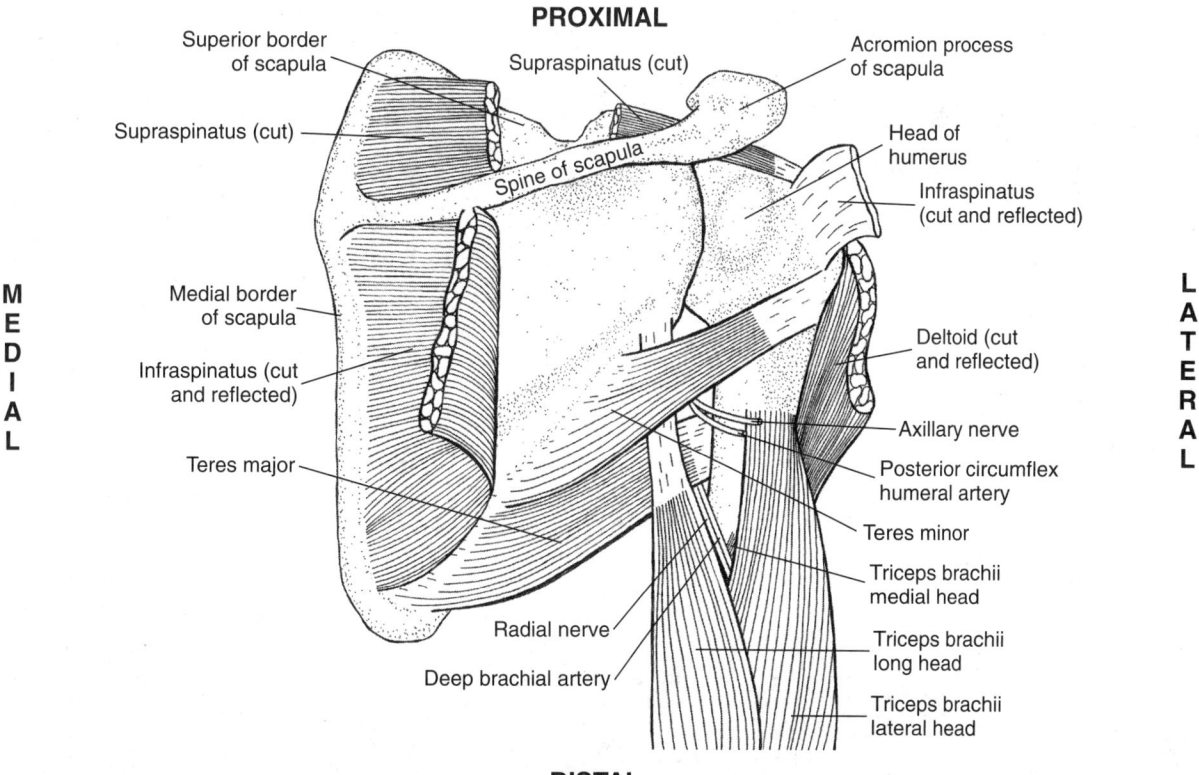

SUPRASPINATUS
(OF THE ROTATOR CUFF GROUP)

soo-pra-spy-**nay**-tus

Action
Abduction of the arm at the shoulder joint

Innervation
The suprascapular nerve

Arterial Supply
The suprascapular artery

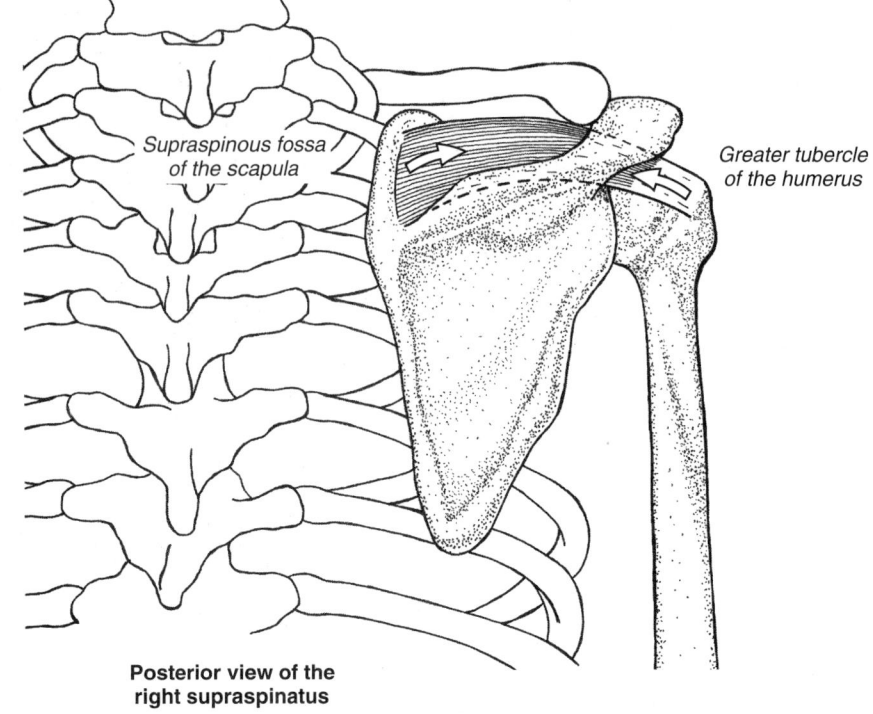

Posterior view of the right supraspinatus

INFRASPINATUS
(OF THE ROTATOR CUFF GROUP)

in-fra-spy-**nay**-tus

Action
Lateral rotation of the arm at the shoulder joint

Innervation
The suprascapular nerve

Arterial Supply
The suprascapular artery

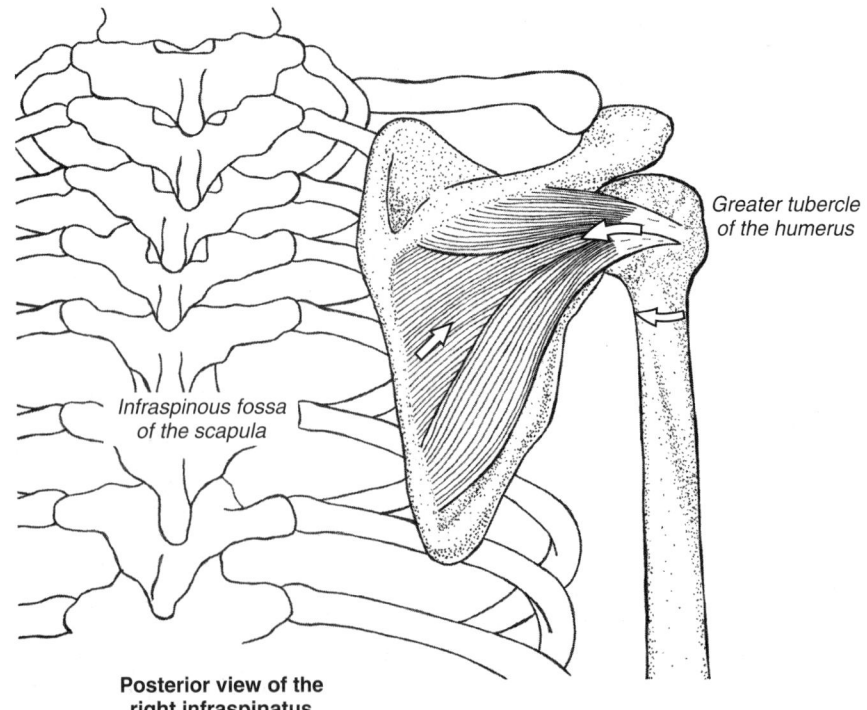

Posterior view of the right infraspinatus

THE MUSCULAR SYSTEM Muscles of the Scapula/Arm

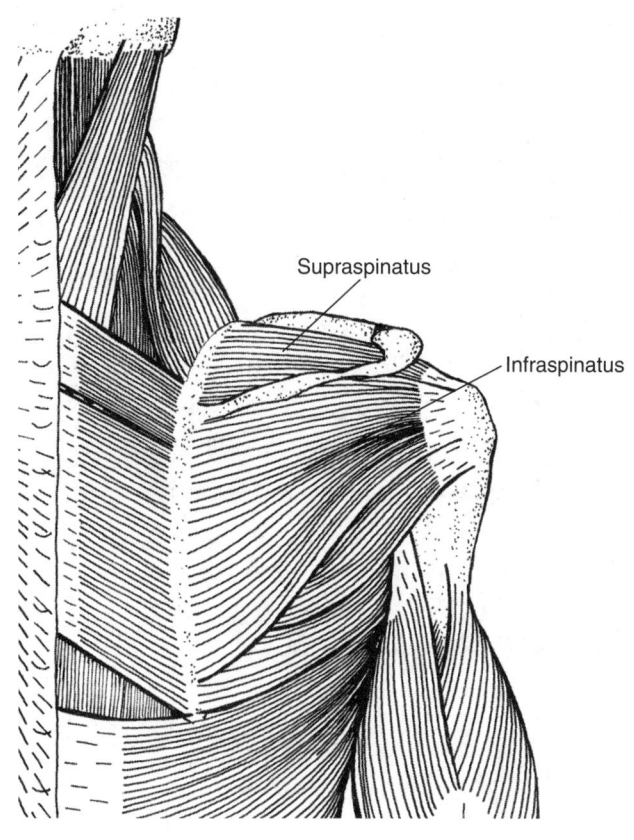

> **DID YOU KNOW?**
> The distal tendon of the supraspinatus is the most commonly injured tendon of the rotator cuff group.

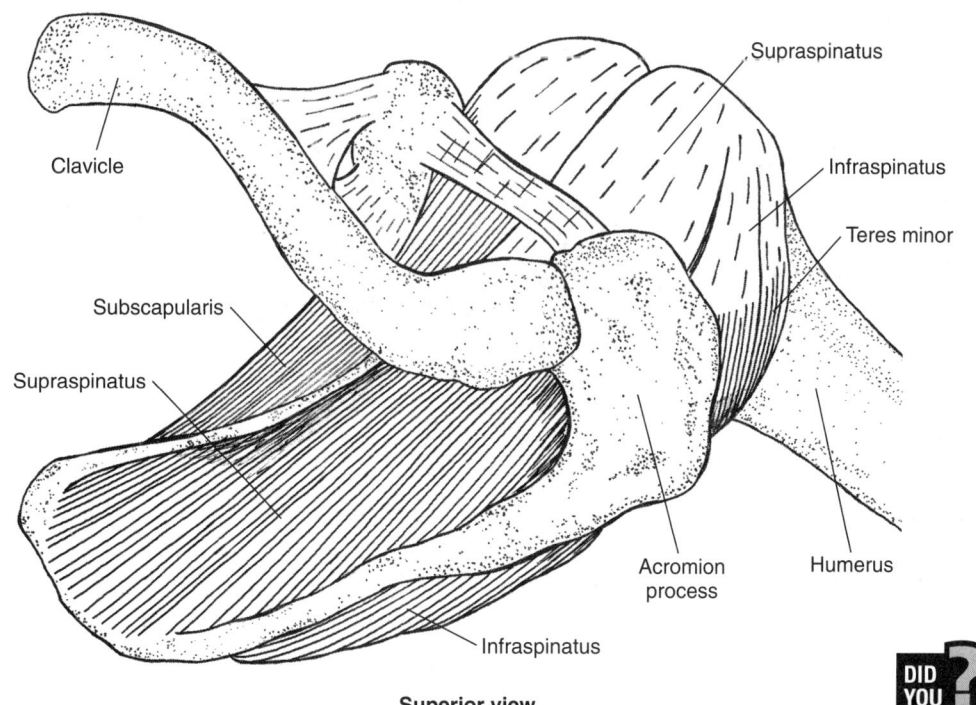

Superior view

> **DID YOU KNOW?**
> There is usually a thick layer of fascia overlying the infraspinatus.

TERES MINOR
(OF THE ROTATOR CUFF GROUP)

te-reez my-nor

Action
Lateral rotation of the arm at the shoulder joint
Adduction of the arm at the shoulder joint

Innervation
The axillary nerve

Arterial Supply
The circumflex scapular artery

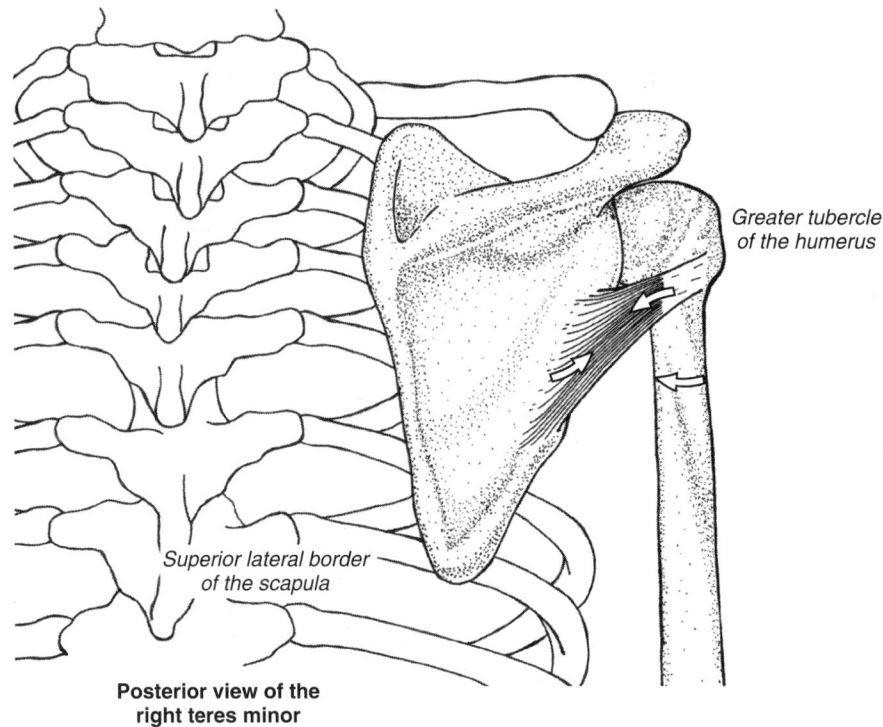

Posterior view of the right teres minor

SUBSCAPULARIS
(OF THE ROTATOR CUFF GROUP)

sub-skap-u-la-ris

Action
Medial rotation of the arm at the shoulder joint

Innervation
The upper and lower subscapular nerves

Arterial Supply
The circumflex scapular artery and the dorsal scapular and suprascapular arteries

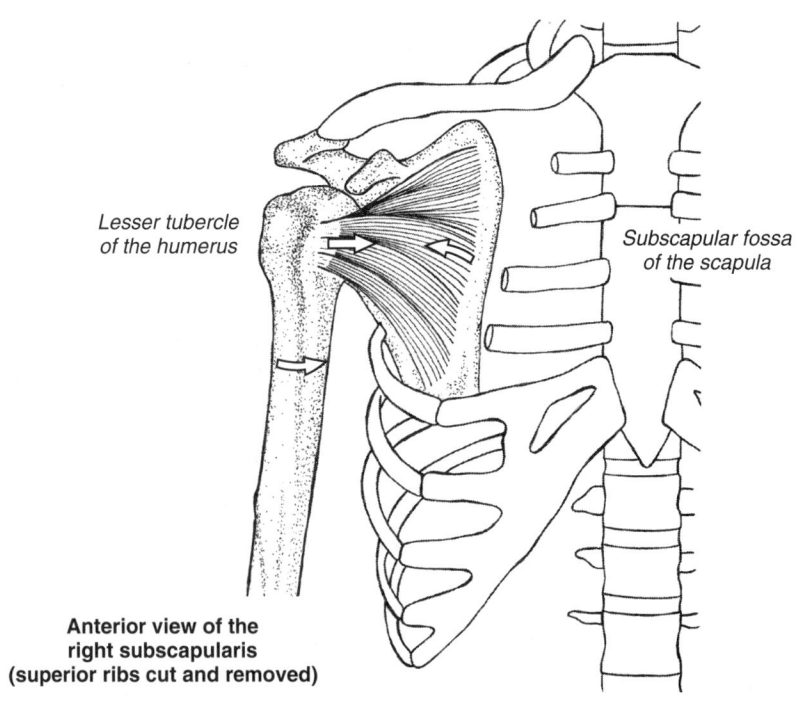

Anterior view of the right subscapularis (superior ribs cut and removed)

THE MUSCULAR SYSTEM Muscles of the Scapula/Arm

Teres minor

DID YOU KNOW

The teres minor often blends with the infraspinatus.

Subscapularis

DID YOU KNOW

The subscapularis is the only muscle of the rotator cuff group that attaches onto the lesser tubercle of the humerus.

TERES MAJOR
te-reez may-jor

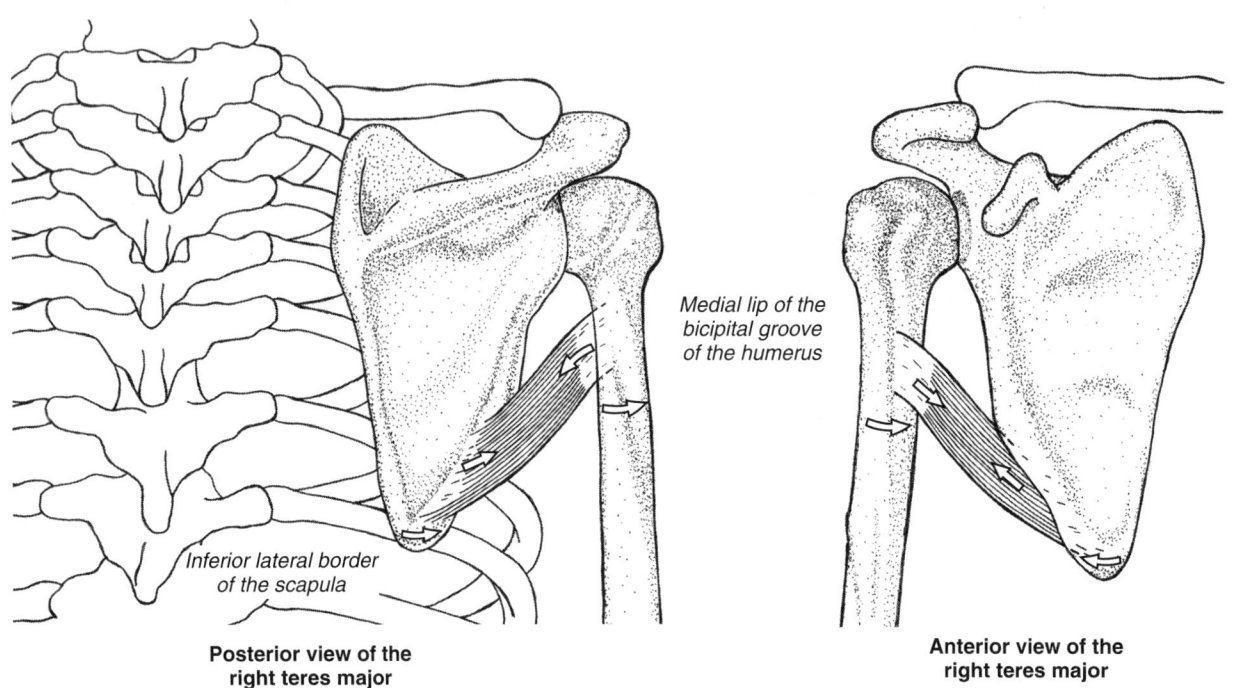

Posterior view of the right teres major

Anterior view of the right teres major

Actions
Medial rotation of the arm at the shoulder joint
Adduction of the arm at the shoulder joint
Extension of the arm at the shoulder joint
Upward rotation of the scapula at the scapulocostal joint

Innervation
The lower subscapular nerve

Arterial Supply
The circumflex scapular artery

THE MUSCULAR SYSTEM Muscles of the Scapula/Arm

Teres major

The teres major can do all three actions of the arm at the shoulder joint (extension, adduction, and medial rotation) that the latissimus dorsi can. Therefore, these muscles often work together.

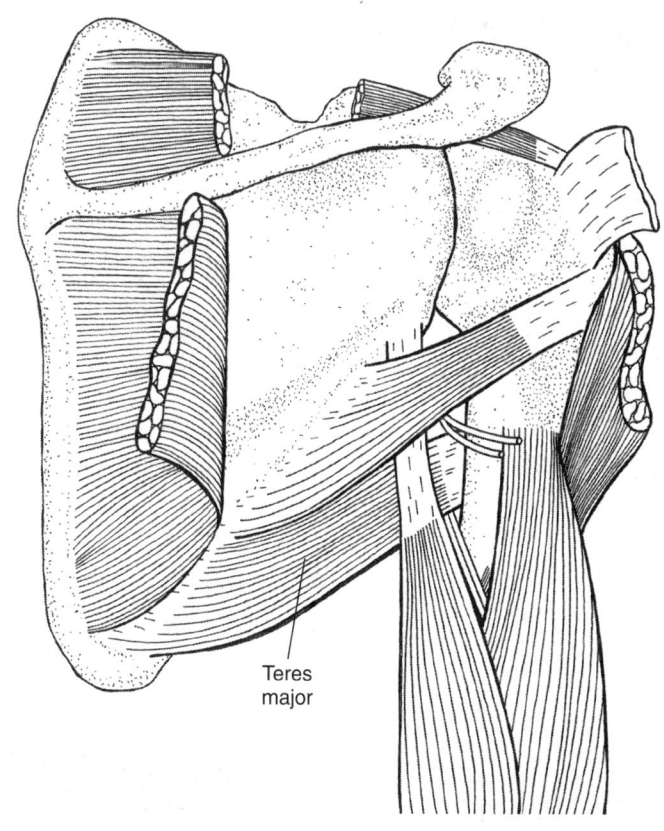

Teres major

THE MUSCULAR SYSTEM Muscles of the Scapula/Arm

DELTOID
del-toid

Actions
Abduction of the arm at the shoulder joint (entire muscle)
Flexion of the arm at the shoulder joint (anterior deltoid)
Extension of the arm at the shoulder joint (posterior deltoid)
Medial rotation of the arm at the shoulder joint (anterior deltoid)
Lateral rotation of the arm at the shoulder joint (posterior deltoid)
Downward rotation of the scapula at the scapulocostal joint (entire muscle)
Ipsilateral rotation of the trunk at the shoulder joint (anterior deltoid)
Contralateral rotation of the trunk at the shoulder joint (posterior deltoid)

Innervation
The axillary nerve

Arterial Supply
The anterior and posterior circumflex humeral arteries

Lateral view of the right deltoid

THE MUSCULAR SYSTEM: Muscles of the Scapula/Arm

 DID YOU KNOW?

The name "deltoid" tells us that it has a triangular shape like the Greek letter delta (Δ).

CORACOBRACHIALIS
kor-a-ko-**bray**-key-**al**-is

Coracoid process of the scapula

Medial shaft of the humerus

Anterior view of the right coracobrachialis

Actions
Flexion of the arm at the shoulder joint
Adduction of the arm at the shoulder joint

Innervation
The musculocutaneous nerve

Arterial Supply
The muscular branches of the brachial artery

THE MUSCULAR SYSTEM — Muscles of the Scapula/Arm

DID YOU KNOW?

The name coracobrachialis tells us that this muscle attaches from the coracoid process of the scapula to the brachium (arm). That in turn, tells us that it crosses the shoulder joint so its actions must be at the shoulder joint.

Coracobrachialis

Coracobrachialis

BICEPS BRACHII
by-seps bray-key-eye

Actions
Flexion of the forearm at the elbow joint (entire muscle)
Supination of the forearm at the radioulnar joints (entire muscle)
Flexion of the arm at the shoulder joint (entire muscle)
Abduction of the arm at the shoulder joint (long head)
Adduction of the arm at the shoulder joint (short head)

Innervation
The musculocutaneous nerve

Arterial Supply
The muscular branches of the brachial artery

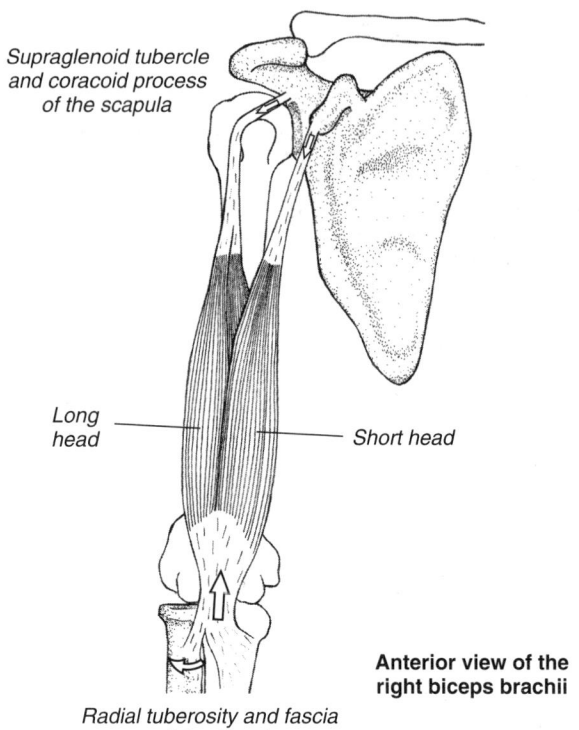

Anterior view of the right biceps brachii

BRACHIALIS
bray-key-al-is

Action
Flexion of the forearm at the elbow joint

Innervation
The musculocutaneous nerve

Arterial Supply
Muscular branches of the brachial artery

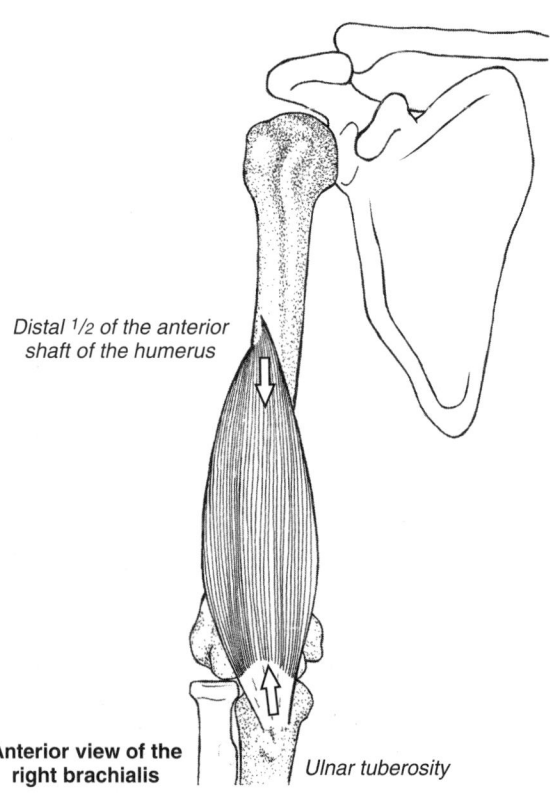

Anterior view of the right brachialis

THE MUSCULAR SYSTEM Muscles of the Scapula/Arm

 DID YOU KNOW

The bicipital groove of the humerus is so named because the long head of the biceps brachii courses through it.

 DID YOU KNOW

The brachialis is a strong and fairly large muscle, which accounts for much of the contour of the biceps brachii being so visible. Behind every great biceps brachii is a great brachialis ☺.

TRICEPS BRACHII
try-seps bray-key-eye

Actions
Extension of the forearm at the elbow joint (entire muscle)
Adduction of the arm at the shoulder joint (long head)
Extension of the arm at the shoulder joint (long head)

Innervation
The radial nerve

Arterial Supply
The deep brachial artery

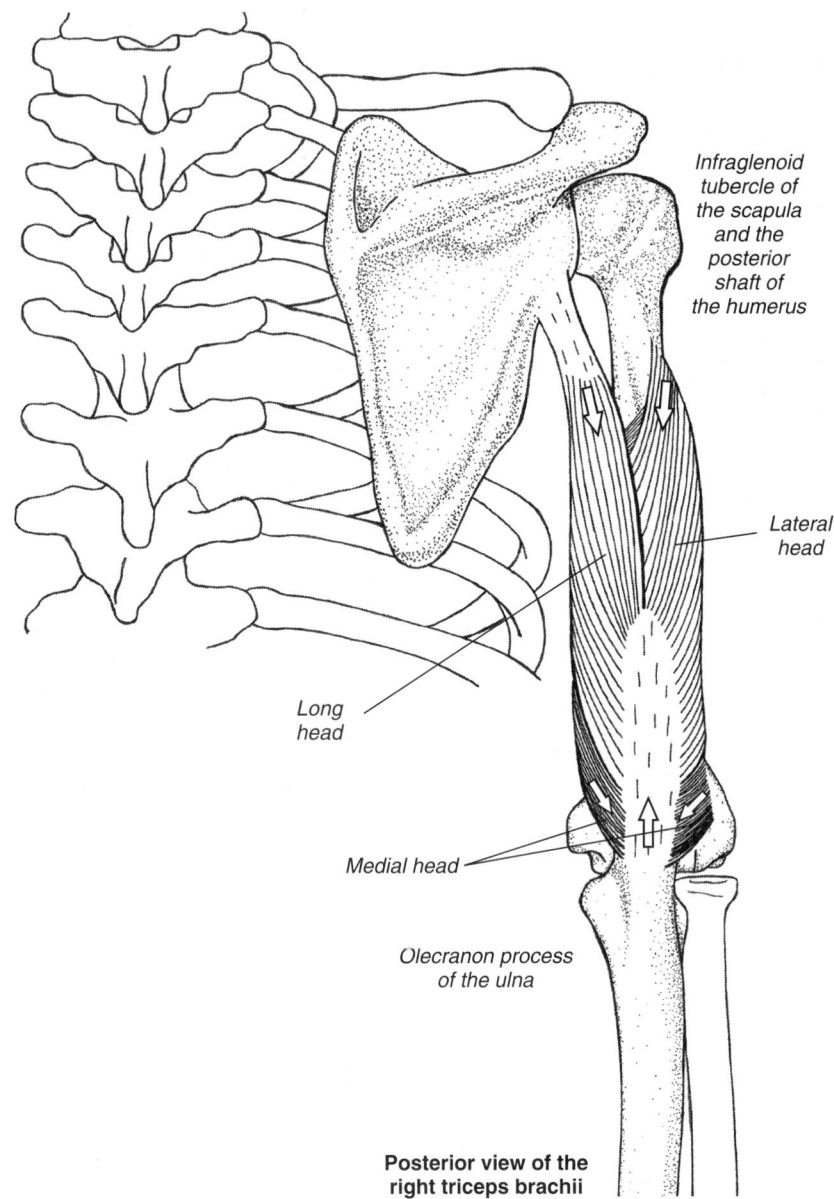

Infraglenoid tubercle of the scapula and the posterior shaft of the humerus

Lateral head

Long head

Medial head

Olecranon process of the ulna

Posterior view of the right triceps brachii

THE MUSCULAR SYSTEM Muscles of the Scapula/Arm

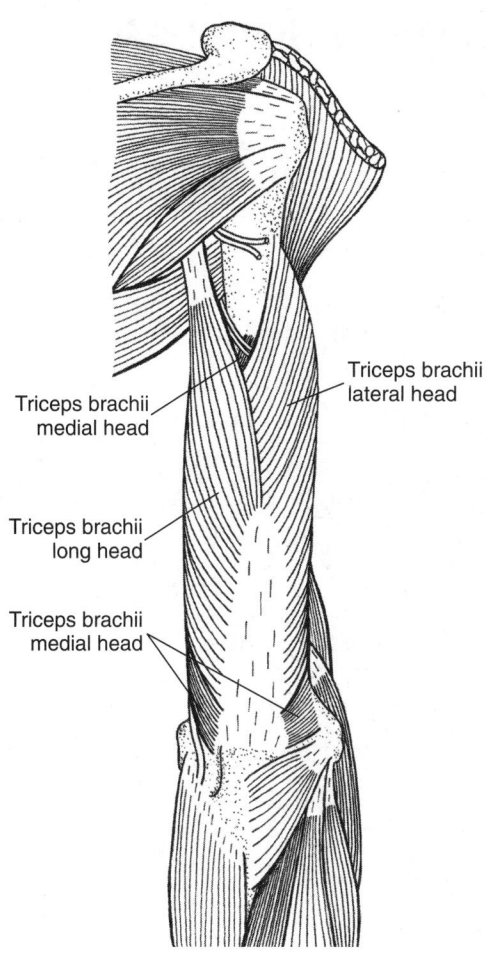

Triceps brachii medial head
Triceps brachii lateral head
Triceps brachii long head
Triceps brachii medial head

DID YOU KNOW

The triceps brachii has three heads, the lateral, medial, and long heads; only the long head crosses and therefore can move the shoulder joint.

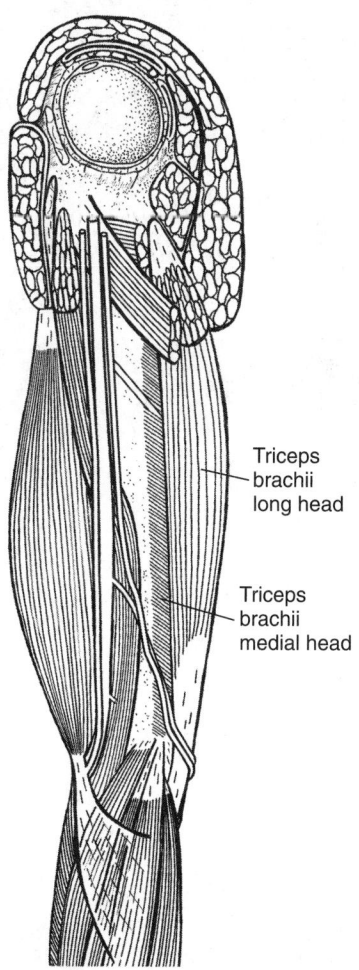

Triceps brachii long head
Triceps brachii medial head

THE MUSCULAR SYSTEM Muscles of the Scapula/Arm

ANTERIOR VIEW OF THE RIGHT SHOULDER

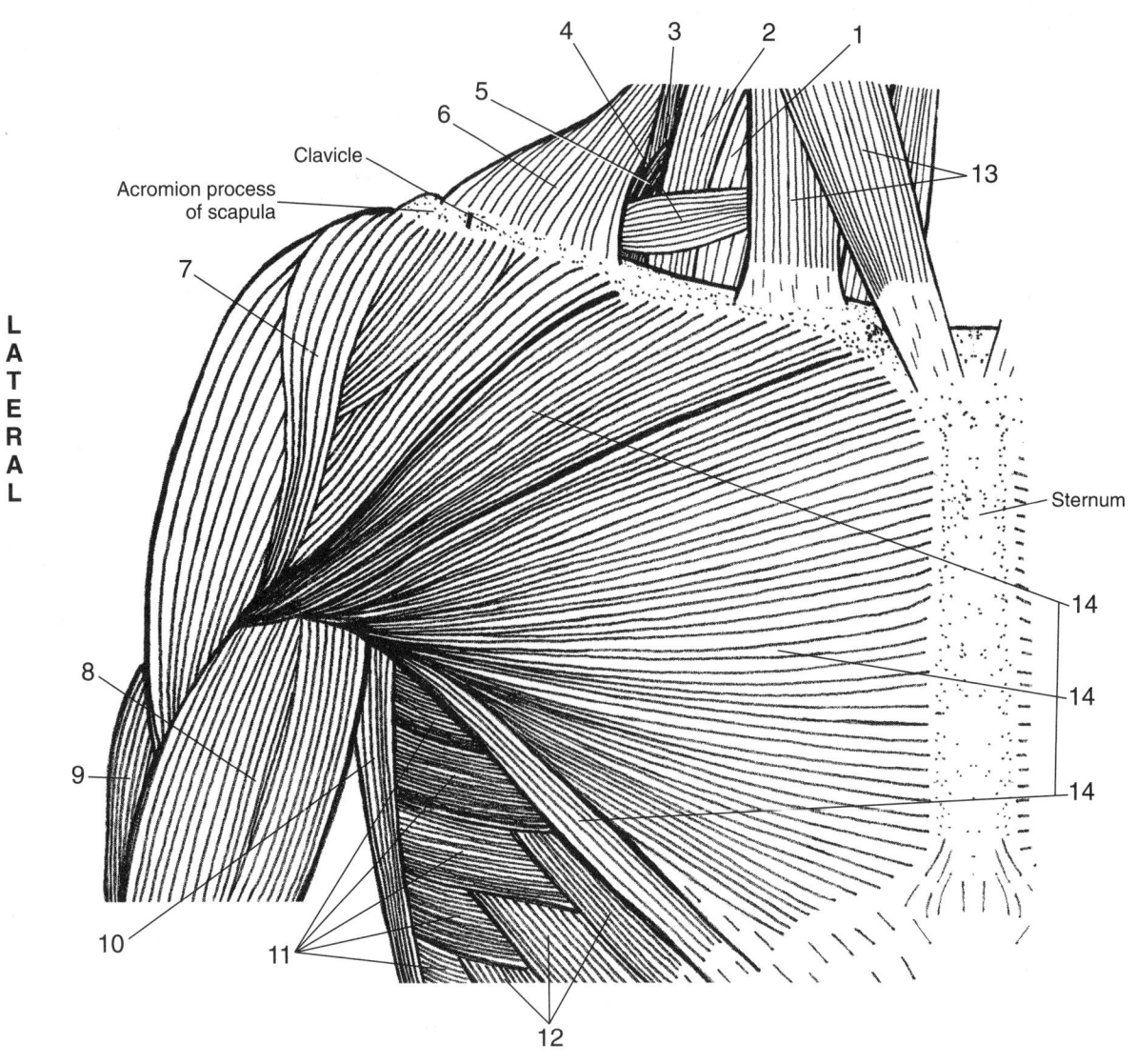

Answers to labeling exercises are on p. 468.

THE MUSCULAR SYSTEM Muscles of the Scapula/Arm 317

POSTERIOR VIEW OF THE SHOULDERS
(SUPERFICIAL AND INTERMEDIATE)

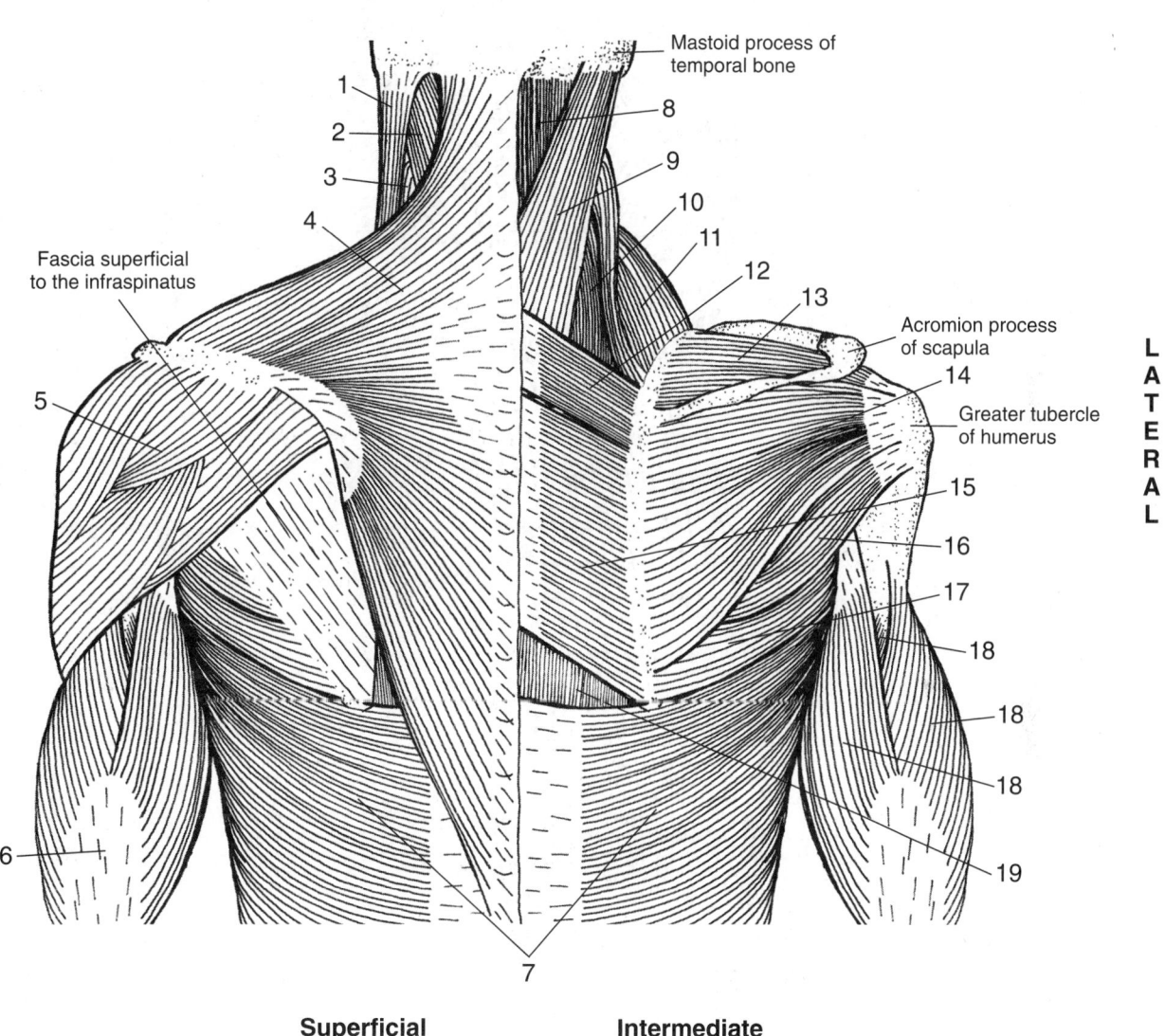

Superficial　　**Intermediate**

THE MUSCULAR SYSTEM — Muscles of the Scapula/Arm

ANTERIOR VIEW OF THE RIGHT ARM (SUPERFICIAL)

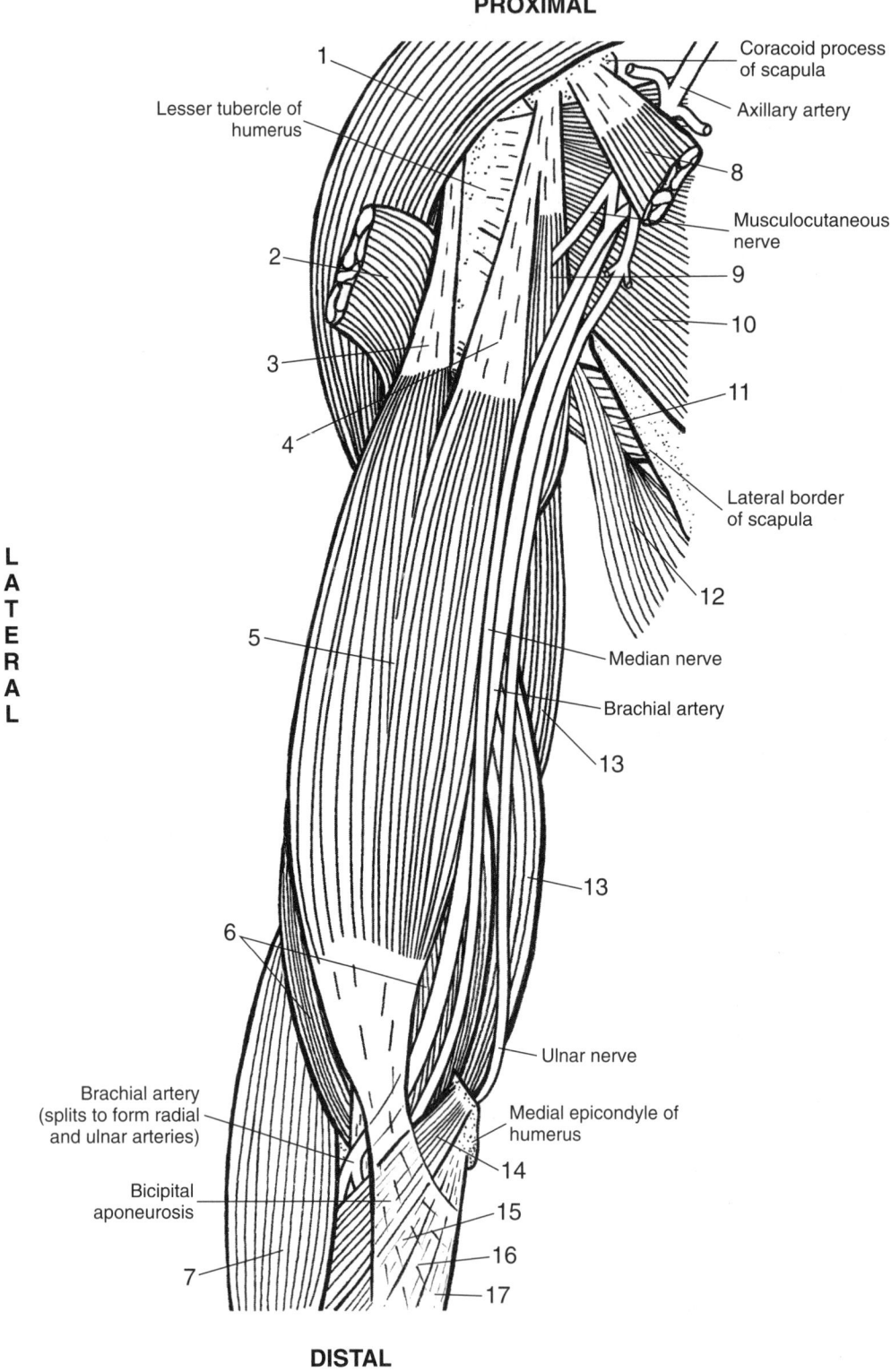

THE MUSCULAR SYSTEM Muscles of the Scapula/Arm

ANTERIOR VIEW OF THE RIGHT ARM (DEEP)

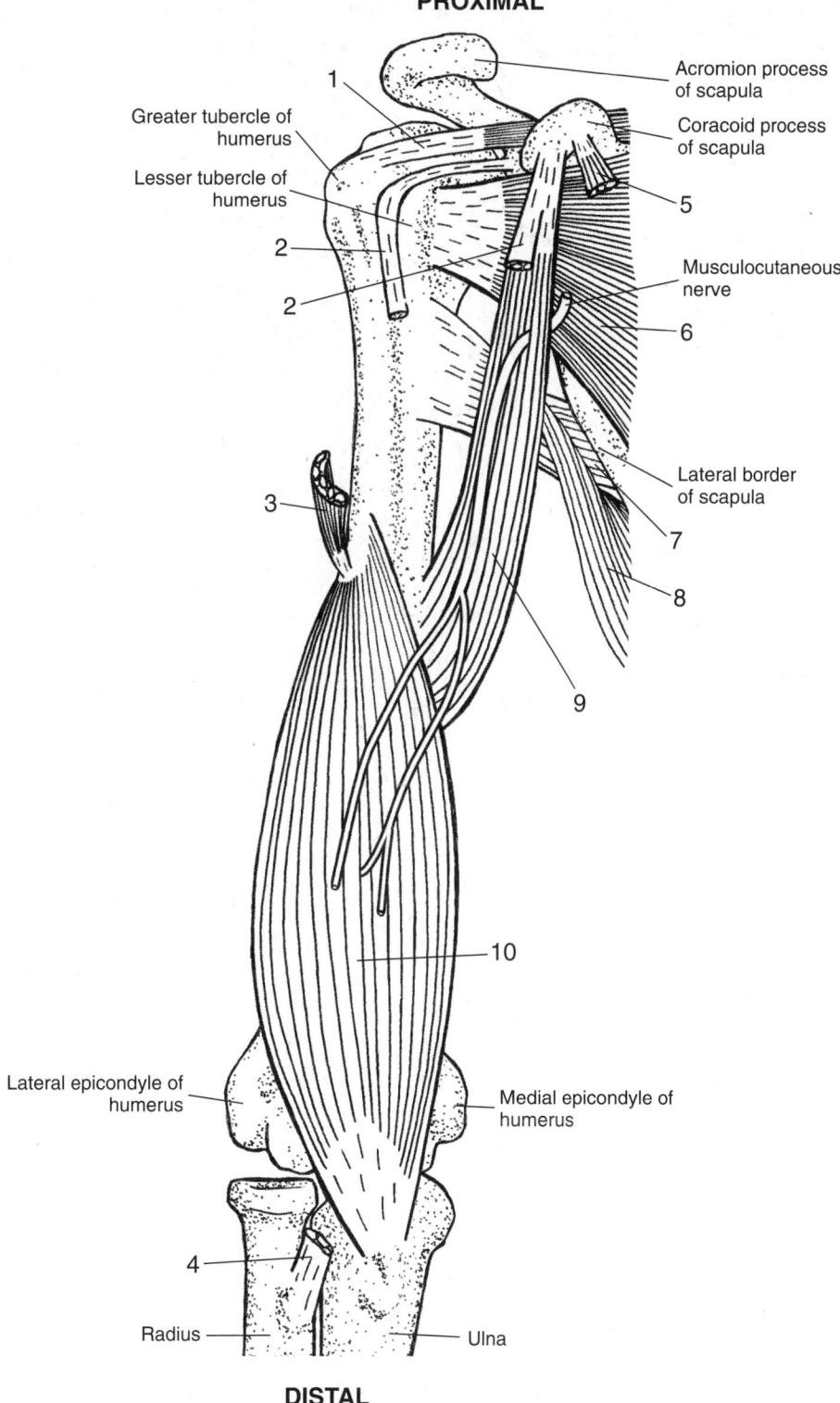

320 THE MUSCULAR SYSTEM — Muscles of the Scapula/Arm

MEDIAL VIEW OF THE RIGHT ARM

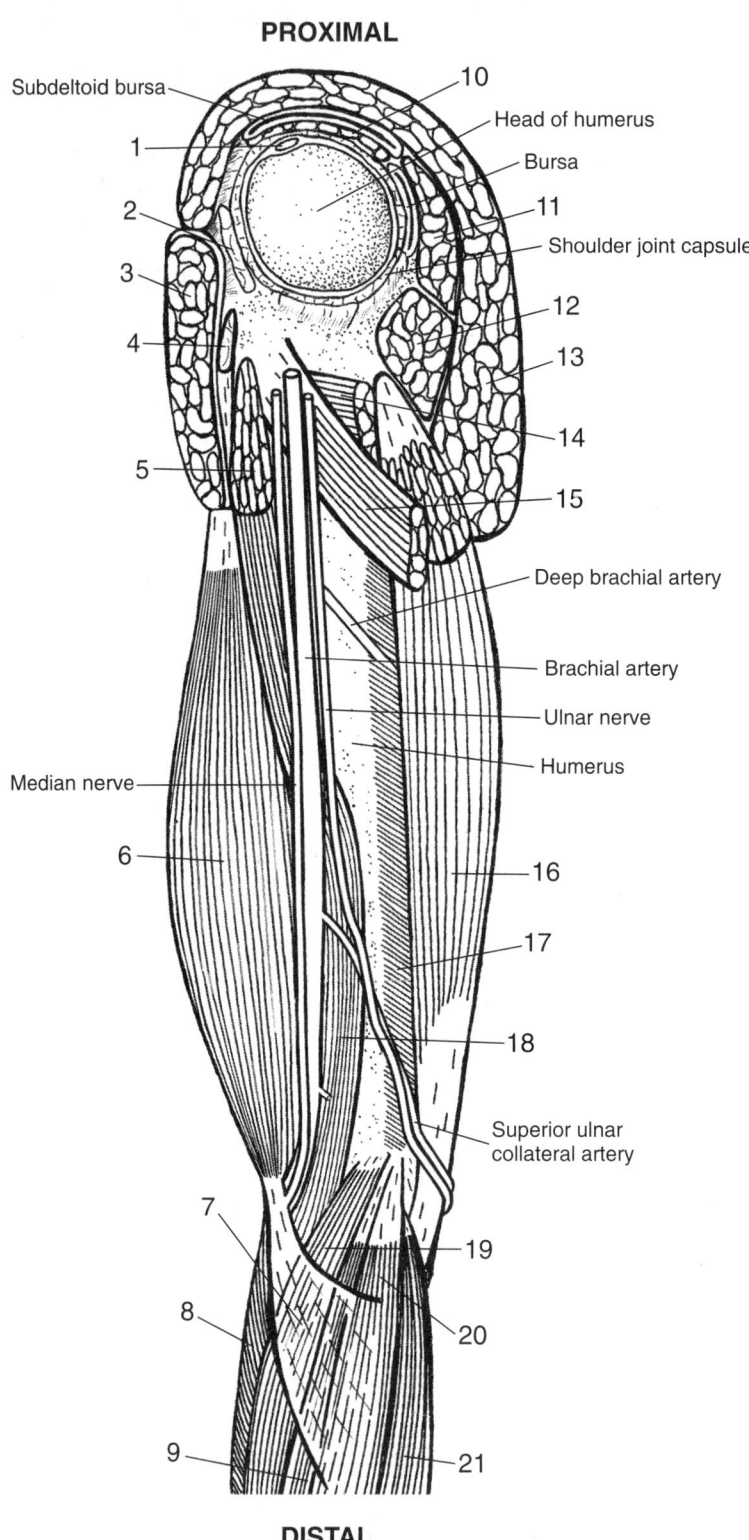

THE MUSCULAR SYSTEM Muscles of the Scapula/Arm

LATERAL VIEW OF THE RIGHT ARM

PROXIMAL

POSTERIOR

ANTERIOR

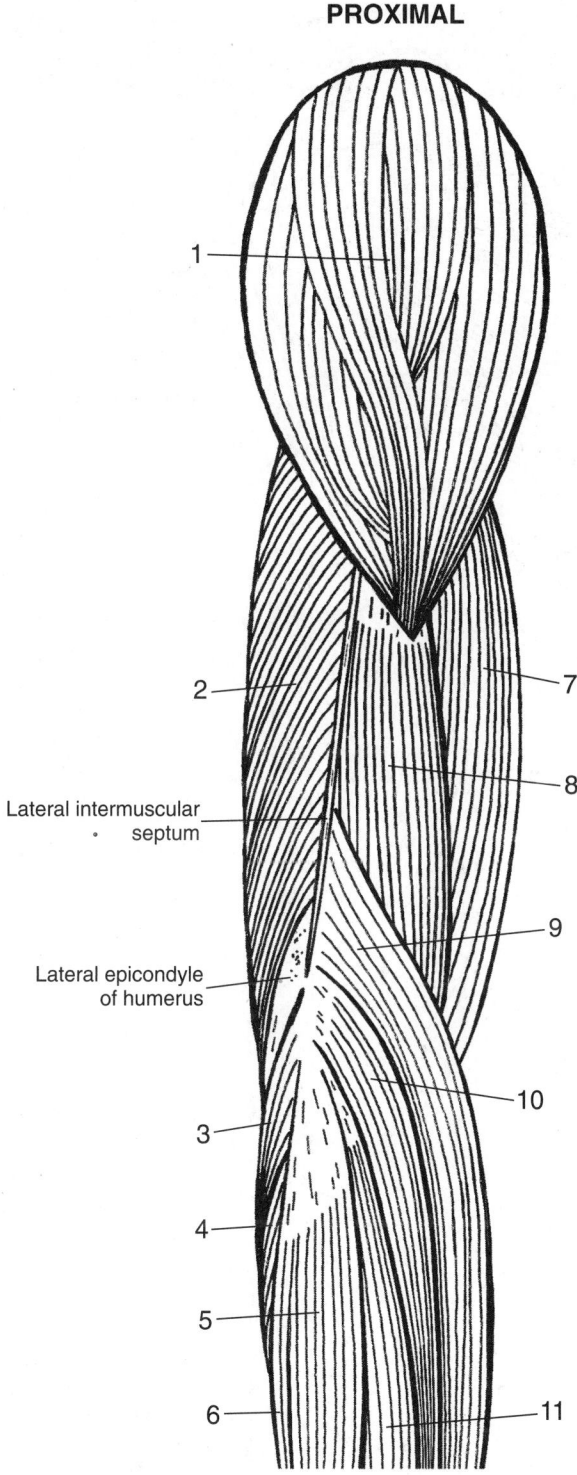

1 —
2 —
Lateral intermuscular septum
Lateral epicondyle of humerus
3 —
4 —
5 —
6 —
7 —
8 —
9 —
10 —
11 —

DISTAL

322 THE MUSCULAR SYSTEM Muscles of the Scapula/Arm

POSTERIOR VIEW OF THE RIGHT ARM

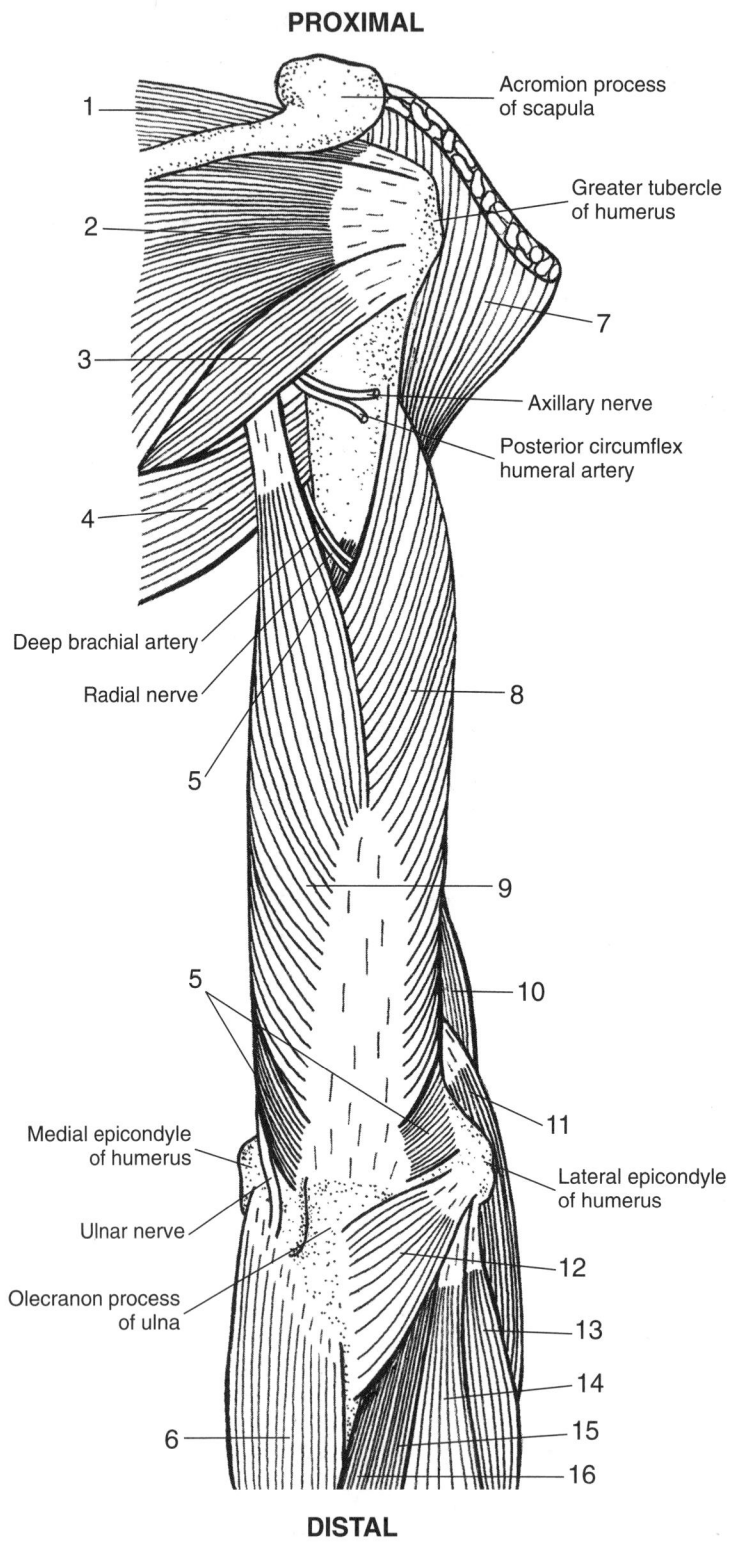

THE MUSCULAR SYSTEM Muscles of the Scapula/Arm

ANTERIOR VIEW OF THE RIGHT GLENOHUMERAL JOINT

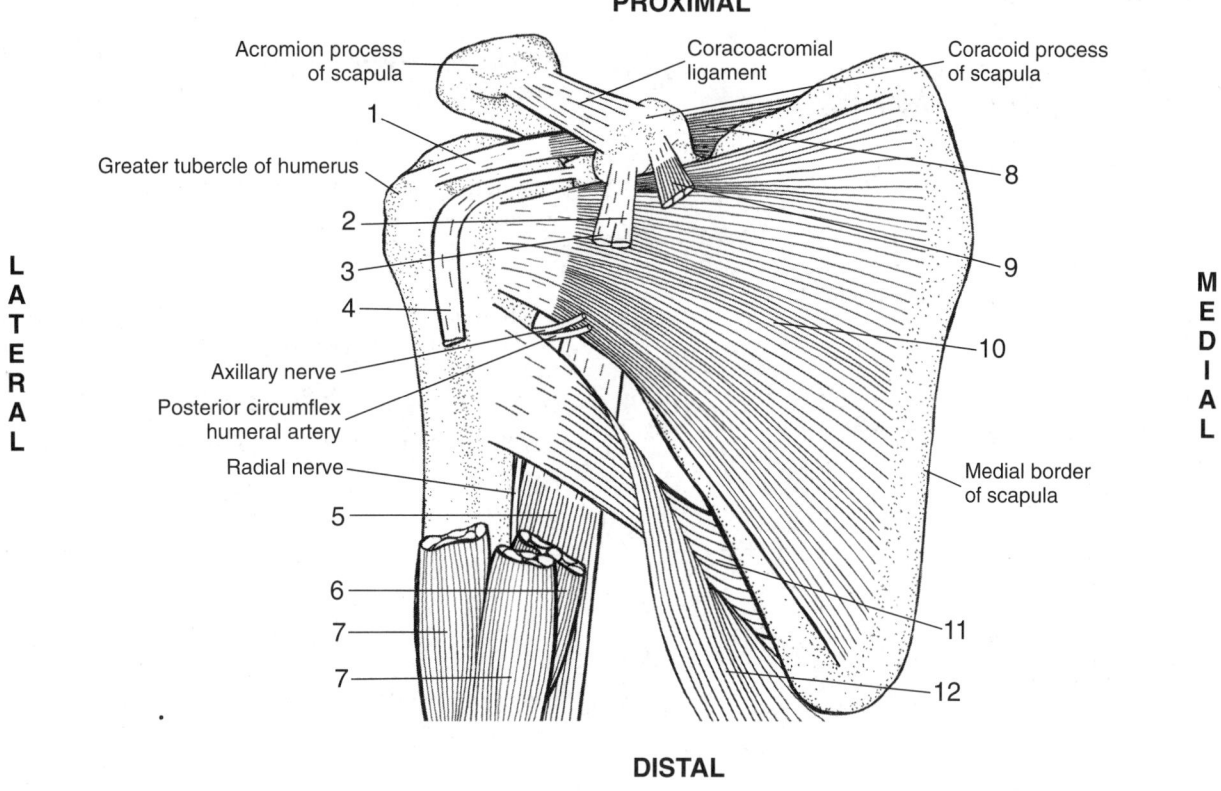

POSTERIOR VIEW OF THE RIGHT GLENOHUMERAL JOINT

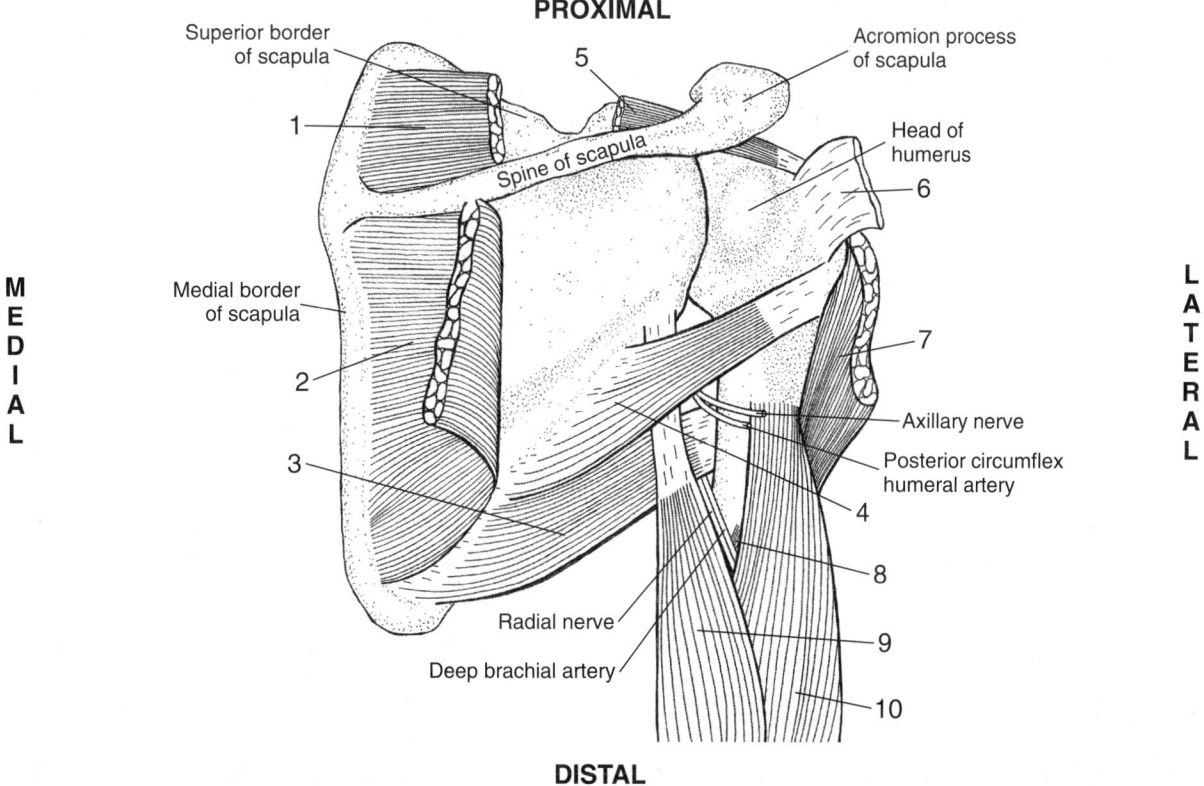

Review Questions

Muscles of the Scapula/Arm
Answers to these questions are found on page 468.

1. Name an antagonist to the brachialis.

2. Is the short head of the biceps brachii synergistic with or antagonistic to the coracobrachialis?

3. From the anterior perspective, is the coracobrachialis superficial or deep to the subscapularis?

4. What joint action would lengthen and stretch the infraspinatus?

5. How is the deltoid synergistic with the supraspinatus?

6. The long head of the triceps brachii passes between which two muscles?

7. From a posterior perspective, where is the teres major compared to the long head of the triceps brachii?

8. Which is the deepest head of the triceps brachii?

9. How are the anterior and posterior fibers of the deltoid antagonistic to each other?

10. Which portion of the deltoid attaches to the lateral clavicle?

11. The distal attachments of the supraspinatus and infraspinatus are deep to what muscle?

12. Name three muscles that attach to the coracoid process of the scapula.

13. Name a rotator cuff muscle that is synergistic to the teres major.

14. Which head of the triceps brachii will be stretched if the shoulder joint is flexed?

15. Where is the scapular attachment of the teres major relative to the teres minor?

16. Is the pronator teres synergistic with or antagonistic to the triceps brachii?

17. What muscle is immediately anterior to the triceps brachii on the lateral side?

18. Will passive lateral rotation of the arm at the shoulder joint shorten or lengthen the teres minor?

19. If the forearm is pronated at the radioulnar joints, will the brachialis be shortened or lengthened?

20. If the arm is passively flexed at the shoulder joint, will the coracobrachialis be shortened or lengthened?

21. From the anterior perspective, is the coracobrachialis superficial or deep to the deltoid?

22. From the anterior perspective, which is deeper, the biceps brachii or the brachialis?

23. Are the biceps brachii and brachialis synergistic with or antagonistic to each other?

24. What humeral joint actions would lengthen and stretch the teres major?

25. Besides the teres major, what other muscle attaches to the medial lip of the bicipital groove of the humerus?

26. Which rotator cuff muscle runs deep to the acromion process of the scapula?

27. From which perspective is the greatest amount of the brachialis superficial?

28. How many joints does the biceps brachii cross?

29. What two other muscles share the same distal attachment with the infraspinatus?

30. If the elbow joint is passively extended, will the triceps brachii be shortened or lengthened?

31. What four muscles comprise the rotator cuff group?

32. Are the teres minor and teres major synergistic or antagonistic to each other?

33. What rotator cuff muscle is synergistic with the teres minor?

34. How are the anterior fibers and posterior fibers of the deltoid synergistic with each other?

35. Name three muscles that attach to the greater tubercle of the humerus.

36. Which portion of the pectoralis major is adjacent to the deltoid?

37. What joint actions at the shoulder joint would stretch the coracobrachialis?

38. Is the infraspinatus superior or inferior to the supraspinatus?

39. Where is the teres minor relative to the teres major?

40. What muscle from the pelvis and back shares the same humeral joint actions with the teres major?

41. What two muscles attach to the lateral clavicle, acromion process, and spine of the scapula?

42. What muscle is named for being triangular in shape?

THE MUSCULAR SYSTEM — Muscles of the Forearm

ANTERIOR VIEW OF THE RIGHT FOREARM (SUPERFICIAL)

THE MUSCULAR SYSTEM Muscles of the Forearm   327

ANTERIOR VIEW OF THE RIGHT FOREARM (INTERMEDIATE)

PROXIMAL

- Biceps brachii
- Brachial artery (splits to form radial and ulnar arteries)
- Brachialis
- Radial nerve
- Head of the radius
- Brachialis tendon
- Biceps brachii tendon
- Supinator
- Brachioradialis
- Pronator teres (cut)
- Flexor pollicis longus
- Abductor pollicis longus
- Pronator quadratus
- Radial artery
- Flexor carpi radialis (cut)
- Palmaris longus cut and in reflected fibers of transverse fibers of palmar aponeurosis
- Thenar musculature

- Median nerve
- Triceps brachii medial head
- Pronator teres humeral head (cut and reflected)
- Medial epicondyle of humerus
- Brachialis
- Flexor carpi radialis (cut)
- Palmaris longus (cut)
- Pronator teres ulnar head (cut)
- Flexor digitorum profundus
- Flexor carpi ulnaris
- Flexor digitorum superficialis
- Median nerve
- Ulnar artery
- Ulnar nerve
- Flexor digitorum profundus
- Flexor retinaculum (transverse carpal ligament)
- Hypothenar musculature

Lateral / Radial

Ulnar / Medial

DISTAL

THE MUSCULAR SYSTEM Muscles of the Forearm

ANTERIOR VIEW OF THE RIGHT FOREARM (DEEP)

THE MUSCULAR SYSTEM — Muscles of the Forearm

POSTERIOR VIEW OF THE RIGHT FOREARM (SUPERFICIAL)

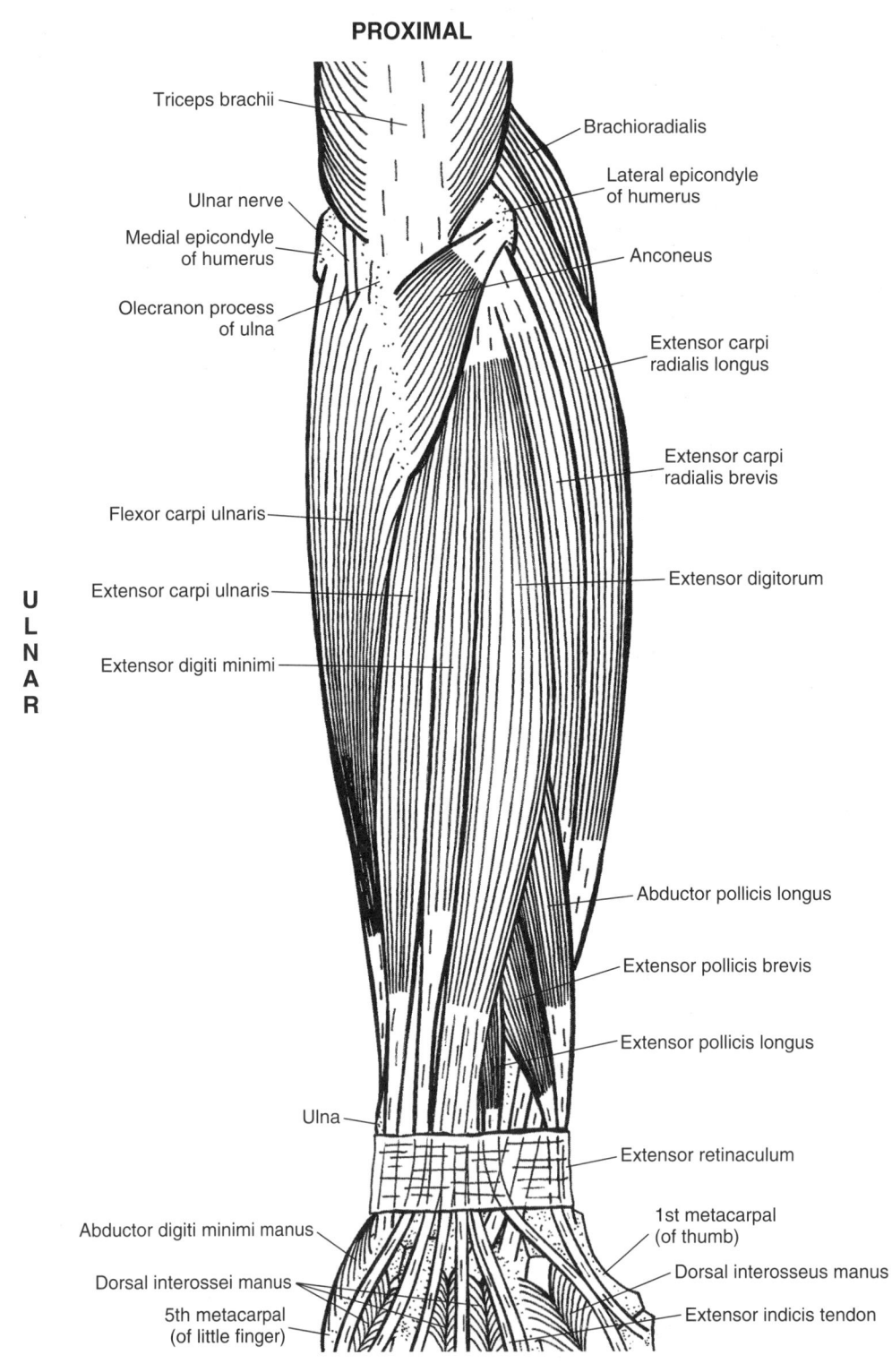

POSTERIOR VIEW OF THE RIGHT FOREARM (DEEP)

THE MUSCULAR SYSTEM Muscles of the Forearm

POSTERIOR VIEW OF THE RIGHT FOREARM AND HAND (SUPERFICIAL)

THE MUSCULAR SYSTEM: Muscles of the Forearm

POSTERIOR VIEW OF THE RIGHT FOREARM AND HAND (DEEP)

PRONATOR TERES
pro-**nay**-tor **te**-reez

Actions
Pronation of the forearm at the radioulnar joints
Flexion of the forearm at the elbow joint

Innervation
The median nerve

Arterial Supply
The ulnar artery

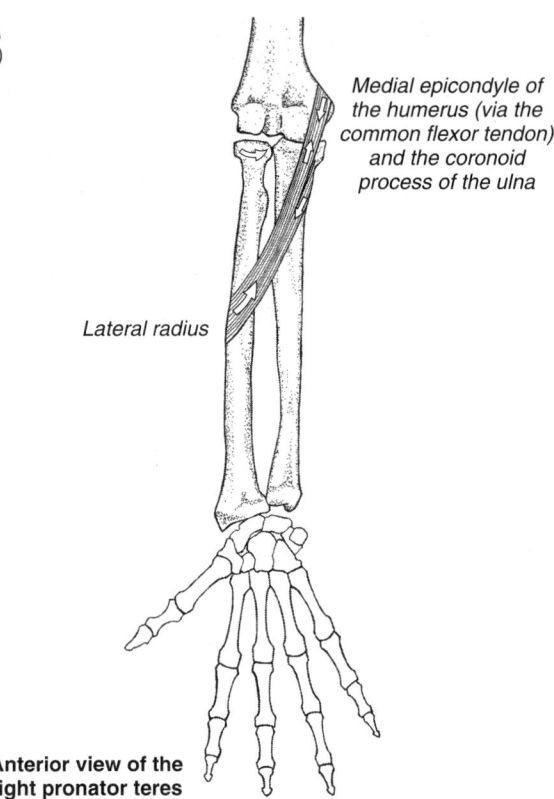

Anterior view of the right pronator teres

PRONATOR QUADRATUS
pro-**nay**-tor kwod-**ray**-tus

Action
Pronation of the forearm at the radioulnar joints

Innervation
The median nerve

Arterial Supply
The anterior interosseus artery

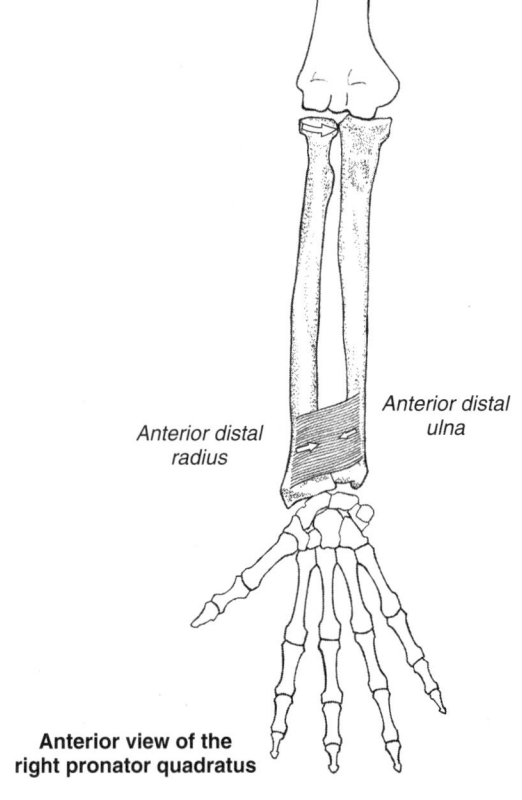

Anterior view of the right pronator quadratus

THE MUSCULAR SYSTEM Muscles of the Forearm

The median nerve runs between the two heads of the pronator teres and can be compressed there, resulting in pronator teres syndrome.

Although it is not very large, the pronator quadratus is considered by most sources to be the prime mover of pronation of the forearm at the radioulnar joints.

FLEXOR CARPI RADIALIS

(OF THE WRIST FLEXOR GROUP)

fleks-or **kar**-pie **ray**-dee-**a**-lis

Actions
Flexion of the hand at the wrist joint
Radial deviation (abduction) of the hand at the wrist joint
Flexion of the forearm at the elbow joint
Pronation of the forearm at the radioulnar joints

Innervation
The median nerve

Arterial Supply
The ulnar and radial arteries

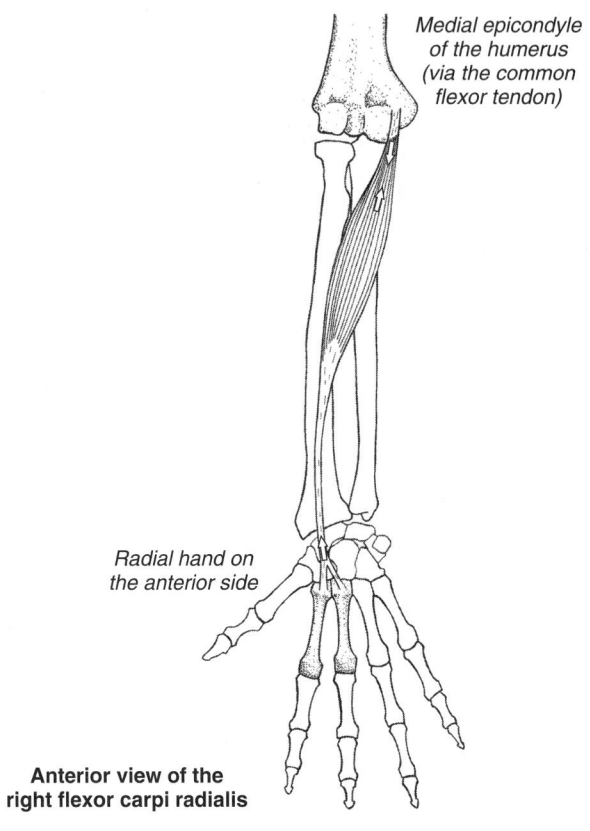

Anterior view of the right flexor carpi radialis

PALMARIS LONGUS

(OF THE WRIST FLEXOR GROUP)

pall-**ma**-ris **long**-us

Actions
Flexion of the hand at the wrist joint
Flexion of the forearm at the elbow joint
Pronation of the forearm at the radioulnar joints
Wrinkles the skin of the palm

Innervation
The median nerve

Arterial Supply
The ulnar artery

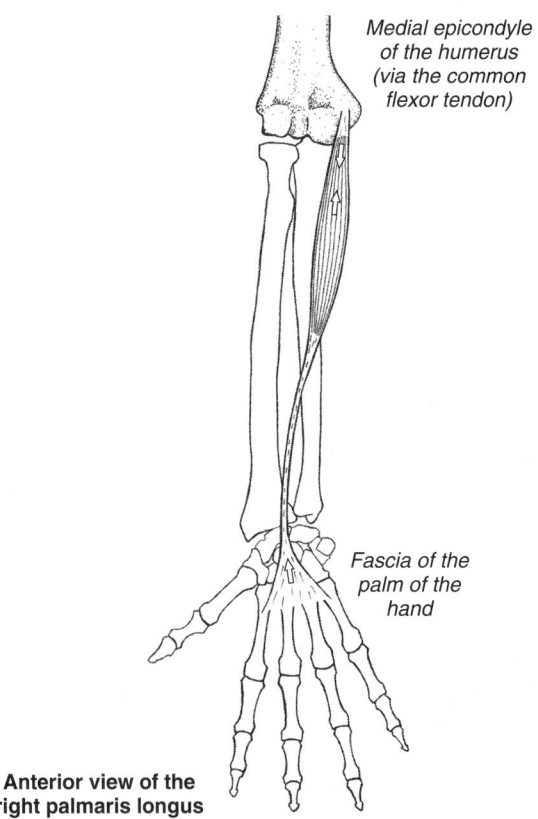

Anterior view of the right palmaris longus

THE MUSCULAR SYSTEM Muscles of the Forearm

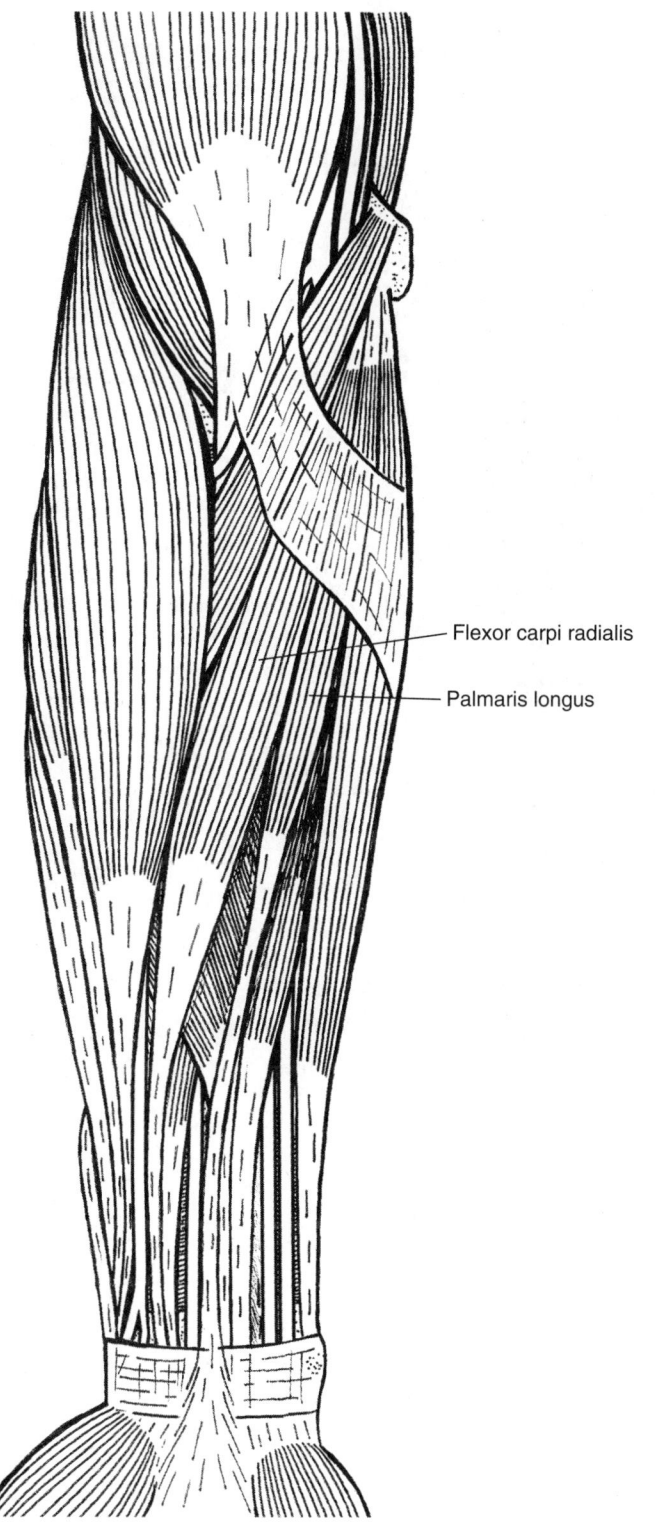

- Flexor carpi radialis
- Palmaris longus

Irritation and inflammation of the medial epicondyle of the humerus and/or the common flexor tendon is known as medial epicondylitis and is usually called "golfer's elbow."

The palmaris longus is often missing, sometimes unilaterally, sometimes bilaterally.

FLEXOR CARPI ULNARIS
(OF THE WRIST FLEXOR GROUP)

fleks-or **kar**-pie ul-**na**-ris

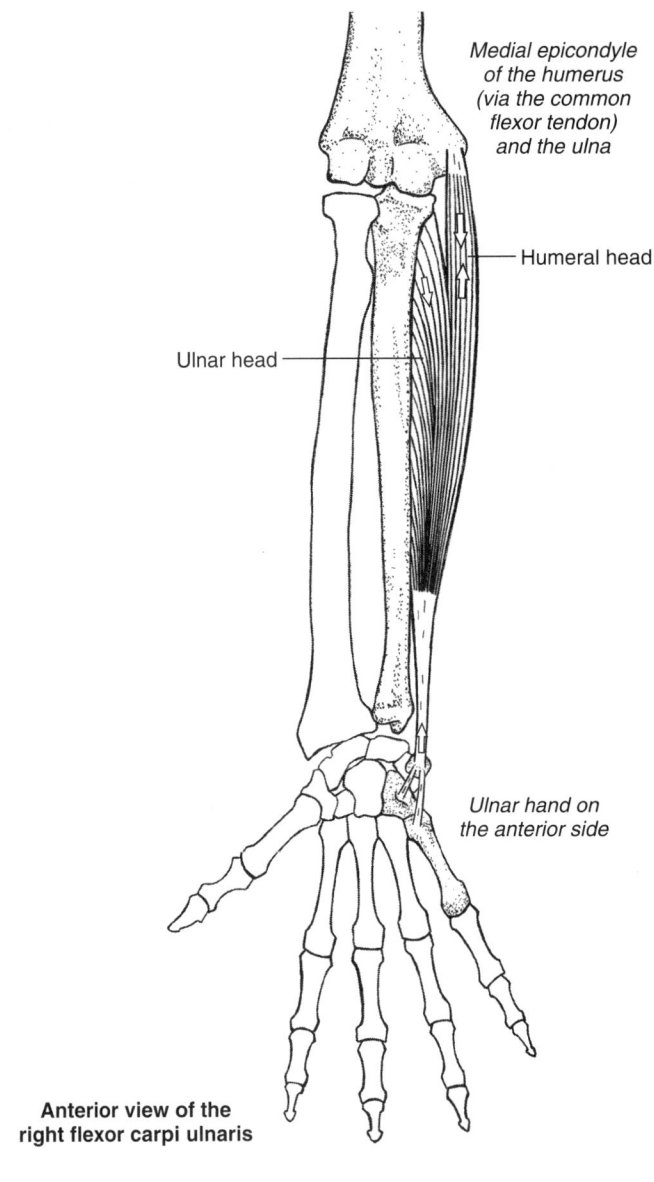

Anterior view of the right flexor carpi ulnaris

Actions
Flexion of the hand at the wrist joint
Ulnar deviation (adduction) of the hand at the wrist joint
Flexion of the forearm at the elbow joint

Innervation
The ulnar nerve

Arterial Supply
The ulnar artery

THE MUSCULAR SYSTEM Muscles of the Forearm   339

Flexor carpi ulnaris

DID YOU KNOW?

All three wrist flexor group muscles (flexor carpi radialis, palmaris longus, and flexor carpi ulnaris) attach onto the medial epicondyle of the humerus via the common flexor tendon. Only the flexor carpi ulnaris has an additional proximal attachment, onto the ulna.

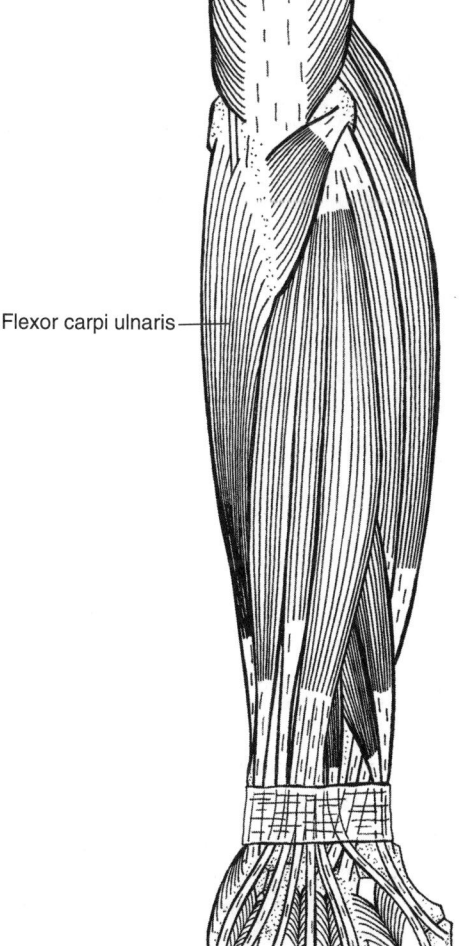

Flexor carpi ulnaris

BRACHIORADIALIS
(OF THE RADIAL GROUP)
bray-key-o-**ray**-dee-**al**-is

Lateral view of the right brachioradialis

Actions
Flexion of the forearm at the elbow joint
Supination of the forearm at the radioulnar joints
Pronation of the forearm at the radioulnar joints

Innervation
The radial nerve

Arterial Supply
Branches of the brachial artery and the radial artery

THE MUSCULAR SYSTEM Muscles of the Forearm   341

DID YOU KNOW?

The brachioradialis can both pronate and supinate the forearm at the radioulnar joints. But, it can only create these actions to a halfway position.

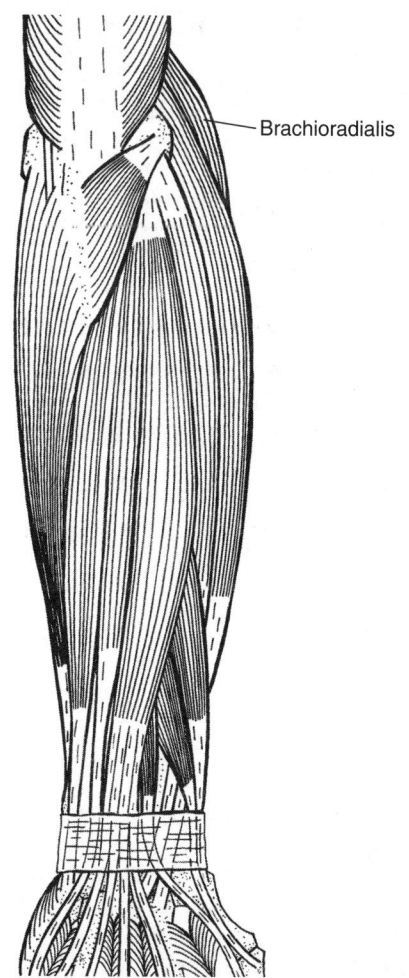

Brachioradialis (left illustration)

Brachioradialis (right illustration)

FLEXOR DIGITORUM SUPERFICIALIS

fleks-or dij-i-**toe**-rum **soo**-per-fish-ee-**a**-lis

Actions
Flexion of fingers #2-5 at the metacarpophalangeal and proximal interphalangeal joints
Flexion of the hand at the wrist joint
Flexion of the forearm at the elbow joint

Innervation
The median nerve

Arterial Supply
The ulnar and radial arteries

Medial epicondyle of the humerus (via the common flexor tendon) and the anterior ulna, and the radius

Anterior view of the right flexor digitorum superficialis

Anterior surfaces of fingers #2-5

FLEXOR DIGITORUM PROFUNDUS

fleks-or dij-i-**toe**-rum pro-**fun**-dus

Actions
Flexion of fingers #2-5 at the metacarpophalangeal and proximal and distal interphalangeal joints
Flexion of the hand at the wrist joint

Innervation
The median and the ulnar nerves

Arterial Supply
The ulnar and radial arteries and the anterior interosseus artery

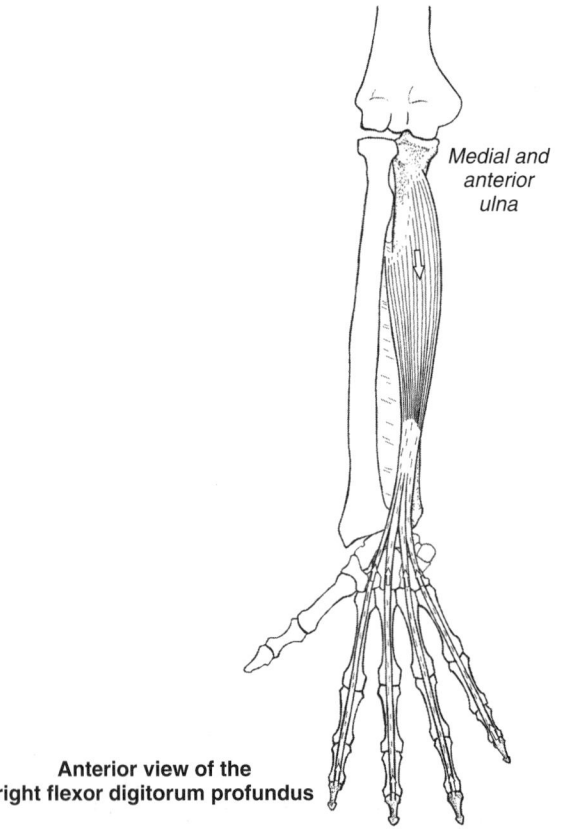

Medial and anterior ulna

Anterior view of the right flexor digitorum profundus

Anterior surfaces of fingers #2-5

THE MUSCULAR SYSTEM Muscles of the Forearm   343

The distal tendons of the flexor digitorum superficialis split to allow passage of the distal tendons of the flexor digitorum profundus to the distal phalanges of fingers #2-5.

The flexor digitorum profundus is the only muscle that can flex the distal phalanges of fingers #2-5 at the distal interphalangeal joints.

FLEXOR POLLICIS LONGUS
fleks-or pol-i-sis long-us

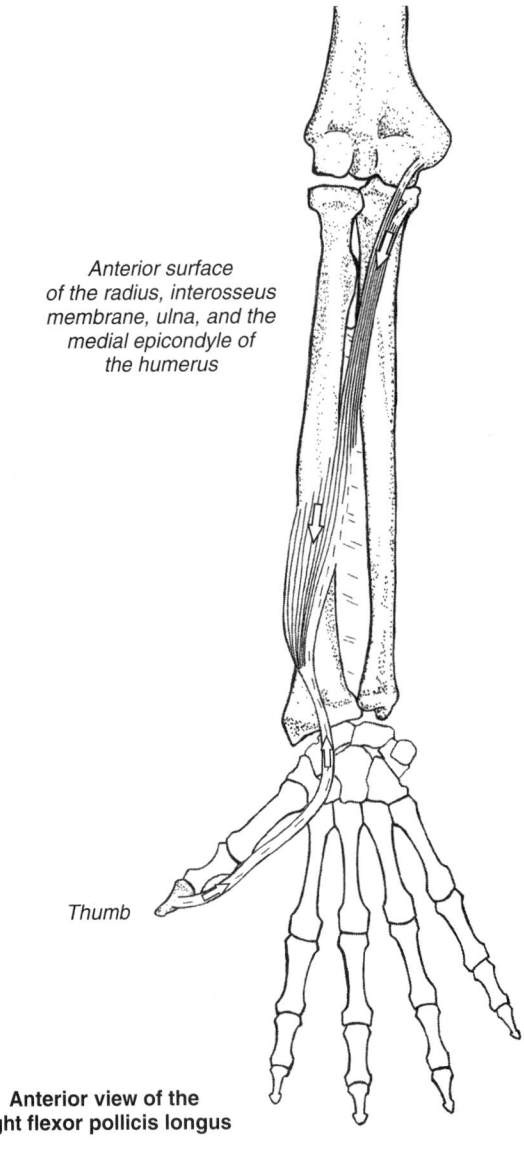

Anterior surface of the radius, interosseus membrane, ulna, and the medial epicondyle of the humerus

Thumb

Anterior view of the right flexor pollicis longus

Actions
Flexion of the thumb at the carpometacarpal, metacarpophalangeal, and interphalangeal joints
Flexion of the hand at the wrist joint
Radial deviation (abduction) of the hand at the wrist joint
Flexion of the forearm at the elbow joint

Innervation
The median nerve

Arterial Supply
The radial artery and the anterior interosseus artery

THE MUSCULAR SYSTEM Muscles of the Forearm

Flexor pollicis longus

DID YOU KNOW? *The flexor pollicis longus has a common variation wherein it is missing its humeroulnar head.*

Flexor pollicis longus (cut)

Flexor pollicis longus tendon (cut)

ANCONEUS
an-**ko**-nee-us

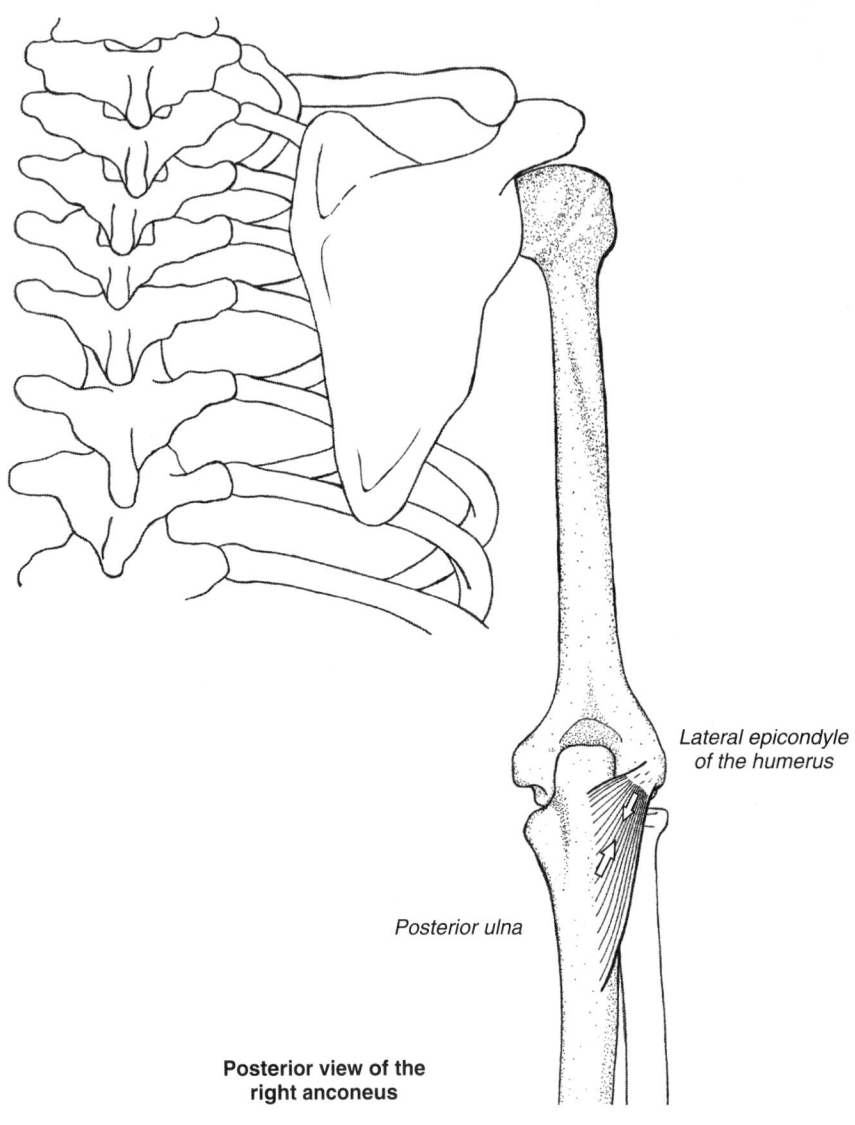

Lateral epicondyle of the humerus

Posterior ulna

Posterior view of the right anconeus

Action	**Innervation**	**Arterial Supply**
Extension of the forearm at the elbow joint	The radial nerve	The deep brachial artery

THE MUSCULAR SYSTEM Muscles of the Forearm

DID YOU KNOW?

The anconeus is easily palpable in the posterior proximal forearm just distal to a point that is halfway between the olecranon process of the ulna and the lateral epicondyle of the humerus.

EXTENSOR CARPI RADIALIS LONGUS

(OF THE WRIST EXTENSOR GROUP AND THE RADIAL GROUP)

eks-**ten**-sor **kar**-pie **ray**-dee-a-lis **long**-us

Actions
Extension of the hand at the wrist joint
Radial deviation (abduction) of the hand at the wrist joint
Flexion of the forearm at the elbow joint
Pronation of the forearm at the radioulnar joints

Innervation
The radial nerve

Arterial Supply
Branches of the brachial artery and the radial artery

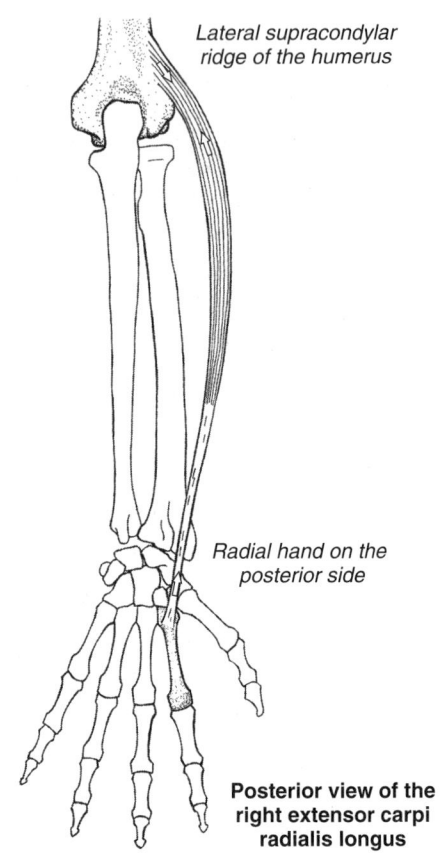

Lateral supracondylar ridge of the humerus

Radial hand on the posterior side

Posterior view of the right extensor carpi radialis longus

EXTENSOR CARPI RADIALIS BREVIS

(OF THE WRIST EXTENSOR GROUP AND THE RADIAL GROUP)

eks-**ten**-sor **kar**-pie **ray**-dee-a-lis **bre**-vis

Actions
Extension of the hand at the wrist joint
Radial deviation (abduction) of the hand at the wrist joint
Flexion of the forearm at the elbow joint

Innervation
The radial nerve

Arterial Supply
Branches of the brachial artery and the radial artery

Lateral epicondyle of the humerus (via the common extensor tendon)

Radial hand on the posterior side

Posterior view of the right extensor carpi radialis brevis

THE MUSCULAR SYSTEM: Muscles of the Forearm

The extensor carpi radialis longus is the only one of the wrist extensor group muscles (extensor carpi radialis longus, extensor carpi radialis brevis, and extensor carpi ulnaris) that attaches onto the lateral supracondylar ridge of the humerus.

Irritation and inflammation of the lateral epicondyle of the humerus and/or the common extensor tendon is known as lateral epicondylitis and is usually called "tennis elbow."

EXTENSOR CARPI ULNARIS
(OF THE WRIST EXTENSOR GROUP)

eks-**ten**-sor **kar**-pie ul-**na**-ris

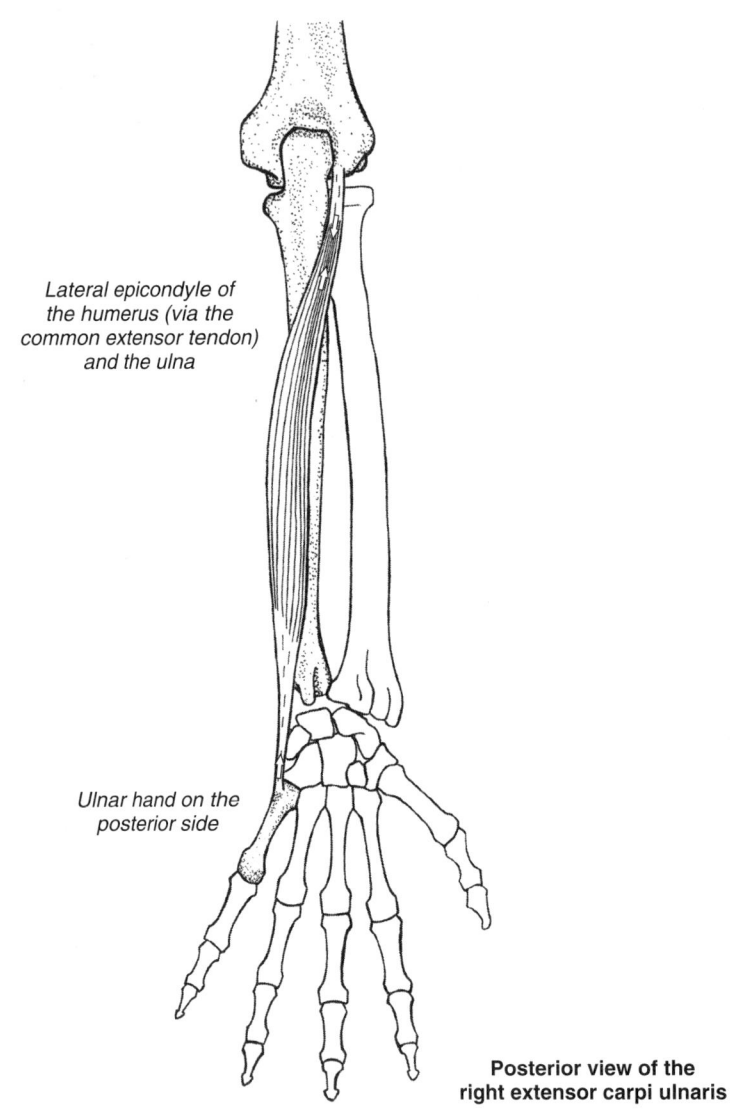

Lateral epicondyle of the humerus (via the common extensor tendon) and the ulna

Ulnar hand on the posterior side

Posterior view of the right extensor carpi ulnaris

Actions	Innervation	Arterial Supply
Extension of the hand at the wrist joint Ulnar deviation (adduction) of the hand at the wrist joint Extension of the forearm at the elbow joint	The radial nerve	The posterior interosseus artery

THE MUSCULAR SYSTEM Muscles of the Forearm   351

Extensor carpi ulnaris

DID YOU KNOW

The extensor carpi ulnaris is the only one of the wrist extensor group muscles (extensor carpi radialis longus, extensor carpi radialis brevis, and extensor carpi ulnaris) that has an additional proximal attachment, onto the ulna.

Extensor carpi ulnaris

EXTENSOR DIGITORUM

eks-**ten**-sor dij-i-**toe**-rum

Actions
Extension of fingers #2-5 at the metacarpophalangeal and proximal and distal interphalangeal joints
Extension of the hand at the wrist joint
Medial rotation of the little finger (finger #5) at the carpometacarpal joint
Extension of the forearm at the elbow joint

Innervation
The radial nerve

Arterial Supply
The posterior interosseus artery

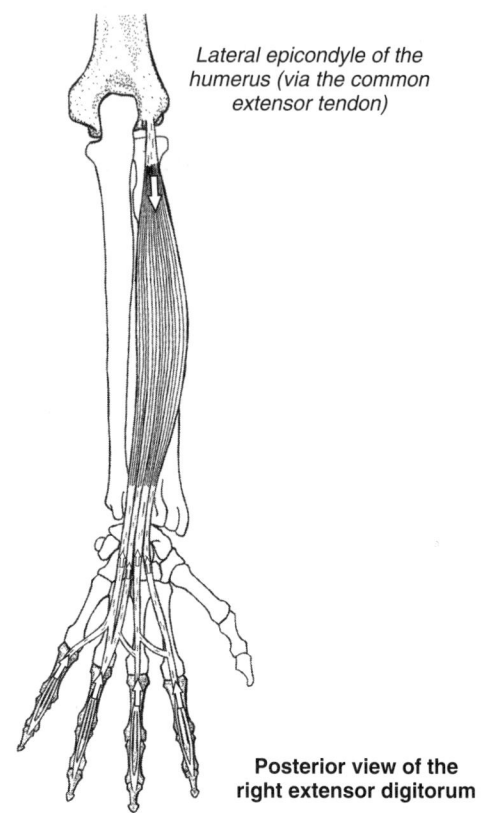

Lateral epicondyle of the humerus (via the common extensor tendon)

Posterior view of the right extensor digitorum

Phalanges of fingers #2-5

EXTENSOR DIGITI MINIMI

eks-**ten**-sor **dij**-i-tee **min**-i-mee

Actions
Extension of the little finger (finger #5) at the metacarpophalangeal and proximal and distal interphalangeal joints
Extension of the hand at the wrist joint
Medial rotation of the little finger (finger #5) at the carpometacarpal joint
Extension of the forearm at the elbow joint

Innervation
The radial nerve

Arterial Supply
The posterior interosseus artery

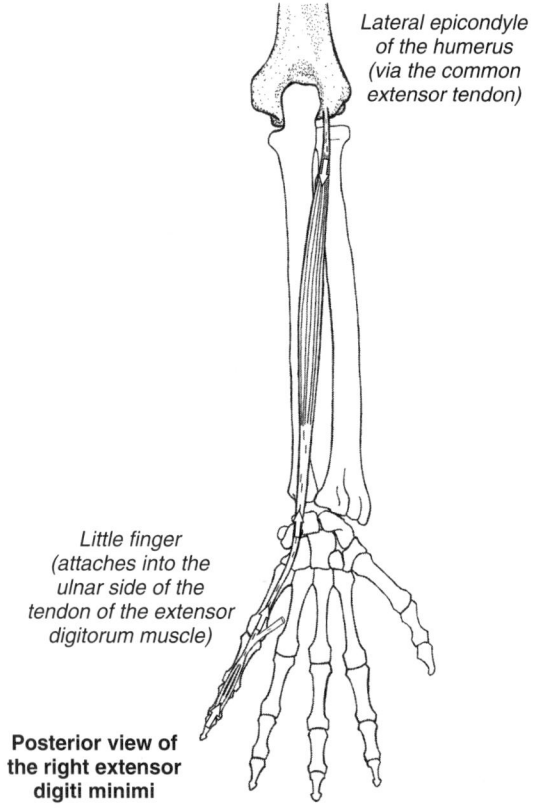

Lateral epicondyle of the humerus (via the common extensor tendon)

Little finger (attaches into the ulnar side of the tendon of the extensor digitorum muscle)

Posterior view of the right extensor digiti minimi

THE MUSCULAR SYSTEM: Muscles of the Forearm

DID YOU KNOW? The distal attachment of the extensor digitorum creates a structure called the dorsal digital expansion, which is an attachment site for many intrinsic muscles of the hand.

DID YOU KNOW? The distal tendon of the extensor digiti minimi joins into the distal tendon of the extensor digitorum that goes to the little finger.

SUPINATOR
sue-pin-**a**-tor

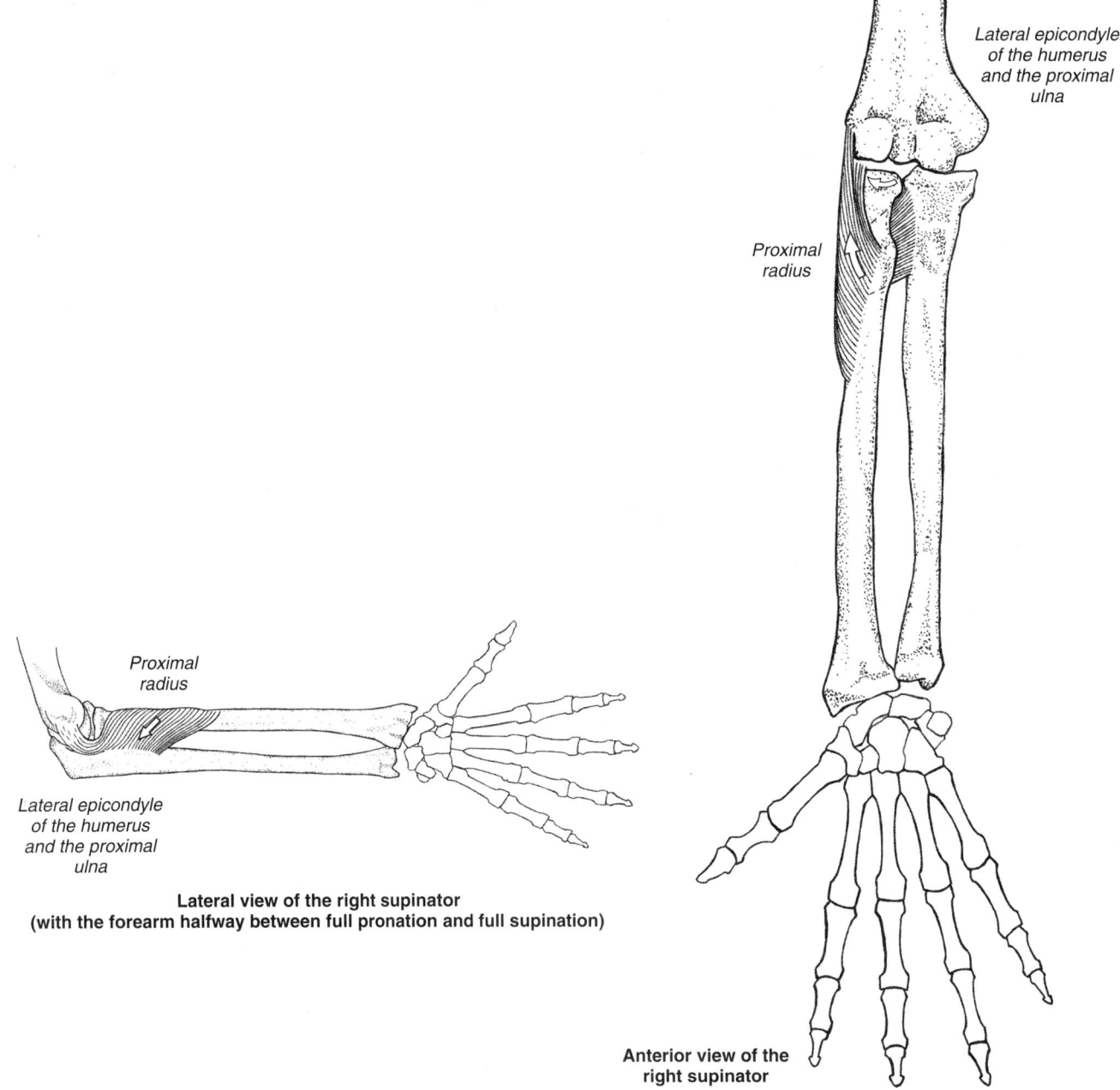

Lateral view of the right supinator
(with the forearm halfway between full pronation and full supination)

Anterior view of the right supinator

Action
Supination of the forearm at the radioulnar joints

Innervation
The radial nerve

Arterial Supply
Branches of the radial artery and the interosseus recurrent and posterior interosseus arteries

THE MUSCULAR SYSTEM Muscles of the Forearm

DID YOU KNOW?

A deep branch of the radial nerve runs between the two layers of the supinator and may be compressed there.

ABDUCTOR POLLICIS LONGUS
(OF THE DEEP DISTAL FOUR GROUP)

ab-**duk**-tor **pol**-i-sis **long**-us

Actions
Abduction of the thumb at the carpometacarpal joint
Extension of the thumb at the carpometacarpal joint
Lateral rotation of the thumb at the carpometacarpal joint
Radial deviation (abduction) of the hand at the wrist joint
Flexion of the hand at the wrist joint
Supination of the forearm at the radioulnar joints

Innervation
The radial nerve

Arterial Supply
The posterior interosseus artery

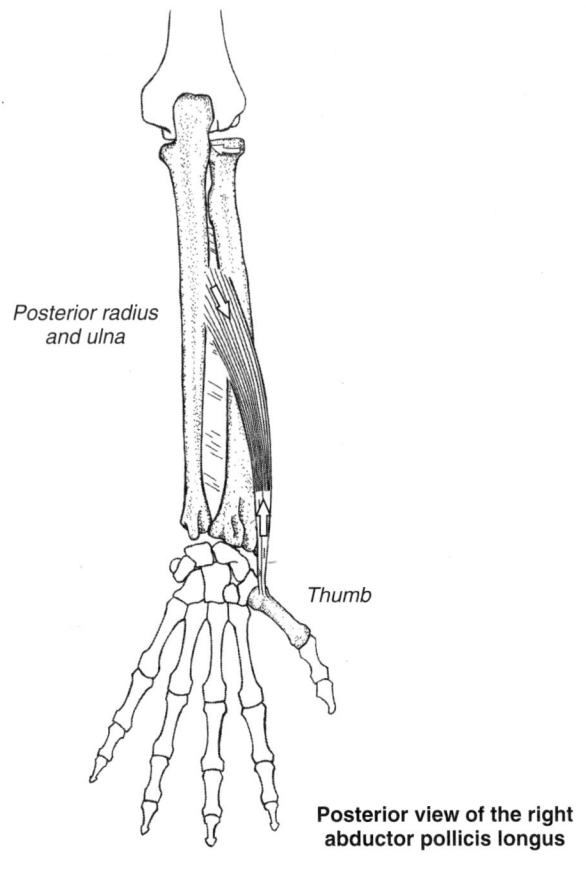

Posterior radius and ulna

Thumb

Posterior view of the right abductor pollicis longus

EXTENSOR POLLICIS BREVIS
(OF THE DEEP DISTAL FOUR GROUP)

eks-**ten**-sor **pol**-i-sis **bre**-vis

Actions
Extension of the thumb at the carpometacarpal and metacarpophalangeal joints
Abduction of the thumb at the carpometacarpal joint
Lateral rotation of the thumb at the carpometacarpal joint
Radial deviation (abduction) of the hand at the wrist joint

Innervation
The radial nerve

Arterial Supply
The posterior interosseus artery

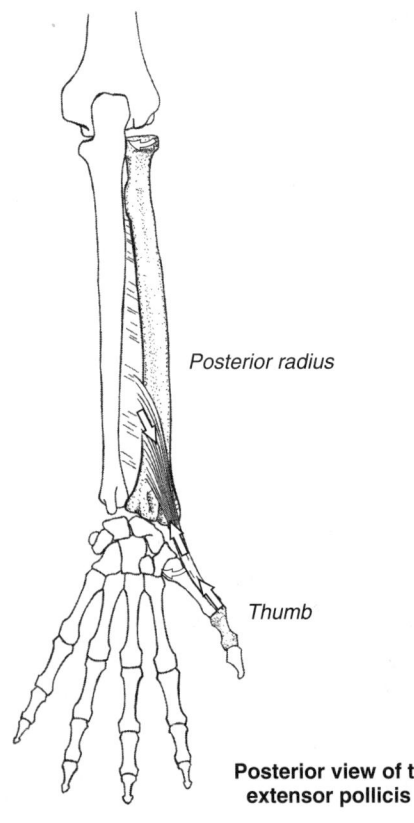

Posterior radius

Thumb

Posterior view of the right extensor pollicis brevis

THE MUSCULAR SYSTEM Muscles of the Forearm

DID YOU KNOW?
The distal tendons of these two muscles form the lateral (radial) border of the anatomic snuffbox.

- Abductor pollicis longus
- Extensor pollicis brevis

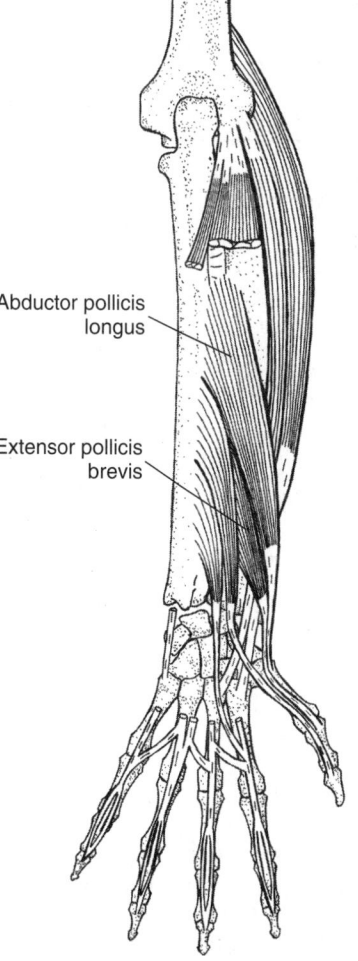

- Abductor pollicis longus
- Extensor pollicis brevis

EXTENSOR POLLICIS LONGUS
(OF THE DEEP DISTAL FOUR GROUP)

eks-**ten**-sor **pol**-i-sis **long**-us

Actions
Extension of the thumb at the carpometacarpal, metacarpophalangeal, and interphalangeal joints
Lateral rotation of the thumb at the carpometacarpal joint
Extension of the hand at the wrist joint
Radial deviation (abduction) of the hand at the wrist joint
Supination of the forearm at the radioulnar joints

Innervation
The radial nerve

Arterial Supply
The posterior interosseus artery

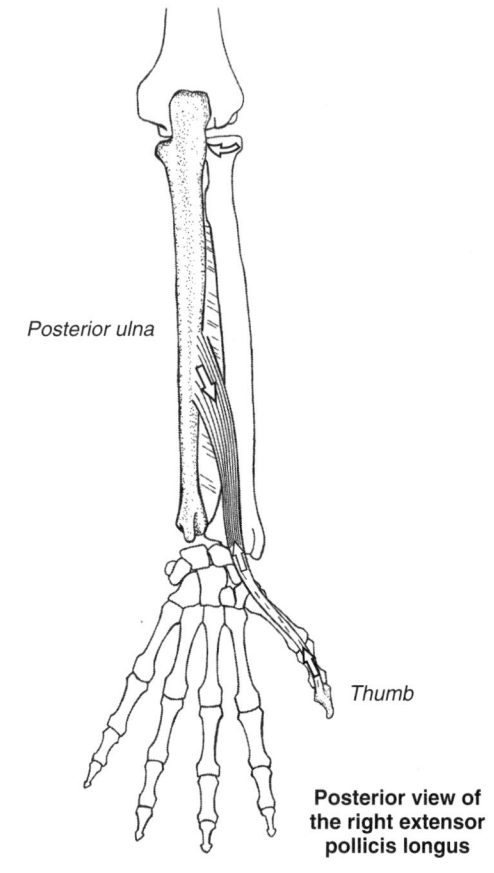

Posterior view of the right extensor pollicis longus

EXTENSOR INDICIS
(OF THE DEEP DISTAL FOUR GROUP)

eks-**ten**-sor **in**-di-sis

Actions
Extension of the index finger (finger #2) at the metacarpophalangeal and proximal and distal interphalangeal joints
Extension of the hand at the wrist joint
Adduction of the index finger (finger #2) at the metacarpophalangeal joint
Supination of the forearm at the radioulnar joints

Innervation
The radial nerve

Arterial Supply
The posterior interosseus artery

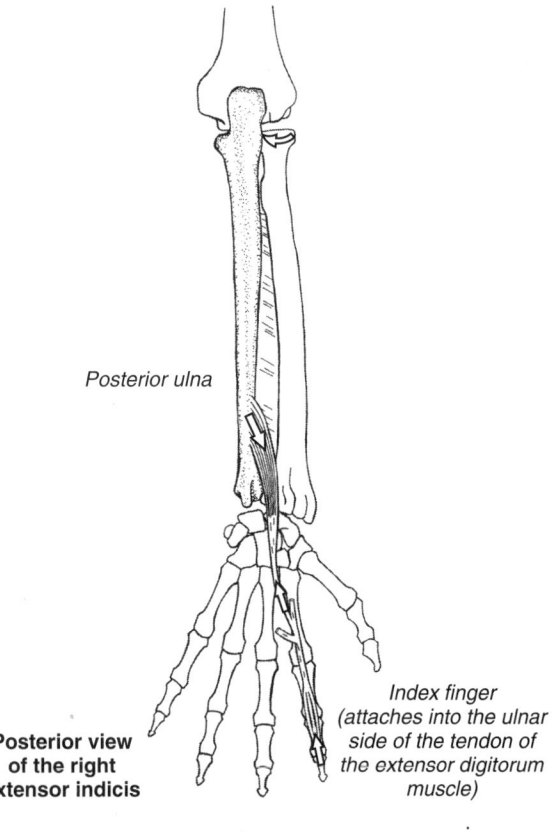

Posterior view of the right extensor indicis

Index finger (attaches into the ulnar side of the tendon of the extensor digitorum muscle)

THE MUSCULAR SYSTEM Muscles of the Forearm   359

Extensor pollicis longus

Extensor indicis tendon

The distal tendon of the extensor pollicis longus forms the medial (ulnar) border of the anatomic snuffbox.

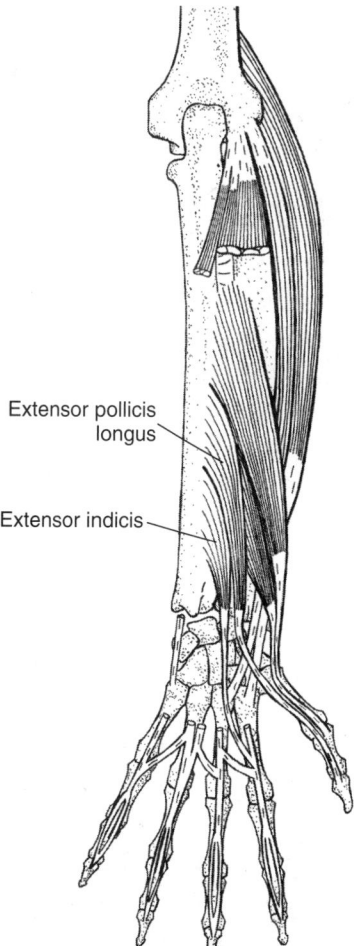

Extensor pollicis longus

Extensor indicis

The extensor indicis aids the extensor digitorum in extending the index finger, which allows us to point out, i.e., indicate things.

THE MUSCULAR SYSTEM Muscles of the Forearm

ANTERIOR VIEW OF THE RIGHT FOREARM (SUPERFICIAL)

PROXIMAL

Median nerve
Brachial artery
Medial epicondyle of humerus

Radial artery

Ulnar artery
Ulnar nerve

Radial artery
Median nerve
Transverse fibers of palmar aponeurosis
Thenar musculature
Hypothenar musculature
Palmar aponeurosis

LATERAL / RADIAL

ULNAR / MEDIAL

DISTAL

THE MUSCULAR SYSTEM Muscles of the Forearm 361

ANTERIOR VIEW OF THE RIGHT FOREARM (INTERMEDIATE)

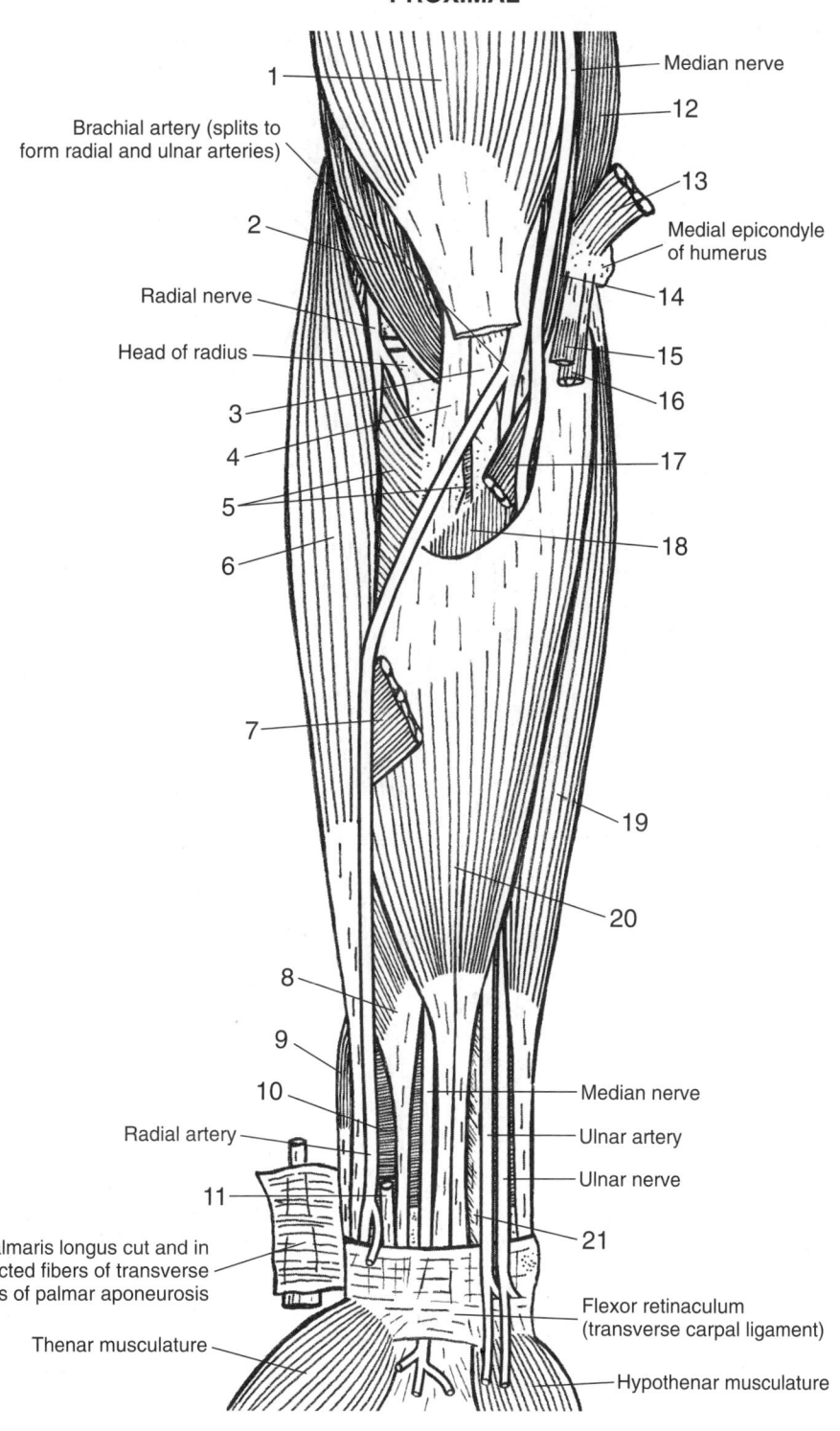

THE MUSCULAR SYSTEM Muscles of the Forearm

ANTERIOR VIEW OF THE RIGHT FOREARM (DEEP)

ANTERIOR VIEWS OF THE PRONATORS AND SUPINATOR OF THE RIGHT RADIUS

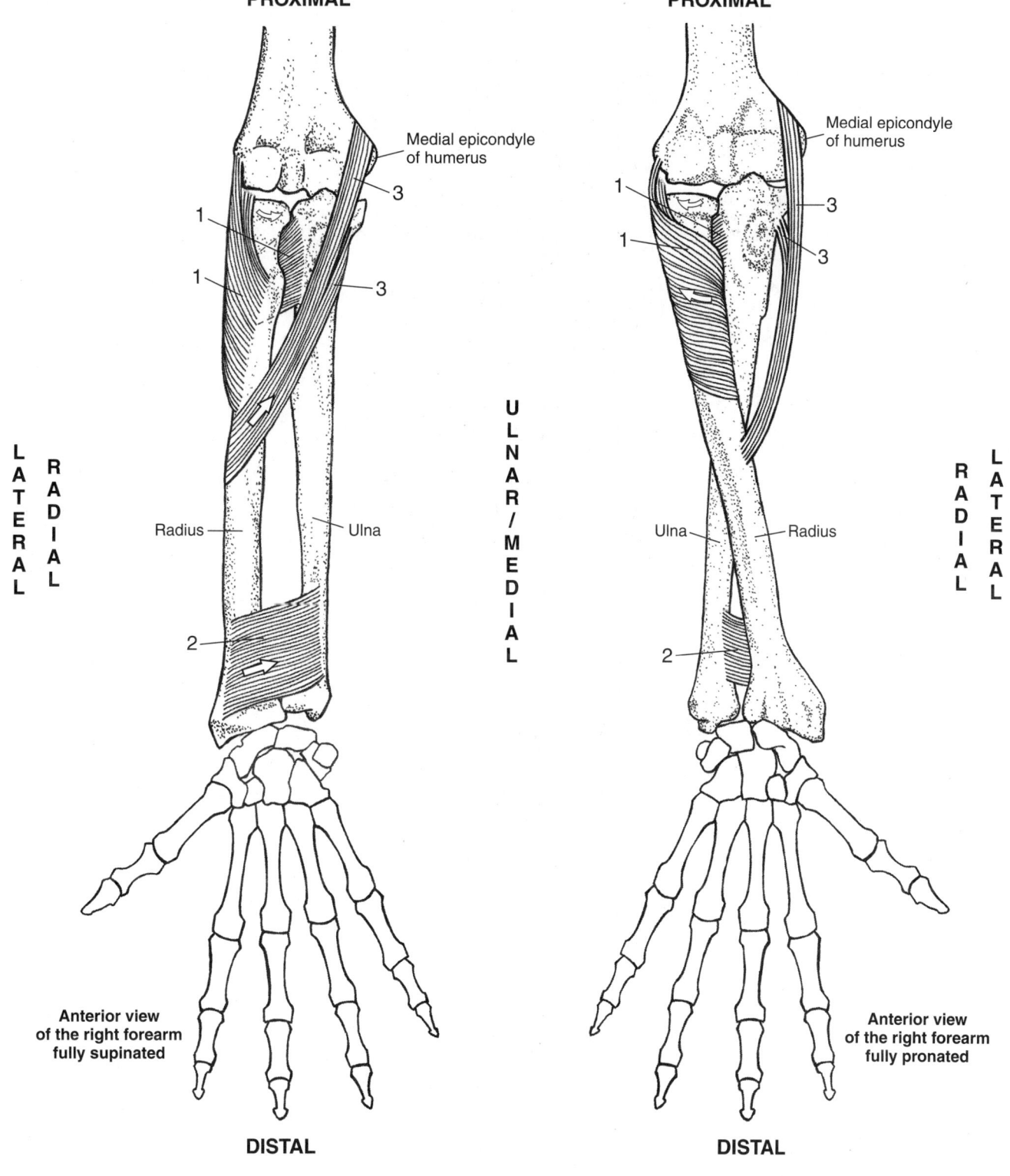

THE MUSCULAR SYSTEM Muscles of the Forearm

POSTERIOR VIEW OF THE RIGHT FOREARM (SUPERFICIAL)

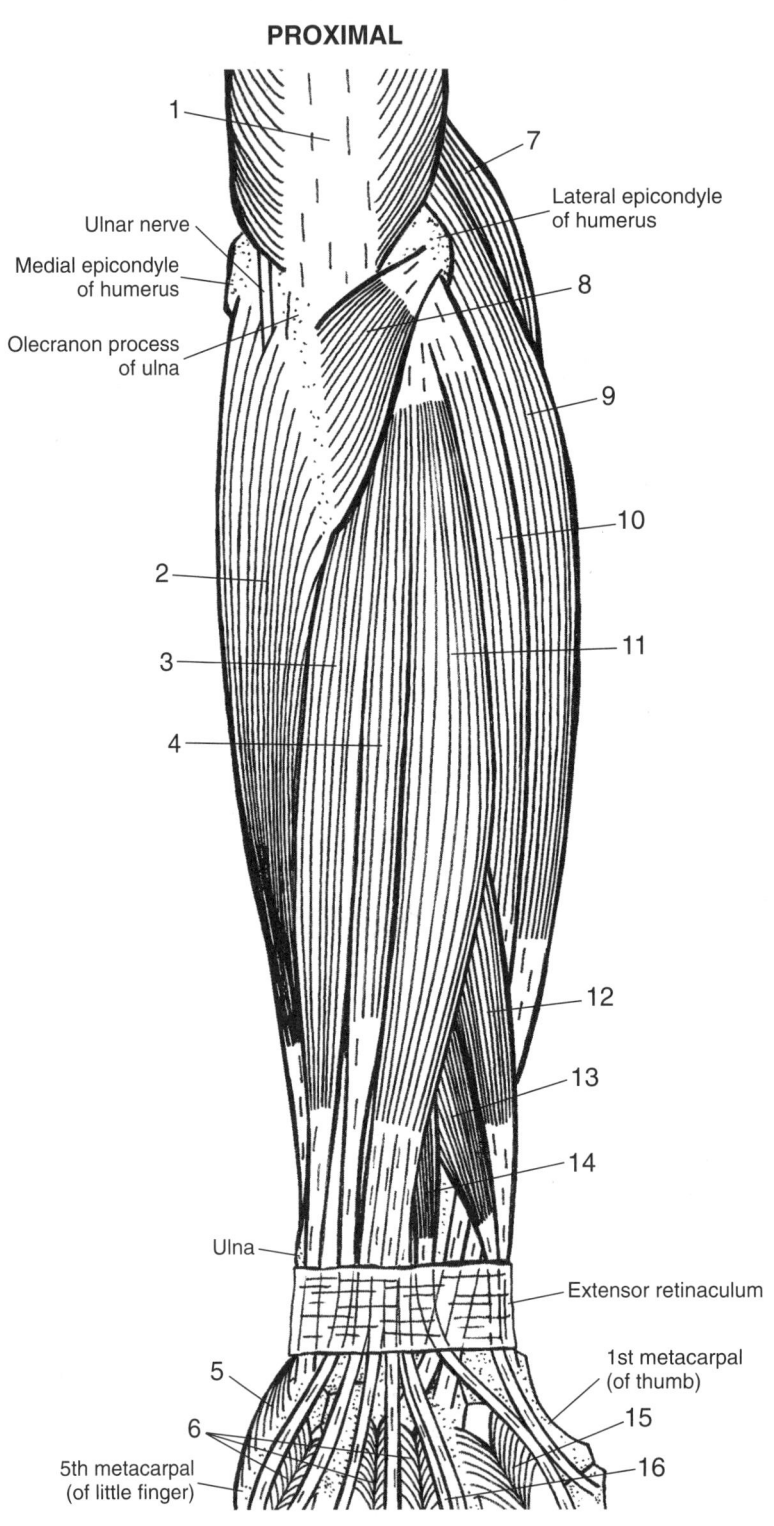

THE MUSCULAR SYSTEM Muscles of the Forearm   365

POSTERIOR VIEW OF THE RIGHT FOREARM (DEEP)

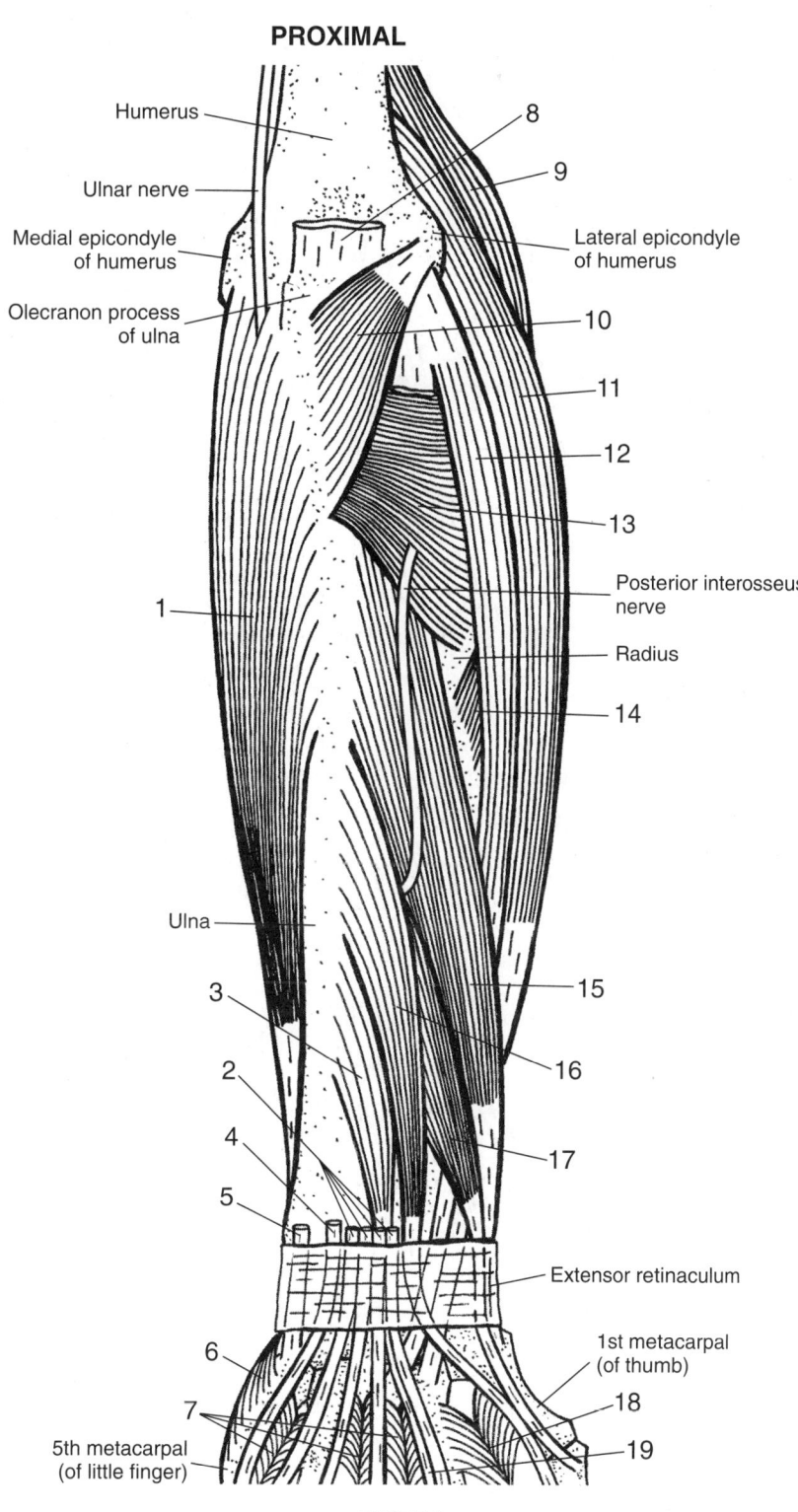

THE MUSCULAR SYSTEM Muscles of the Forearm

POSTERIOR VIEW OF THE RIGHT FOREARM AND HAND (SUPERFICIAL)

THE MUSCULAR SYSTEM Muscles of the Forearm 367

POSTERIOR VIEW OF THE RIGHT FOREARM AND HAND (DEEP)

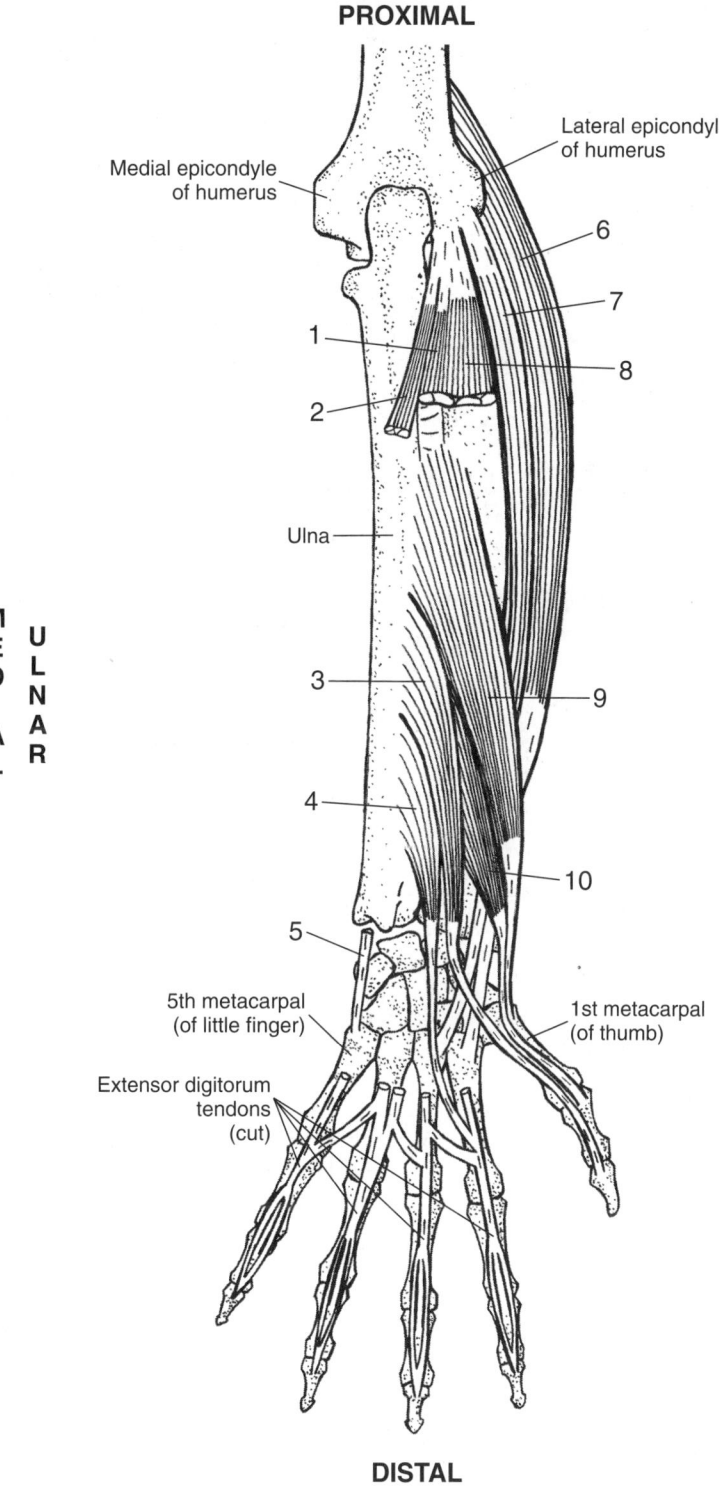

Review Questions

Muscles of the Forearm
Answers to these questions are found on page 469.

1. The distal tendons of what muscle split, allowing passage of the tendons of the flexor digitorum profundus to the distal phalanges?

2. From an anterior perspective, where is the radial attachment of the pronator teres relative to the brachioradialis?

3. Where they overlap, which muscle is deeper, the anconeus or the extensor carpi ulnaris?

4. At the wrist, the distal tendon of the flexor pollicis longus can be found between the distal tendons of which two wrist flexor muscles?

5. The distal attachment of the pronator teres is deep to what muscle?

6. What joint action(s) is/are occurring at the wrist joint when the extensor carpi ulnaris is concentrically contracting?

7. What six muscles attach to the lateral epicondyle of the humerus?

8. The extensors carpi radialis longus and brevis and the extensor carpi ulnaris attach onto which metacarpals?

9. What joint actions would lengthen and stretch the flexor carpi radialis?

10. What is the major antagonist to the flexor digitorum profundus?

11. Why is the flexor carpi radialis antagonistic to the anconeus?

12. How is the brachioradialis synergistic to the supinator?

13. What muscle is immediately medial to the extensor digiti minimi?

14. Where they overlap, which muscle is deeper, the flexor digitorum superficialis or the flexor pollicis longus?

15. What two muscles attach to the lateral supracondylar ridge of the humerus?

16. What joint action would stretch the pronator teres but not the pronator quadratus?

17. From an anterior perspective, which muscle is deeper, the flexor digitorum superficialis or profundus?

18. What nerve runs between the two heads of the pronator teres?

19. Golfer's elbow (also known as medial epicondylitis or medial epicondylosis) involves what tendon of the forearm?

20. What is the only muscle in the body that can flex the thumb at the interphalangeal joint?

21. What muscle is immediately lateral to the extensor carpi radialis brevis?

22. How are the flexor carpi radialis and palmaris longus synergistic with each other?

23. What three muscles comprise the wrist extensor group?

24. What muscle is immediately medial to the extensor carpi ulnaris?

25. What two muscles attach to the lateral epicondyle of the humerus but not via the common extensor tendon?

26. What muscle of the deep distal four group attaches the most proximally?

27. What two muscles attach distally into a tendon of the extensor digitorum?

28. What three muscles border the anatomic snuffbox?

29. The abductor pollicis longus becomes superficial by emerging between what two muscles?

30. How are the extensor pollicis brevis and extensor carpi ulnaris antagonistic to each other?

31. The distal attachment of the supinator is immediately deep to what three muscles?

32. What motion of the hand at the wrist joint might occur when the extensor pollicis brevis concentrically contracts?

33. The proximal attachment of the supinator is deep to what muscle?

34. What is the only muscle of the deep distal four group that does not cross the radioulnar joints?

35. Which four muscles comprise the deep distal four group of the forearm?

36. What muscle is antagonistic to the extensor indicis at the distal interphalangeal joint of the index finger?

37. The distal tendons of what two muscles pass deep to the extensor pollicis longus?

38. What happens to the length of the abductor pollicis longus when the thumb flexes at the carpometacarpal joint?

39. Which muscle of the deep distal four group is the deepest?

40. What muscle is immediately deep to the ulnar head of the flexor carpi ulnaris?

41. What three muscles comprise the radial group?

42. What is the major synergist to the anconeus?

43. What muscle is immediately anterior to the extensor carpi ulnaris?

44. How are the flexor carpi radialis (FCR) and flexor carpi ulnaris (FCU) antagonistic to each other?

THE MUSCULAR SYSTEM — Muscles of the Forearm

45. Which "pronator" muscle shares its proximal attachment with the wrist flexor group?

46. What are the two major antagonists to the supinator?

47. What is the common distal attachment of both the pronator teres and quadratus?

48. What happens to the length of the extensors carpi radialis longus and brevis when the hand radially deviates at the wrist joint?

49. What happens to the length of the extensor digitorum as the hand extends at the wrist joint?

50. What four muscles can flex the thumb at the carpometacarpal joint?

51. What is the common proximal attachment of the flexors carpi radialis and ulnaris, and the palmaris longus?

52. What muscle is immediately proximal to the anconeus?

53. What three muscles comprise the wrist flexor group?

54. Which "pronator" muscle crosses the elbow joint as well as the radioulnar joints?

55. How are the flexor carpi radialis and flexor carpi ulnaris synergistic with each other?

56. What five muscles are deep to the extensors digitorum and digiti minimi?

57. What muscle is immediately posterior to the flexor carpi ulnaris?

58. Name a synergist to the finger actions of the flexor digitorum superficialis.

59. What muscle is immediately medial to the extensor carpi radialis brevis in the proximal forearm?

60. Name a muscle that is synergistic to the supinator.

61. Name three powerful synergists to the brachioradialis' action at the elbow joint.

62. What muscle is antagonistic to all three joint actions of the extensor carpi ulnaris?

63. Which muscle is deeper, the flexor pollicis longus or the pronator quadratus?

64. What are the two major antagonists to the extensor digitorum?

65. What joint action occurs when the supinator eccentrically contracts?

66. What muscles attach to the lateral epicondyle via the common extensor tendon?

67. The belly of what muscle is immediately deep to the bellies of the flexor carpi radialis and palmaris longus?

68. What happens to the length of the brachioradialis if the elbow joint is passively flexed?

69. What muscle is immediately posterior to the brachioradialis?

70. What action(s) at the wrist joint are occurring if the flexor carpi ulnaris is eccentrically contracting?

71. What happens to the length of the extensor digitorum as the fingers flex at the metacarpophalangeal and interphalangeal joints?

72. The distal attachment of what muscle creates the dorsal digital expansion?

73. What happens to the length of the extensors carpi radialis longus and brevis when the hand ulnar deviates at the wrist joint?

74. What happens to the length of the flexor carpi ulnaris when the wrist joint is actively extended?

75. What joint action is occurring when the anconeus is shortening?

76. What happens to the length of the flexor pollicis longus if the hand is flexed at the wrist joint?

77. What joint actions may be occurring if the flexor digitorum superficialis is eccentrically contracting?

78. Which finger flexor muscle of the forearm crosses the distal interphalangeal joints?

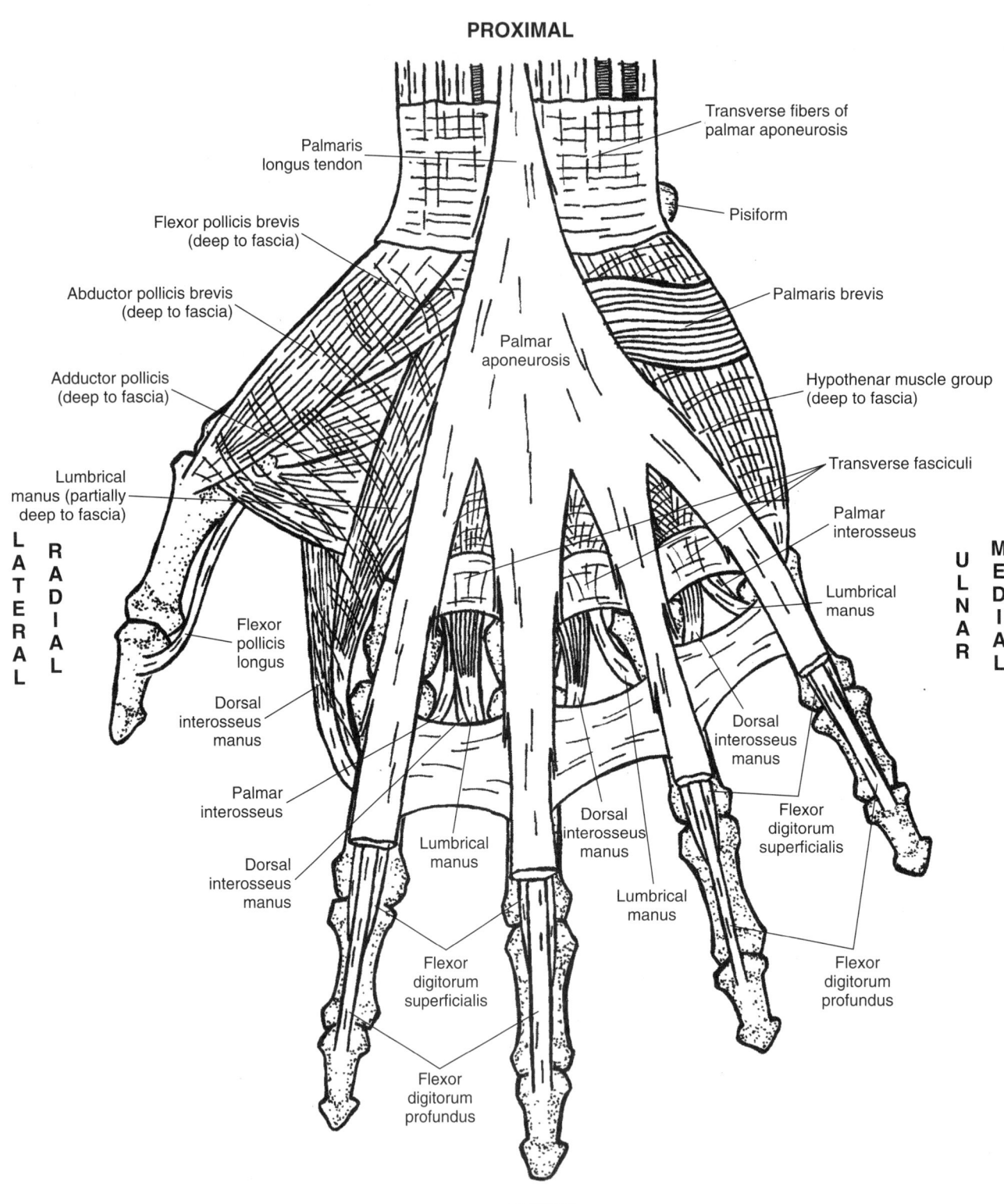

THE MUSCULAR SYSTEM — Muscles of the Hand

PALMAR VIEW OF THE RIGHT HAND (SUPERFICIAL MUSCULAR LAYER)

374 THE MUSCULAR SYSTEM Muscles of the Hand

PALMAR VIEW OF THE RIGHT HAND (DEEP MUSCULAR LAYER)

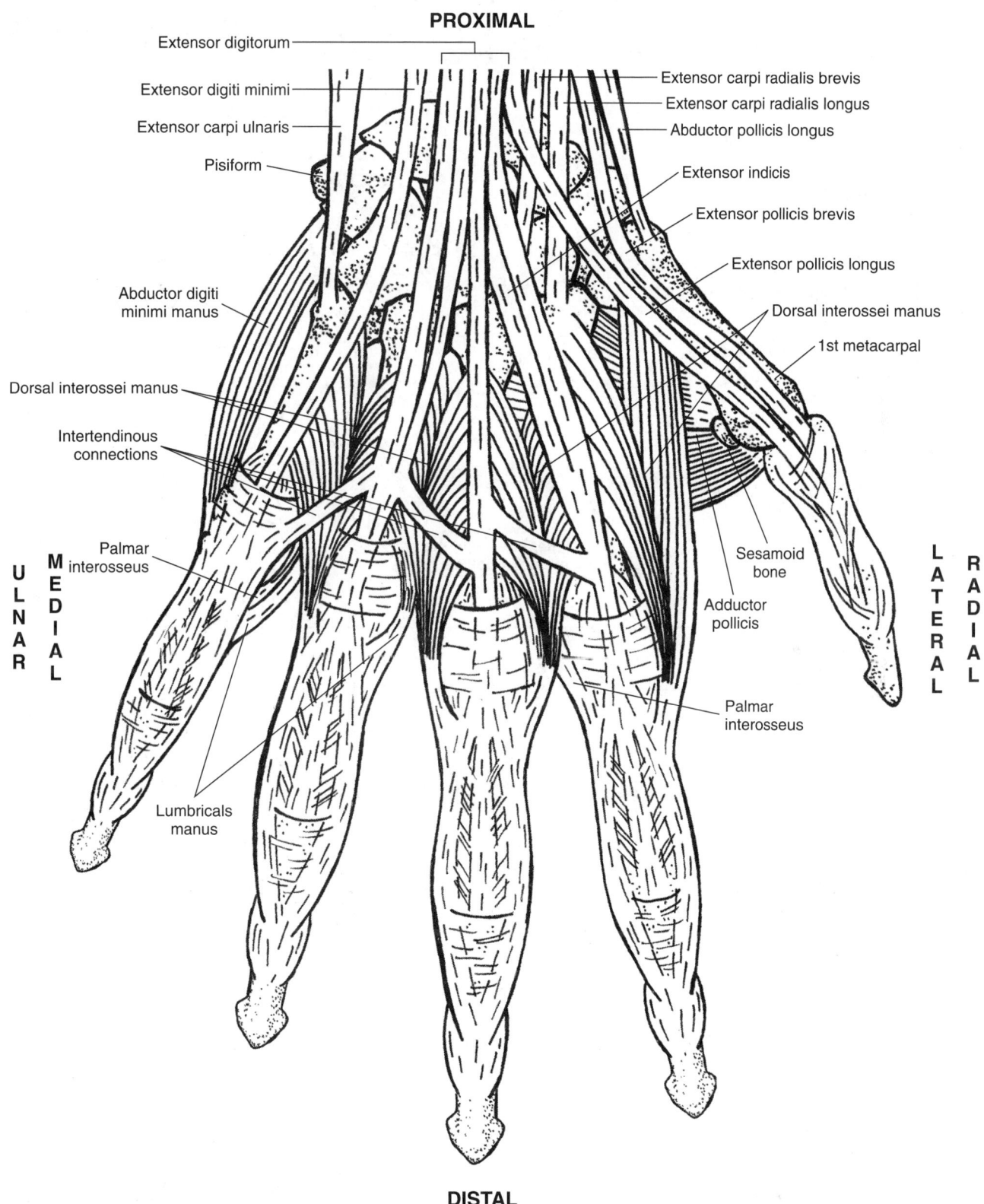

ABDUCTOR POLLICIS BREVIS
(OF THE THENAR EMINENCE)

ab-**duk**-tor **pol**-i-sis **bre**-vis

Actions
Abduction of the thumb at the carpometacarpal joint
Flexion of the thumb at the metacarpophalangeal joint
Extension of the thumb at the carpometacarpal and interphalangeal joints

Innervation
The median nerve

Arterial Supply
Branches of the radial artery

Anterior view of the right abductor pollicis brevis

FLEXOR POLLICIS BREVIS
(OF THE THENAR EMINENCE)

fleks-or **pol**-i-sis **bre**-vis

Actions
Flexion of the thumb at the carpometacarpal and the metacarpophalangeal joints
Abduction of the thumb at the carpometacarpal joint

Innervation
The median and ulnar nerves

Arterial Supply
Branches of the radial artery

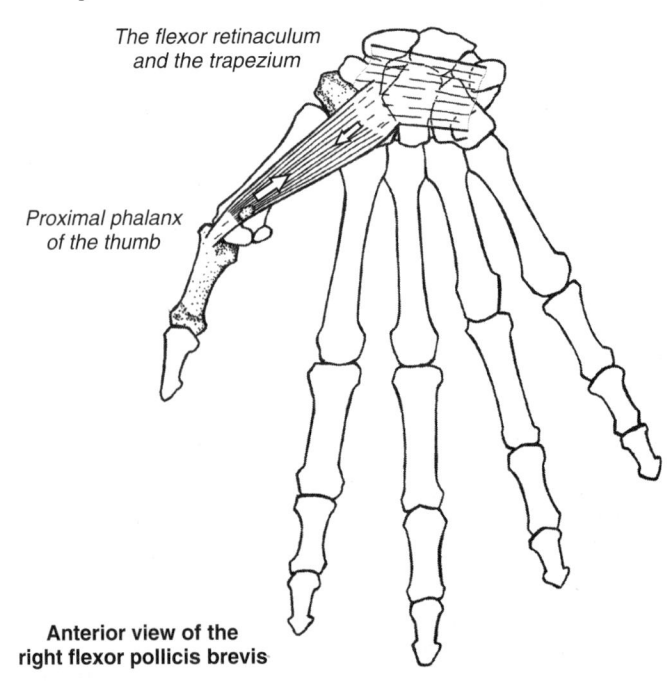

Anterior view of the right flexor pollicis brevis

THE MUSCULAR SYSTEM Muscles of the Hand   377

DID YOU KNOW?

The abductor pollicis brevis is the most superficial of the three muscles of the thenar eminence group.

DID YOU KNOW?

The flexor pollicis brevis of the thenar eminence group has a sesamoid bone in its distal tendon.

OPPONENS POLLICIS
(OF THE THENAR EMINENCE)
op-po-nens pol-i-sis

Actions
Opposition of the thumb at the carpometacarpal joint
Flexion of the thumb at the carpometacarpal joint
Medial rotation of the thumb at the carpometacarpal joint
Abduction of the thumb at the carpometacarpal joint

Innervation
The median and ulnar nerves

Arterial Supply
Branches of the radial artery

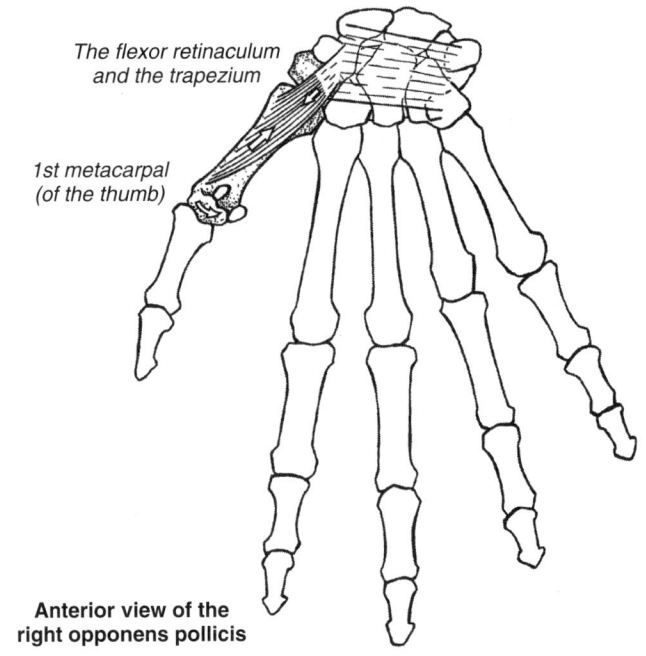

Anterior view of the right opponens pollicis

OPPONENS DIGITI MINIMI
(OF THE HYPOTHENAR EMINENCE)
op-po-nens dij-i-tee min-i-mee

Actions
Opposition of the little finger (finger #5) at the carpometacarpal joint
Flexion of the little finger (finger #5) at the carpometacarpal joint
Adduction of the little finger (finger #5) at the carpometacarpal joint
Lateral rotation of the little finger (finger #5) at the carpometacarpal joint

Innervation
The ulnar nerve

Arterial Supply
Branches of the ulnar artery

Anterior view of the right opponens digiti minimi

THE MUSCULAR SYSTEM Muscles of the Hand 379

DID YOU KNOW?

The opponens pollicis is the only muscle of the thenar eminence group that attaches onto the metacarpal of the thumb instead of the proximal phalanx of the thumb.

DID YOU KNOW?

The thumb is not the only opposable finger; the opponens digiti minimi of the hypothenar group opposes the little finger.

THE MUSCULAR SYSTEM — Muscles of the Hand

ABDUCTOR DIGITI MINIMI MANUS
(OF THE HYPOTHENAR EMINENCE)

ab-**duk**-tor **dij**-i-tee **min**-i-mee **man**-us

Actions
Abduction of the little finger (finger #5) at the carpometacarpal and metacarpophalangeal joints

Extension of the little finger (finger #5) at the proximal and distal interphalangeal joints

Innervation
The ulnar nerve

Arterial Supply
Branches of the ulnar artery

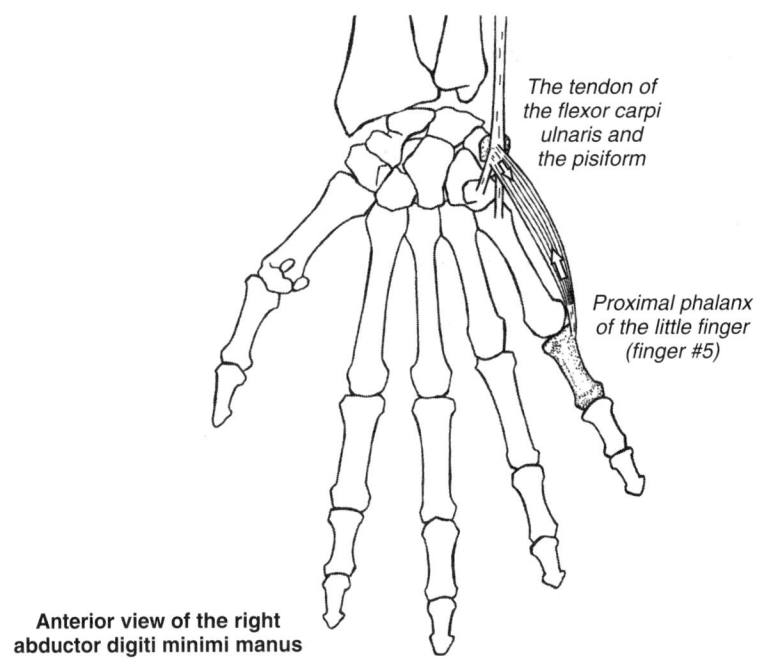

The tendon of the flexor carpi ulnaris and the pisiform

Proximal phalanx of the little finger (finger #5)

Anterior view of the right abductor digiti minimi manus

FLEXOR DIGITI MINIMI MANUS
(OF THE HYPOTHENAR EMINENCE)

fleks-or **dij**-i-tee **min**-i-mee **man**-us

Action
Flexion of the little finger (finger #5) at the metacarpophalangeal joint

Innervation
The ulnar nerve

Arterial Supply
Branches of the ulnar artery

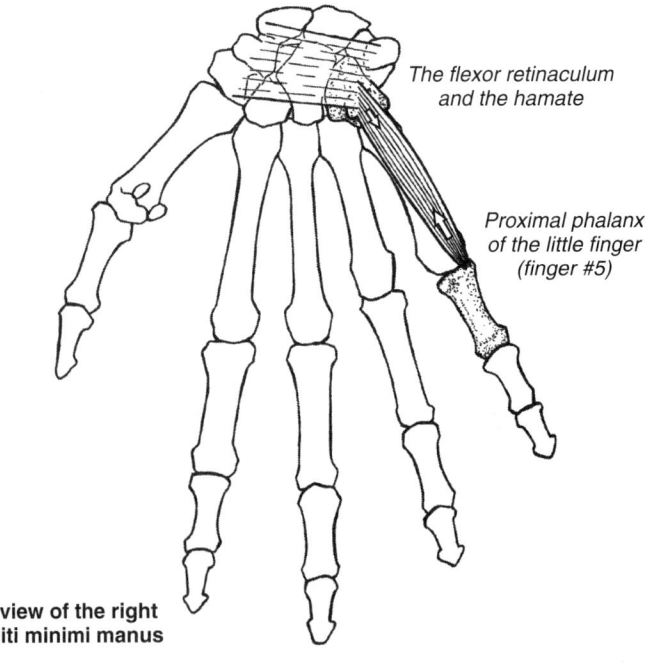

The flexor retinaculum and the hamate

Proximal phalanx of the little finger (finger #5)

Anterior view of the right flexor digiti minimi manus

THE MUSCULAR SYSTEM Muscles of the Hand   381

Abductor digiti minimi manus

Flexor digiti minimi manus

The abductor digiti minimi manus is the most superficial of the three muscles of the hypothenar eminence group.

Abductor digiti minimi manus (cut)

Flexor digiti minimi manus (cut)

The flexor digiti minimi manus of the hypothenar eminence group is often known simply as the flexor digiti minimi or the flexor digiti minimi brevis.

PALMARIS BREVIS
pall-ma-ris bre-vis

The flexor retinaculum and the palmar aponeurosis

Dermis of the ulnar (medial) border of the hand

Anterior view of the right palmaris brevis

Action	Innervation	Arterial Supply
Wrinkles the skin of the palm	The ulnar nerve	The ulnar artery and the superficial palmar branch of the radial artery

THE MUSCULAR SYSTEM Muscles of the Hand

Did you know?

The palmaris brevis' action of wrinkling the skin of the palm contributes to the strength and security of gripping an object in your hand.

Palmaris brevis

ADDUCTOR POLLICIS
(OF THE CENTRAL COMPARTMENT)
ad-**duk**-tor **pol**-i-sis

Actions
Adduction of the thumb at the carpometacarpal joint
Flexion of the thumb at the carpometacarpal and metacarpophalangeal joints
Extension of the thumb at the interphalangeal joint

Innervation
The ulnar nerve

Arterial Supply
Branches of the radial artery

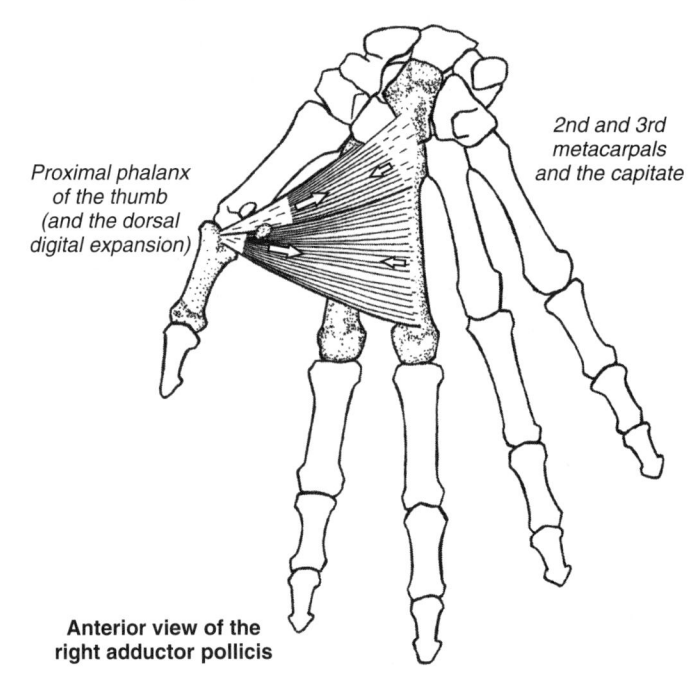

Anterior view of the right adductor pollicis

LUMBRICALS MANUS
(OF THE CENTRAL COMPARTMENT)
(There are four lumbrical manus muscles, named #1, #2, #3, and #4.)
lum-bri-kuls **man**-us

Actions
Extension of fingers #2-5 at the proximal and distal interphalangeal joints
Flexion of fingers #2-5 at the metacarpophalangeal joint

Innervation
The median and ulnar nerves

Arterial Supply
Branches of the radial and ulnar arteries

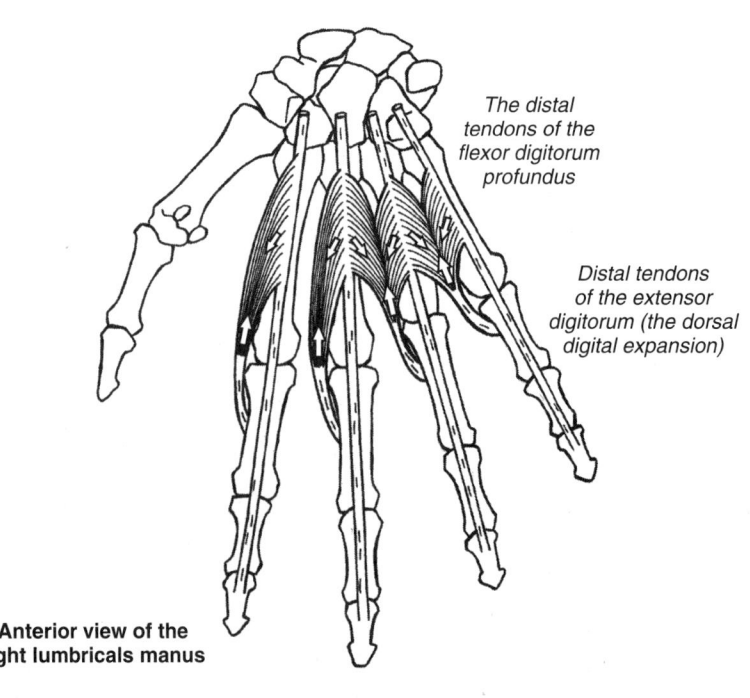

Anterior view of the right lumbricals manus

THE MUSCULAR SYSTEM Muscles of the Hand 385

Adductor pollicis (deep to fascia)

Lumbricals manus

There is a sesamoid bone in the distal tendon of the oblique head of the adductor pollicis.

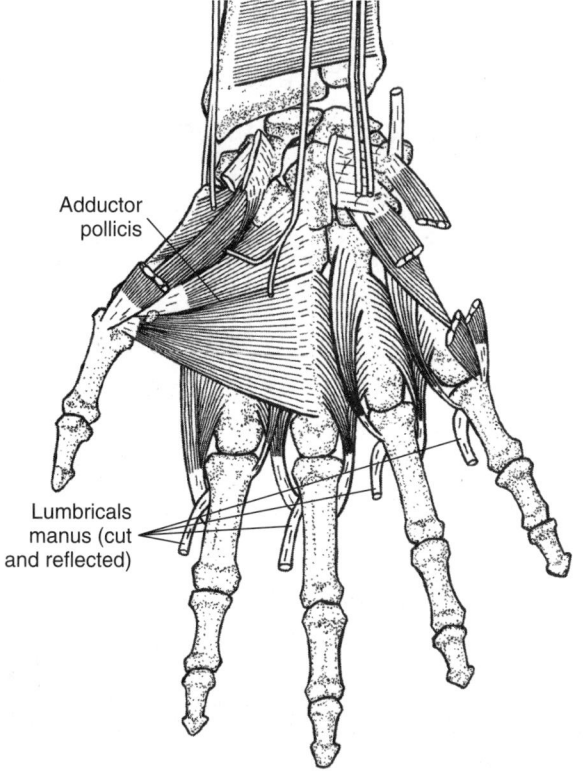

Adductor pollicis

Lumbricals manus (cut and reflected)

The actions of the lumbricals manus (flexion of the proximal phalanges at the metacarpophalangeal joints and extension of the middle and distal phalanges at the interphalangeal joints) puts the hand in the shape of the letter "**L**", as in **L**umbricals ☺.

PALMAR INTEROSSEI
(OF THE CENTRAL COMPARTMENT)
(There are three palmar interossei, named #1, #2, and #3.)

pal-mar in-ter-oss-ee-i

Actions
Adduction of fingers #2, #4, and #5 at the metacarpo-phalangeal joint
Flexion of fingers #2, #4, and #5 at the metacarpophalangeal joint
Extension of fingers #2, #4, and #5 at the proximal and distal interphalangeal joints

Innervation
The ulnar nerve

Arterial Supply
Branches of the radial and ulnar arteries

The metacarpal of fingers #2, #4, and #5

Proximal phalanx of fingers #2, #4, and #5 on the "middle finger side" (and the dorsal digital expansion)

Anterior view of the right palmar interossei

DORSAL INTEROSSEI MANUS
(OF THE CENTRAL COMPARTMENT)
(There are four dorsal interossei manus muscles, named #1, #2, #3, and #4.)

dor-sul in-ter-oss-ee-i man-us

Actions
Abduction of fingers #2, #3, and #4 at the metacarpophalangeal joint
Flexion of fingers #2, #3, and #4 at the metacarpophalangeal joint
Extension of fingers #2, #3, and #4 at the proximal and distal interphalangeal joints

Innervation
The ulnar nerve

Arterial Supply
Branches of the radial and ulnar arteries

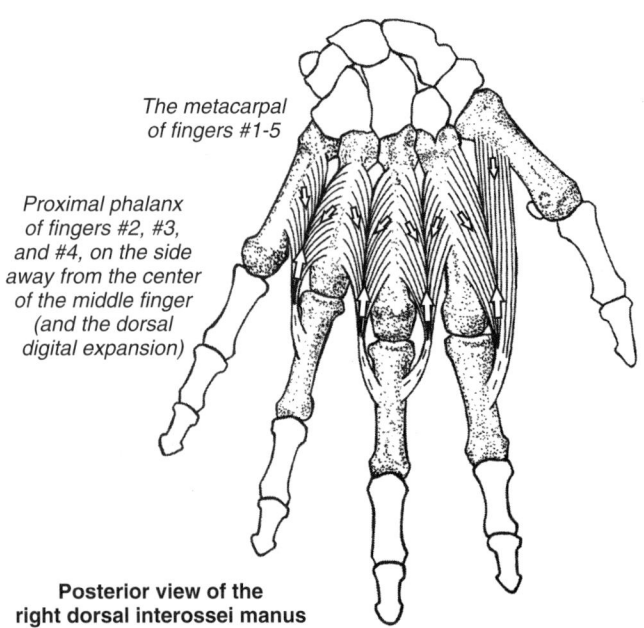

The metacarpal of fingers #1-5

Proximal phalanx of fingers #2, #3, and #4, on the side away from the center of the middle finger (and the dorsal digital expansion)

Posterior view of the right dorsal interossei manus

THE MUSCULAR SYSTEM Muscles of the Hand

 DID YOU KNOW?

The main action of the dorsal interossei manus is abduction of the fingers at the metacarpophalangeal joints. The main action of the palmar interossei is adduction of the fingers at the metacarpophalangeal joints. The mnemonic to remember these actions is **DAB PAD**; **D**orsals **AB**duct, **P**almars **AD**duct.

THE MUSCULAR SYSTEM Muscles of the Hand

PALMAR VIEW OF THE RIGHT HAND (SUPERFICIAL)

Answers to labeling exercises are on p. 470.

THE MUSCULAR SYSTEM Muscles of the Hand

PALMAR VIEW OF THE RIGHT HAND
(SUPERFICIAL MUSCULAR LAYER)

THE MUSCULAR SYSTEM Muscles of the Hand

PALMAR VIEW OF THE RIGHT HAND
(DEEP MUSCULAR LAYER)

THE MUSCULAR SYSTEM Muscles of the Hand

DORSAL VIEW OF THE RIGHT HAND

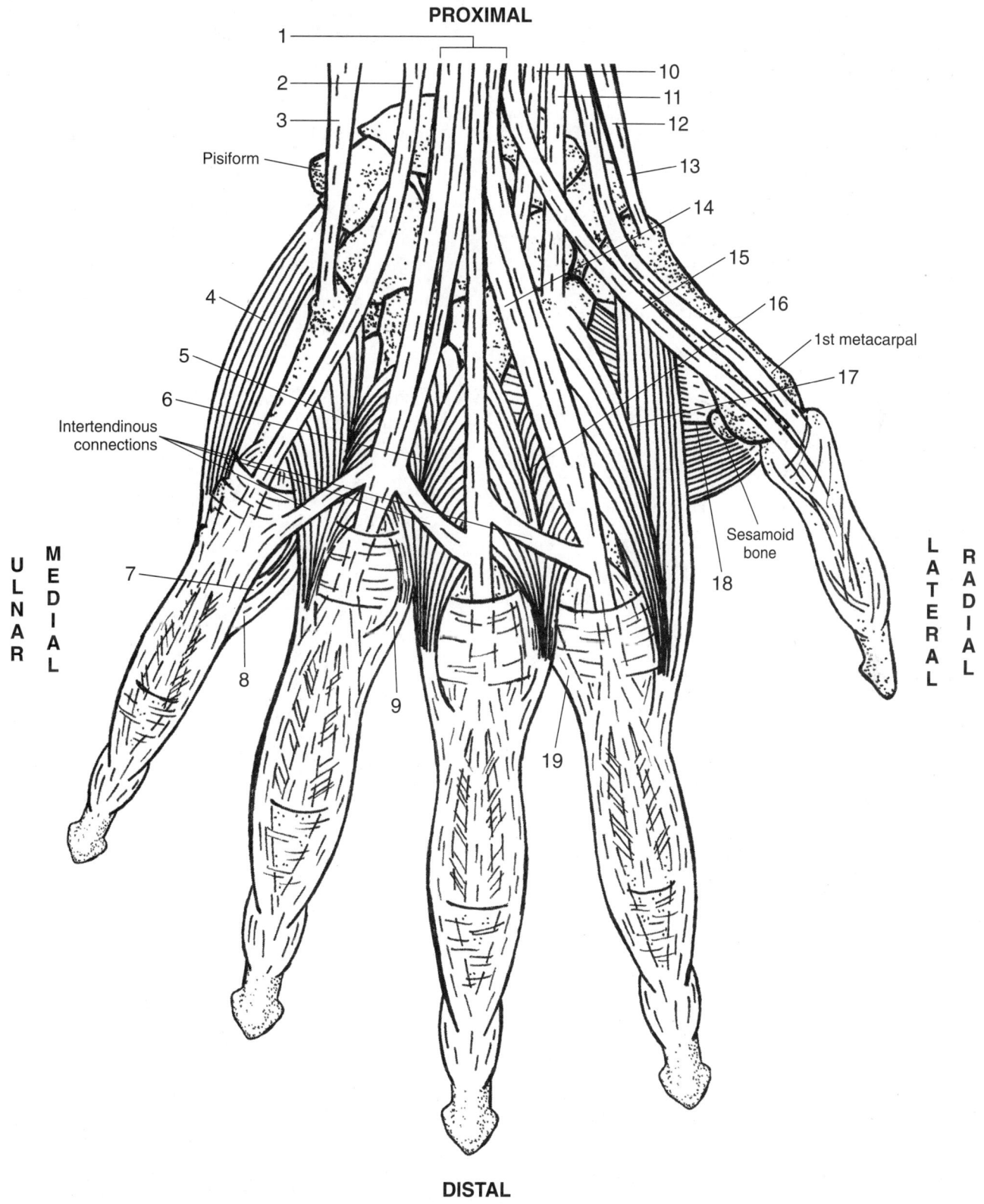

Review Questions

Muscles of the Hand
Answers to these questions are found on page 470.

1. What are the three major groups of intrinsic muscles of the hand?

2. What intrinsic hand muscles are antagonistic to the carpometacarpal action of the adductor pollicis?

3. Which intrinsic hand muscles attach into the dorsal digital expansion?

4. How are the palmar interossei and dorsal interossei manus synergistic with each other?

5. The palmaris brevis is superficial to what group of intrinsic hand muscles?

6. What muscle is synergistic with the palmaris brevis?

7. What muscle is deep to the opponens digiti minimi?

8. What joint action(s) is/are occurring when the flexor pollicis brevis is concentrically contracting?

9. All three muscles of the thenar group attach to which carpal bone?

10. What muscle makes up the majority of the thumb web?

11. Where is the flexor retinaculum located relative to the palmaris brevis?

12. What intrinsic hand muscles comprise the central compartment group?

13. What are the three muscles of the thenar group?

14. What intrinsic muscles of the hand do abduction of the thumb at the carpometacarpal joint?

15. From an anterior perspective, which are deeper, the lumbricals manus or the palmar interossei?

16. What is unusual about the attachments of the palmaris brevis?

17. What intrinsic hand muscles are synergistic to the opponens pollicis?

18. How are the opponens digiti minimi and abductor digiti minimi manus antagonistic to each other?

19. During what functional activity does the palmaris brevis usually contract?

20. What joint action occurs when the flexor digiti minimi manus isometrically contracts?

21. Which thenar group muscle has a sesamoid bone in its distal tendon?

22. From an anterior perspective, where is the adductor pollicis relative to the lumbricals manus?

23. Which is the most superficial muscle of the thenar group?

24. Which intrinsic hand muscles flex fingers at the metacarpophalangeal joints and extend fingers at the interphalangeal joints?

25. If the thumb is passively extended at the carpometacarpal joint, what happens to the length of the flexor pollicis brevis?

26. Which two carpals are attached onto by hypothenar muscles?

27. What joint action occurs when the flexor digiti minimi manus eccentrically contracts?

28. What muscles are deep to the palmaris brevis?

29. What type of rotation does the opponens digiti minimi do?

30. What happens to the length of the abductor pollicis brevis when the adductor pollicis is concentrically contracting and moving the carpometacarpal joint?

31. From a posterior perspective, which are deeper, the palmar interossei or the dorsal interossei manus?

32. What are the three intrinsic hand muscles of the hypothenar group?

33. What is similar about the distal attachments of the opponens pollicis and opponens digiti minimi?

34. Do the lumbricals manus flex and/or extend the fingers?

35. What muscle is immediately superficial to the opponens digiti minimi?

36. How are the palmar interossei and dorsal interossei manus antagonistic to each other?

Other Skeletal Muscles 3

GET READY TO EXPLORE:

Anterior Views of the Other Muscles of the Abdomen, 396

Views of the Muscles of the Perineum, 397

Views of the Muscles of the Tongue, 398

View of the Muscles of the Palate, 399

View of the Muscles of the Pharynx, 400

Views of the Muscles of the Larynx, 401

Views of the Muscles of the Larynx, 402

Views of the Extrinsic Muscles of the Right Eye, 403

View of the Muscles of the Tympanic Cavity, 404

Answers to labeling exercises are on p. 470.

More review activities on Evolve at http://evolve.elsevier.com/Muscolino/muscular/

395

OTHER SKELETAL MUSCLES

ANTERIOR VIEWS OF THE OTHER MUSCLES OF THE ABDOMEN

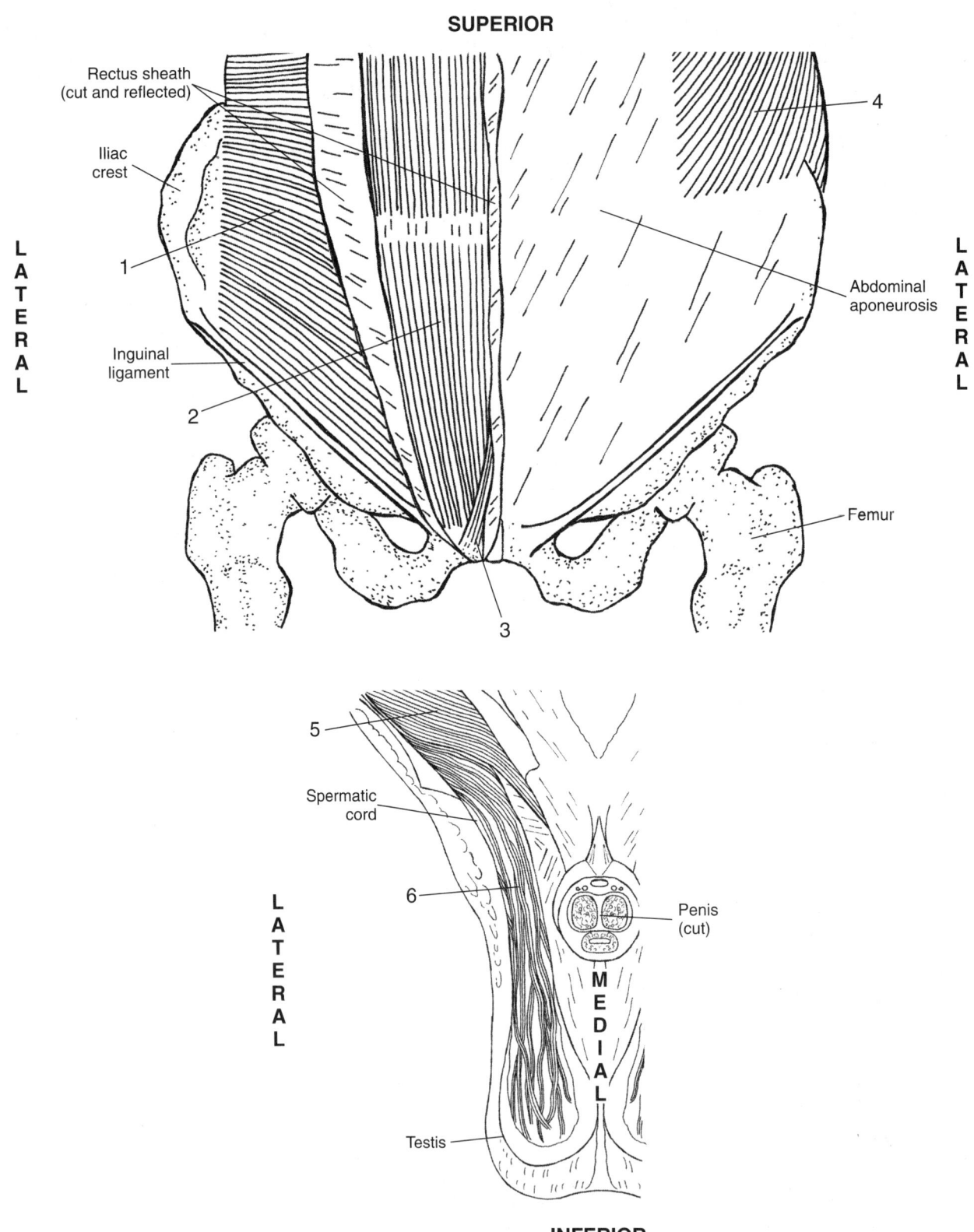

OTHER SKELETAL MUSCLES 397

VIEWS OF THE MUSCLES OF THE PERINEUM

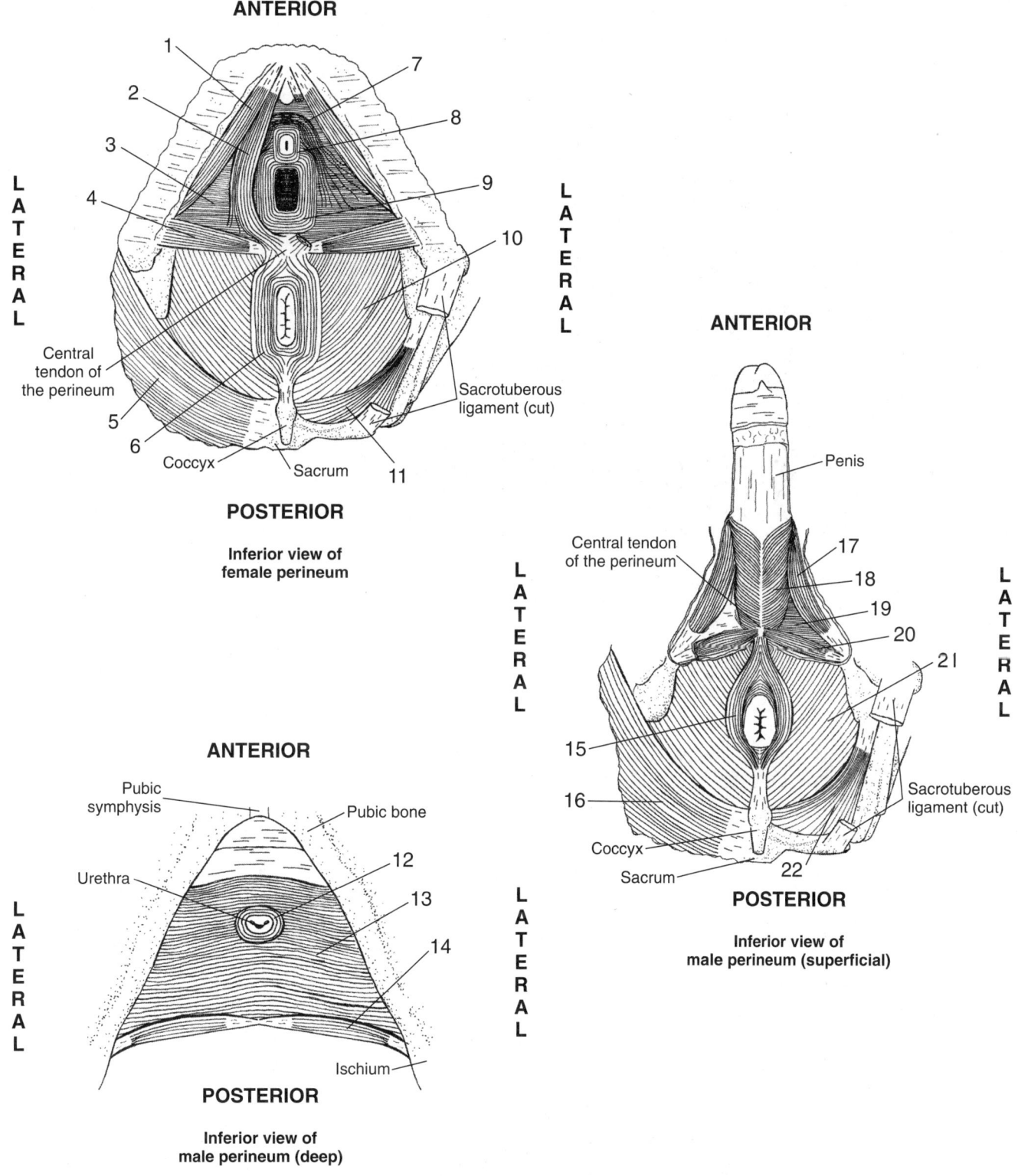

VIEWS OF THE MUSCLES OF THE TONGUE

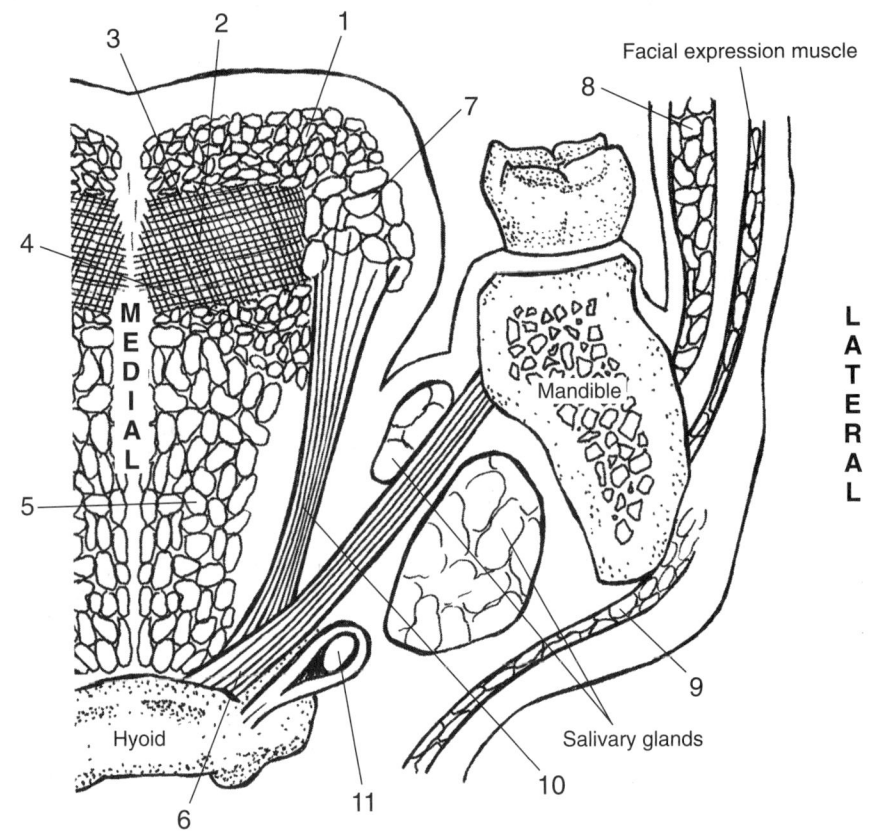

Anterior view (frontal plane section)

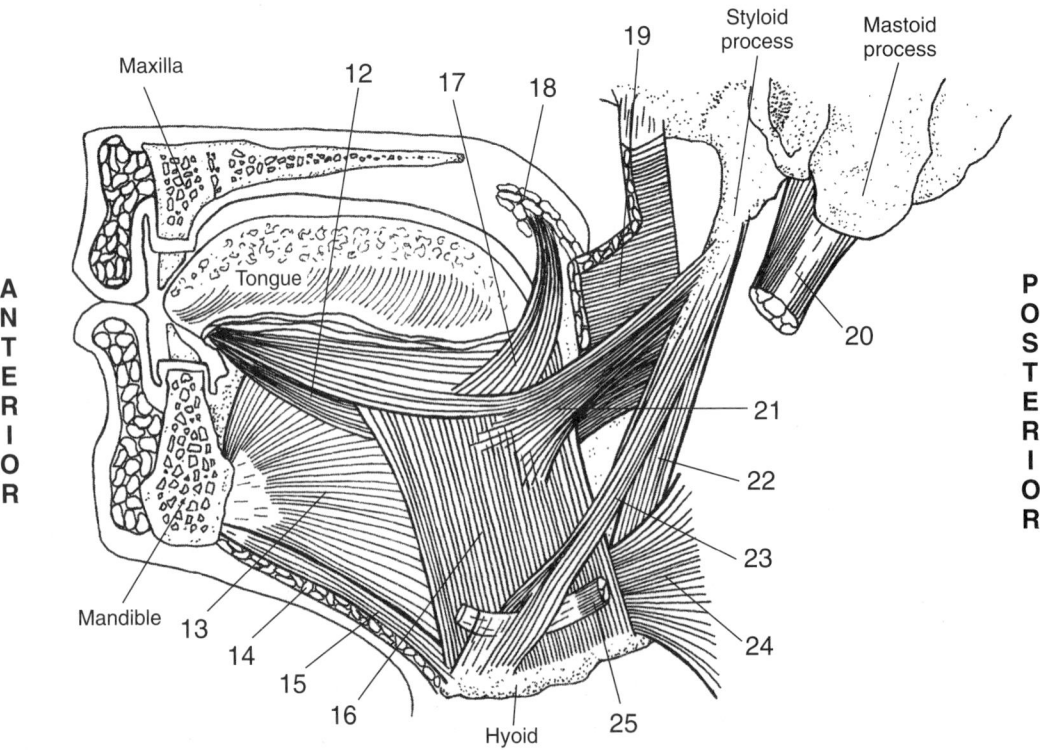

Lateral view (sagittal plane section)

OTHER SKELETAL MUSCLES

VIEW OF THE MUSCLES OF THE PALATE

Medial view (sagittal plane section)

OTHER SKELETAL MUSCLES

VIEW OF THE MUSCLES OF THE PHARYNX

Posterior view
(opened up on the right side)

OTHER SKELETAL MUSCLES 401

VIEWS OF THE MUSCLES OF THE LARYNX

Lateral view

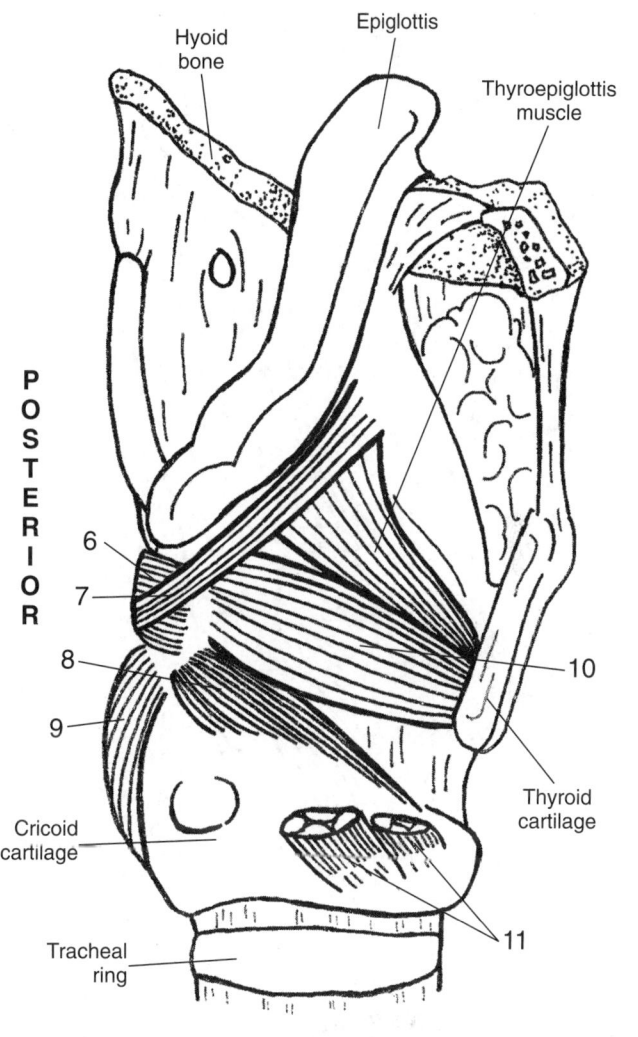

Lateral view (dissected)

VIEWS OF THE MUSCLES OF THE LARYNX

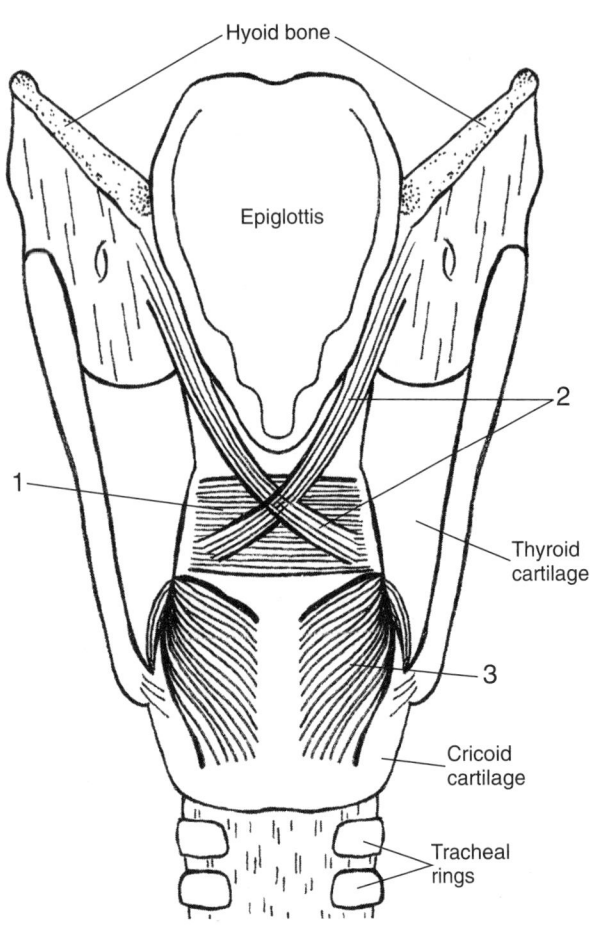

OTHER SKELETAL MUSCLES 403

VIEWS OF THE EXTRINSIC MUSCLES OF THE RIGHT EYE

Lateral view

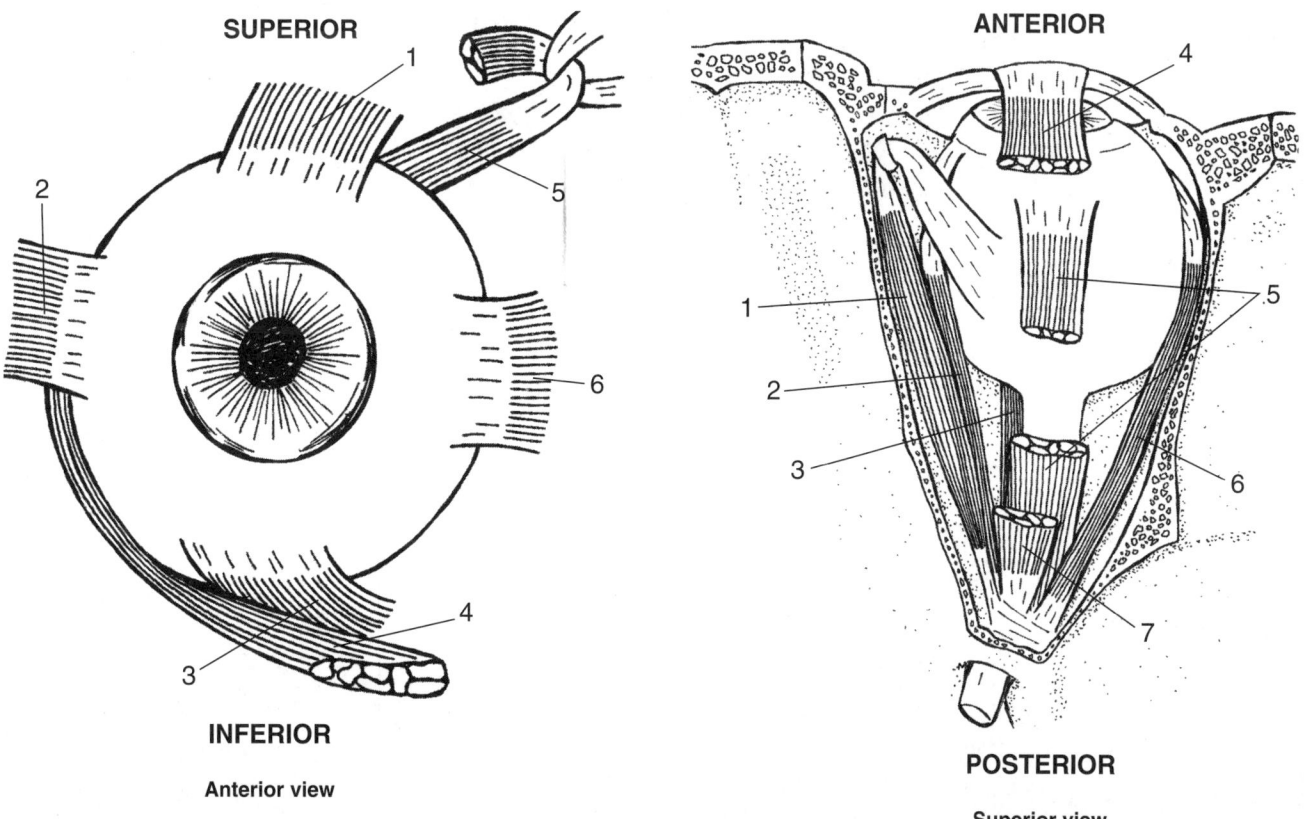

Anterior view

Superior view

OTHER SKELETAL MUSCLES

VIEW OF THE MUSCLES OF THE TYMPANIC CAVITY

Medial view (within the temporal bone)

The Nervous System 4

GET READY TO EXPLORE:

Cranial Nerves, 406

View of Spinal Nerve Organization, 407

View of the Cervical Plexus, 408

View of the Brachial Plexus, 409

View of the Lumbar Plexus, 410

View of the Sacral and Coccygeal Plexuses, 411

Views of Innervation to the Right Lower Extremity, 412

Anterior View of Innervation to the Right Upper Extremity, 413

Answers to labeling exercises are on p. 471.

More review activities on Evolve at http://evolve.elsevier.com/Muscolino/muscular/

THE NERVOUS SYSTEM

CRANIAL NERVES

ANTERIOR

POSTERIOR

Inferior view of the brain

THE NERVOUS SYSTEM

VIEW OF SPINAL NERVE ORGANIZATION

Cross section view of the spinal cord through a cervical vertebra—spinal nerve diagram

THE NERVOUS SYSTEM

VIEW OF THE CERVICAL PLEXUS

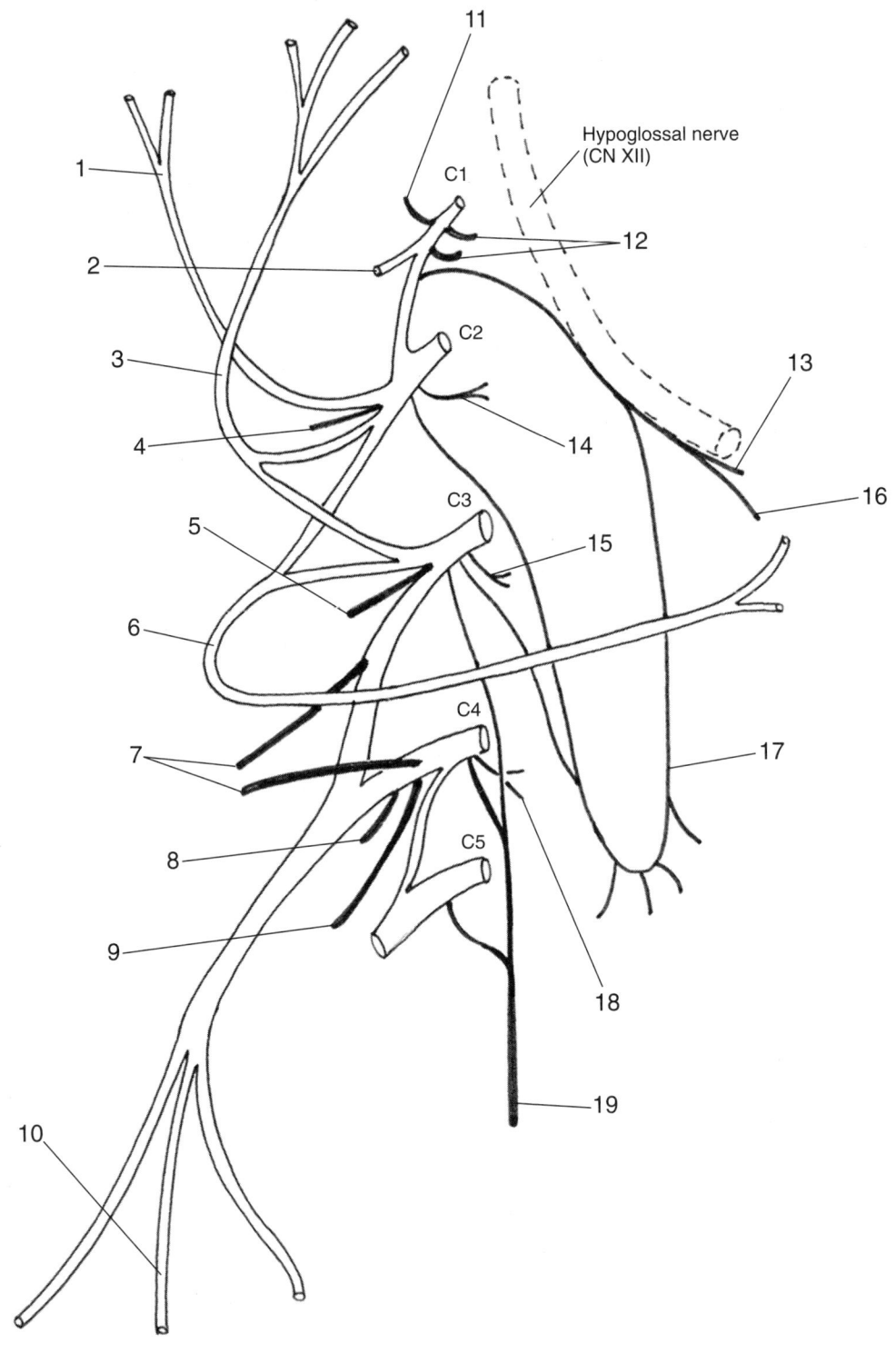

THE NERVOUS SYSTEM

VIEW OF THE BRACHIAL PLEXUS

VIEW OF THE LUMBAR PLEXUS

VIEW OF THE SACRAL AND COCCYGEAL PLEXUSES

THE NERVOUS SYSTEM

VIEWS OF INNERVATION TO THE RIGHT LOWER EXTREMITY

THE NERVOUS SYSTEM

ANTERIOR VIEW OF INNERVATION TO THE RIGHT UPPER EXTREMITY

The Arterial System 5

GET READY TO EXPLORE:

Lateral View of Arterial Supply to the Head and Neck, 416

Anterior View of Arterial Supply to the Trunk and Pelvis, 417

Anterior View of Arterial Supply to the Right Lower Extremity, 418

Anterior View of Arterial Supply to the Right Upper Extremity, 419

Answers to labeling exercises are on p. 471.

More review activities on Evolve at http://evolve.elsevier.com/Muscolino/muscular/

416 THE ARTERIAL SYSTEM

LATERAL VIEW OF ARTERIAL SUPPLY TO THE HEAD AND NECK

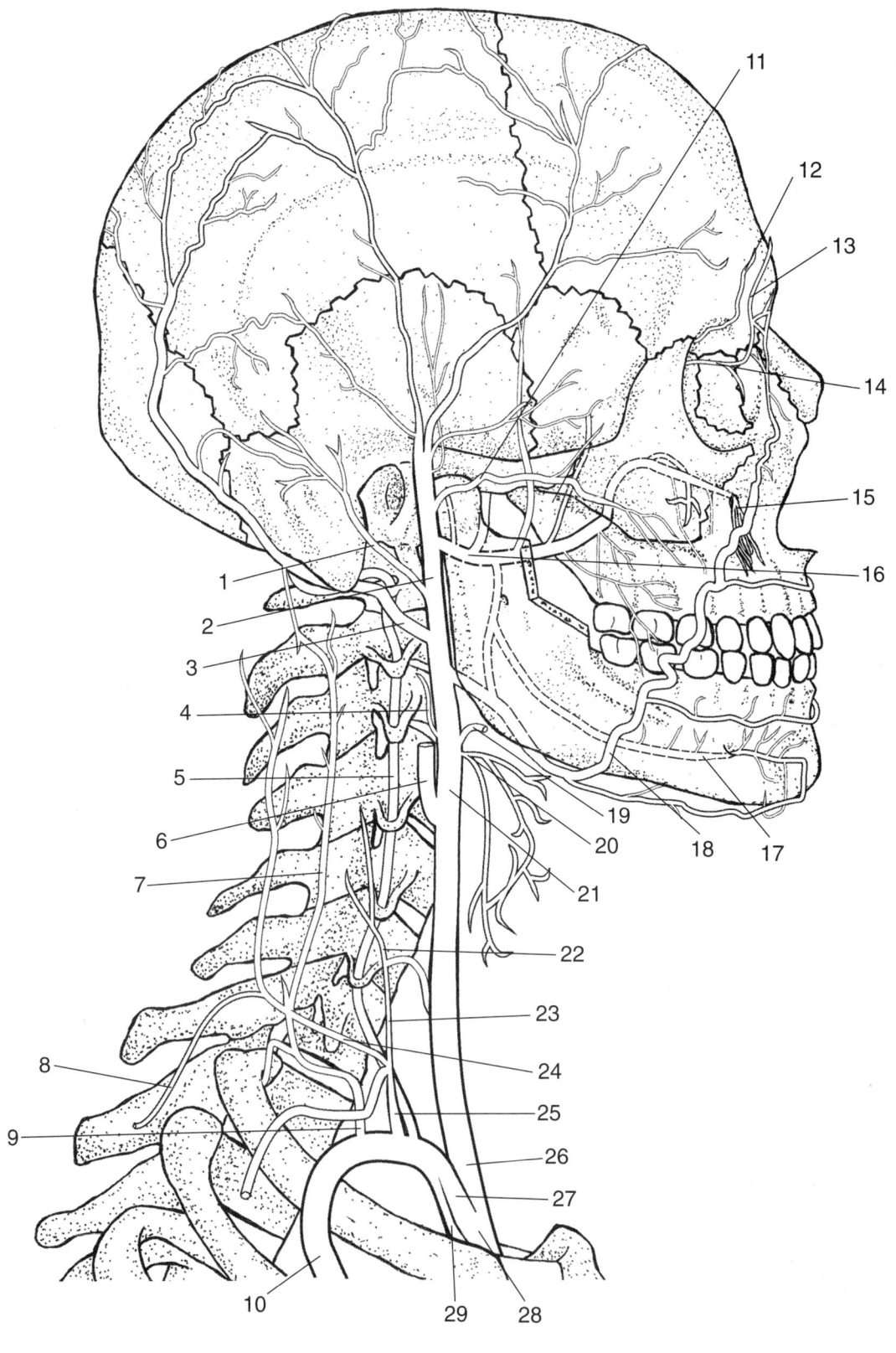

THE ARTERIAL SYSTEM 417

ANTERIOR VIEW OF ARTERIAL SUPPLY TO THE TRUNK AND PELVIS

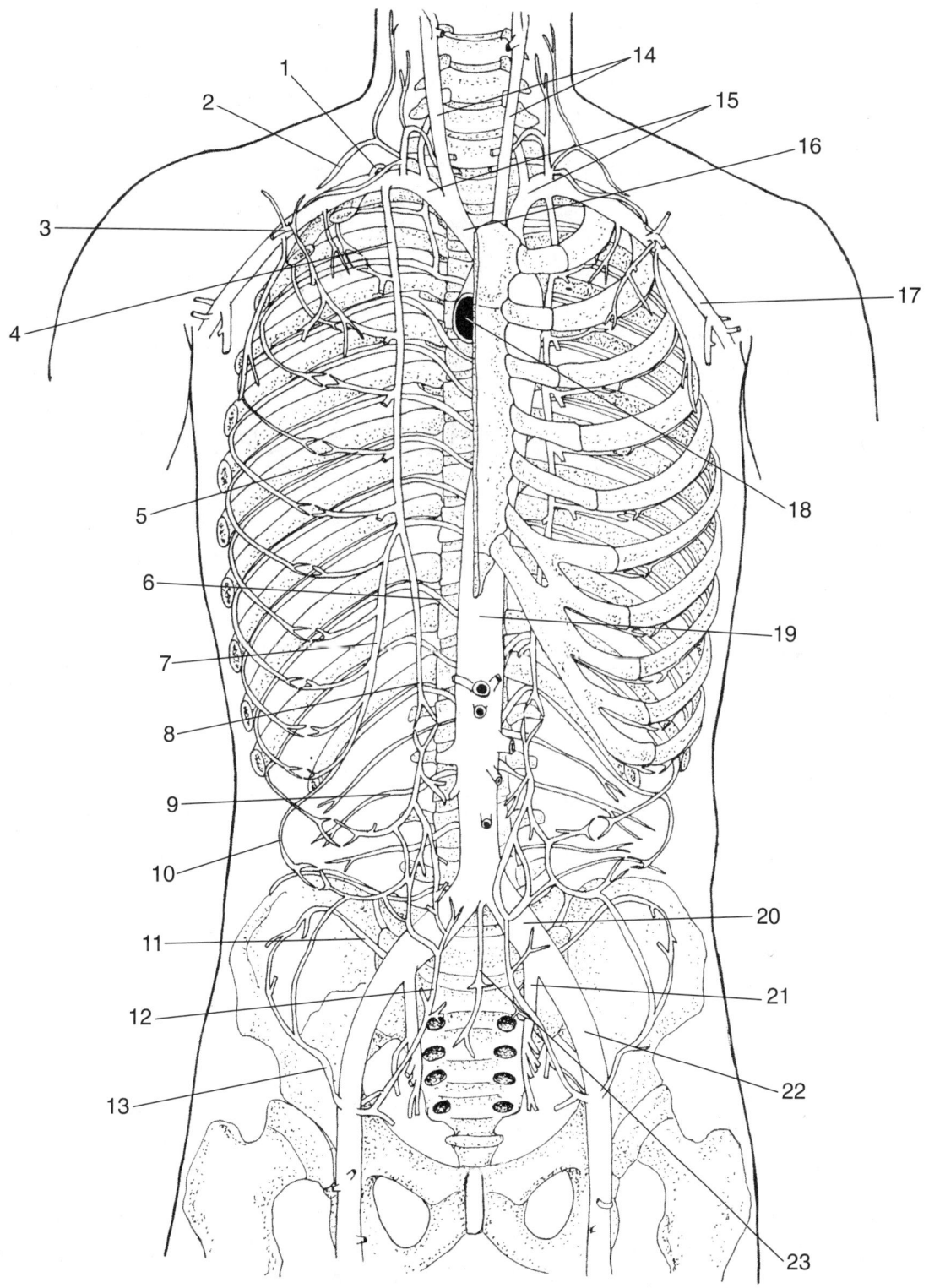

418 THE ARTERIAL SYSTEM

ANTERIOR VIEW OF ARTERIAL SUPPLY TO THE RIGHT LOWER EXTREMITY

THE ARTERIAL SYSTEM

ANTERIOR VIEW OF ARTERIAL SUPPLY TO THE RIGHT UPPER EXTREMITY

Tissue Structure and Other Systems of the Body 6

GET READY TO EXPLORE:

The Cell, 426

Bone Tissue, 428

Muscle Tissue, 430

Nerve Tissue, 434

Joints, 436

Integumentary System, 438

Cardiac System (The Heart), 440

Venous System, 442

Lymphatic System, 444

Respiratory System, 446

Urinary System, 448

Gastrointestinal System, 450

Immune System, 452

Endocrine System, 454

Sensory System, 456

Reproductive System, 459

Answers to labeling exercises are on p. 472.

More review activities on Evolve at http://evolve.elsevier.com/Muscolino/muscular/

BRIEF OVERVIEW OF THE SYSTEMS OF THE BODY

The Cell

The cell is the basic structural and functional building block of the human body. While cells are diverse in structure (and function), there are certain essential elements of most cells. Cells essentially have two parts, an inner nucleus and the surrounding cytoplasmic fluid; both of these two structures have a semipermeable membrane around them. The nucleus contains DNA (the genetic blueprint) and the nucleolus (which makes ribosomes). In the cytoplasm, there are many organelles (small organs), each with a particular function. These organelles are held in place by fine filaments that are found in the cytoplasm; these filaments create a skeletal structure for the cell called the *cytoskeleton*.

The major cytoplasmic organelles are: ribosomes (they function to synthesize proteins), mitochondria (they turn glucose and oxygen into ATP molecules for energy), endoplasmic reticulum (there are two types, "rough" and "smooth"; they function as a transport system within the cell), golgi apparatus (which functions to refine and transport proteins), and lysosomes (which digest and break down intracellular substances).

There are also organelles that can be located on the outside membrane of the cell. These structures are called *cilia* and *flagella*, both of which function to create movement, either of the cell itself, or of substances along the surface of the cell. Usually, a cell has either one long flagellum or numerous shorter cilia.

Integumentary System

An integument is a covering; hence the integumentary system covers the body. The integumentary system is comprised of the cutaneous membrane, (i.e., the skin, and the accessory organs of the skin). The skin has two layers to it: the outer epidermis, which is stratified squamous epithelium, and the deeper dermis, which is fibrous connective tissue. The accessory organs are the hair follicles, arrector pili muscles, sebaceous glands, and eccrine and apocrine sweat glands. The main function of the skin is to provide a barrier between the inside of our body and the outside world. This barrier prevents pathogens (disease-causing microorganisms) from entering the body and keeps moisture and body contents from escaping. The skin also functions to help regulate internal body temperature by two processes: (1) sweating; and (2) dermal blood vessel dilation, which regulates the amount of blood that flows to the skin for exchange of heat with the outside world. Deep to the skin is subcutaneous fascia.

Cardiovascular System

The cardiovascular system is made up of the cardiac system and the vascular system. The cardiac system is comprised of the heart; the vascular system is comprised of blood vessels (i.e., the arteries, capillaries, and the veins).

The heart is essentially a double pump, having a left side and a right side (each side having two chambers: an atrium and a ventricle). The heart's left side pumps oxygen-rich/carbon dioxide–poor blood into vessels that bring the blood out to the cells and tissues of the body; this is called the *systemic circulation*. At the cellular/tissue level, these vessels give their oxygen (and other nutrients) to the cells so that the vital processes of metabolism can occur. These vessels also pick up carbon dioxide (and other waste products) from the cells and transport these substances back to the right side of the heart. The heart's right side then pumps this oxygen-poor/carbon dioxide–rich blood to the lungs, where it is oxygenated and loses much of its carbon dioxide; this is called the *pulmonic circulation*. This oxygen-rich/carbon dioxide–poor blood then returns back to the left side of the heart where it can be pumped out to the cells and tissues of the body once again.

It is the vessels of the cardiovascular system that carry the blood that is pumped by the heart. There are three types of blood vessels: arteries, capillaries, and veins.

Arteries carry blood away from the heart. As they do so, arteries branch and diminish in size, eventually becoming capillaries. Capillaries are thinwalled vessels that do the essential job of exchange of oxygen and carbon dioxide (and other nutrients and waste products) with the intercellular fluid around the cells. Capillaries then converge with each other to form veins, which carry the blood back to the heart. NOTE: Arteries in the systemic circulation carry "oxygenated" blood; arteries in the pulmonic circulation carry "deoxygenated" blood; veins in the systemic circulation carry "deoxygenated" blood; veins in the pulmonic circulation carry "oxygenated" blood. Hence, the cardiovascular system is a double circulation. The systemic circulation is created by the left side of the heart pumping to the cells/tissues of the body and the return of this blood to the right side of the heart; the pulmonic circulation is created by the right side of the heart pumping to the lungs and the return of this blood to the left side of the heart.

Lymphatic System

Not all the fluid of the systemic blood that is pumped out to the tissues of the body by the arteries is returned back to the heart by the veins. A small amount of the fluid that leaves the capillaries at the tissue level is left behind in the tissues. If this extra intercellular tissue fluid is not removed, a build-up of fluid (swelling) will occur in the tissues of the body. It is the job of the lymphatic system to return this fluid back to the heart. The lymphatic system does this by carrying this fluid in lymphatic vessels (where it is termed "lymph") back toward the heart. It actually deposits the lymph into a large vein; from there the venous system returns this fluid back to the right side of the heart. Along the way, the lymph in lymphatic vessels travels through lymph nodes that are high in white blood cells that filter the blood, attacking any foreign disease-causing pathogens. Hence, the lymphatic system has two purposes: to return extra tissue fluid back to the heart and to filter possible pathogens from the blood.

Respiratory System

Oxygen is one of the most important nutrients that the cardiovascular system circulates to the tissues of the body. It is the job of the respiratory system to bring oxygen into the body and place this oxygen into the cardiovascular system. The respiratory system may be divided into the passageways that carry oxygen to the lungs when we breathe in (inspiration), and the lungs themselves. The passageways include: the nose, nasal cavity, mouth, pharynx, larynx, and the trachea. The lungs contain the bronchial tree and the alveolar sacs. It is in the lungs that the blood that comes from the right side of the heart (pulmonic circulation) picks up oxygen to return to the left side of the heart where it can be pumped to the cells and tissues of the body (systemic circulation). The lungs also pick up the waste product carbon dioxide from the blood; this carbon dioxide is then transported out of the lungs to the outside world through the aforementioned passageways when we breathe out (expiration). Hence, the respiratory system has two purposes: to carry oxygen into the body and place it into the blood, and to eliminate carbon dioxide from the blood and carry it out of the body.

Urinary System

As the cardiovascular system circulates blood throughout the body, waste products from cellular metabolism accumulate within the blood. It is the job of the two kidneys of the urinary system to filter these waste products from the blood. The waste products that the kidneys filter from the blood form urine, which leaves each kidney through a long muscular tube called a *ureter*; the two ureters carry the urine to the urinary bladder. The urine is stored in the urinary bladder until a sufficient amount is present. The urine is then expelled from the urinary bladder through the urethra to the outside world. This process of expelling urine is called *urination* or *micturition*.

Gastrointestinal System

As we have said, the cells of the body must be constantly supplied with nutrients by the bloodstream. Other than oxygen that comes from the lungs, these nutrients come from the gastrointestinal system. The gastrointestinal system is comprised of two parts: a long passageway called the *alimentary canal* that begins at the mouth and ends at the anus, and the accessory organs that secrete substances (primarily enzymes) into the alimentary canal. The alimentary canal consists of the mouth, pharynx, esophagus, stomach, small intestine, and large intestine. The accessory organs are the salivary glands, pancreas, liver, and gall bladder. The gastrointestinal system essentially functions as follows: food enters at the mouth; as the food travels through the alimentary canal, whatever is digested and absorbed is taken into the bloodstream for use in the body (i.e., nutrients that the bloodstream carries to the cells); whatever substances are not digested and absorbed continue through the alimentary canal and exit through the anus as feces. The liver also functions to filter unwanted chemicals of the body (both created by metabolism and ingested from external sources) from the blood.

Immune System

"Immunity" means freedom. It is the function of your immune system to keep you free from disease. The immune system does this by fighting foreign microorganisms such as bacteria and viruses (pathogens) that might cause infection and disease. The most important cells of your body that do this are macrophages and a type of white blood cell called *lymphocytes*. There are two main types of lymphocytes, T-lymphocytes and B-lymphocytes (also known as *T cells* and *B cells*); each one of them attacks pathogens in a different manner. T-lymphocytes directly attack the pathogens, engaging in cell to cell contact, secreting substances that are toxic to the pathogen; further, T-lymphocytes help to activate B-lymphocytes. B-lymphocytes secrete antibodies (immunoglobulins) that attack the pathogens. Macrophages destroy pathogens by the process of phagocytosis, in which the pathogens are ingested into the macrophage and broken down by the lysosomes of the macrophage.

Endocrine System

The endocrine system is composed of structures that secrete hormones into the bloodstream. The major endocrine glands are the hypothalamus, pituitary, thyroid, parathyroid, adrenal, pancreas, testes, and ovaries. Other endocrine glands are the pineal and thymus. Generally, the hormones of the hypothalamus control the hormone production of the pituitary and the hormones of the pituitary then control the hormone secretions of other glands such as the thyroid, adrenal, testes, and ovaries. The function of hormones is to act as chemical messengers that regulate the metabolic processes of the body. The endocrine system is also intimately linked to the nervous system of the body; indeed the hypothalamus and pituitary (as well as the pineal gland) are structures of the brain.

Sensory System

The sensory system is the system of receptors in the body that allows us to sense the external world around us as well as sense the internal environment of our body. The senses are usually divided into the somatic senses and special senses. Somatic senses are touch, pressure, temperature, pain, and stretch receptors. Somatic sensory receptors are primarily located in the skin and around the joints. Special senses are smell, taste, vision, hearing, and equilibrium. Special sensory receptors are located in the nasal cavity, mouth, eyes, and ears. All sensory stimuli travel to the central nervous system where they are processed and interpreted. Given these sensory stimuli, the central nervous system determines the appropriate response(s) for our health, enjoyment, and safety.

Nervous System

The nervous system is the master controller of the body. The cells of the nervous system are called *nerve cells* or *neurons*. These neurons carry their messages by the transmission of electrical impulses. There are five types of neuroglial cells that support the neurons in various ways.

Structurally, the nervous system can be divided into the central nervous system (CNS) and the peripheral nervous system (PNS). The central nervous system is in the center of your body; it is comprised of the brain and spinal cord. The brain can be further subdivided into the cerebral hemispheres, cerebellar hemispheres, diencephalon, midbrain, pons, and medulla oblongata. The peripheral nervous system is comprised of all nerves that are located peripheral to the central nervous system; these are the 12 pairs of cranial nerves and the 31 pairs of spinal nerves.

Functionally, the neurons of the nervous system can carry three types of electrical messages: sensory, integrative, and motor. Sensory signals travel through peripheral sensory nerves to the central nervous system. The central nervous system then integrates these sensory stimuli and a response is determined. The order to execute this response, an impulse, then travels through peripheral motor nerves to whatever muscle or gland is being ordered to take action.

The nervous system is a tremendously complex system that controls and coordinates virtually everything in the human body. Further, it is responsible for conscious thought, emotional feeling, memory, and movement, as well as unconscious control of our body.

Reproductive System

The reproductive system has the job of carrying on our species into the future by creating offspring. There are two reproductive systems: the male and female.

The male reproductive system functions to create sperm, maintain them, and then deliver them to the site of fertilization (the reproductive system of the female). The primary structures of the male reproductive system are the testes, which produce the sperm. The accessory organs of the male reproductive system function to maintain and deliver the sperm to the site of fertilization. The accessory reproductive organs can be divided into internal and external structures. The internal accessory reproductive organs are the epididymis, vas deference, seminal vesicle, prostate gland, and the bulbourethral glands. The external accessory reproductive organs are the scrotum and the penis.

The female reproductive system functions to create eggs, maintain and deliver them to the site of fertilization, and if fertilization occurs, provide a favorable environment for the developing offspring to grow, and then deliver the offspring to the outside world. The primary structures of the female reproductive system are the ovaries, which produce the eggs. The accessory organs of the female reproductive system function to carry on the other activities as listed above. The internal accessory reproductive organs are the fallopian tubes, uterus, and the vagina. The external accessory reproductive organs are the labia majora, labia minora, clitoris, vestibular glands, and the vestibular bulb.

Overview of the Interrelationships of the Organ Systems of the Body—The Big Picture

The preceding was a brief overview of the major visceral organ systems of the body, each one described somewhat independently. However, understanding how each system of the body works without understanding the bigger picture of how these systems interrelate to create the smooth operation of the human body as a whole is like understanding what each piece of a jigsaw puzzle looks like without having any sense of what the bigger picture is that the puzzle creates. Toward that end, the following is a glimpse of the bigger picture of how the organ systems of the human interrelate to operate our body. Admittedly, it is a gross simplification, but is still useful for our purposes.

Our body is composed of trillions of cells, each one a living entity that requires two things: 1) nutrients to carry on its functions, and 2) its waste products to be carried away.

These two crucial jobs fall to the cardiovascular system, along with the aid of the lymphatic system (together, these two systems comprise the circulatory system). These two systems circulate fluid (blood and lymph) that carries the nutrients and wastes of the cells of the body. As the circulation of blood occurs, needed nutrients are used up. It is the job of the respiratory system to bring in needed oxygen to the blood and it is the job of the gastrointestinal system to bring in most every other needed nutrient. As the blood circulates, it also builds up waste products of metabolism and other undesired elements, and needs to be filtered. The blood is filtered by the lungs, lymph nodes, kidney, and liver. The integumentary system provides a covering or barrier between the internal contents and the outside world. This barrier is especially important in preventing foreign microorganisms from entering our body and causing infection and disease. When pathogens do find entry into the body, the immune system functions to attack these foreign invaders. The endocrine system secretes hormones into the bloodstream that function to control the metabolism of the body. Sensory receptors gather sensory stimuli and carry these stimuli to the central nervous system of the body. The brain and spinal cord of the central nervous system then integrate and interpret these sensory stimuli and determine what response(s) the body will have. It is the responsibility of the reproductive system to see that our species is continued into the future by the birth of offspring.

For all movement of the body, the musculoskeletal system is involved. The musculoskeletal system is comprised of the bones of the skeleton, the joints located between the bones, and the muscles that move the bones at the joints of the body.

TISSUE STRUCTURE AND OTHER SYSTEMS OF THE BODY

THE CELL

A typical cell.

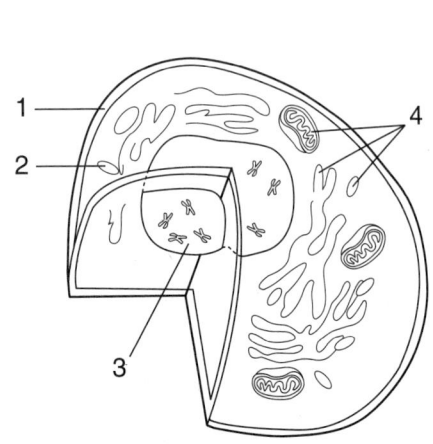

Major components of a cell.

The cytoskeleton.

TISSUE STRUCTURE AND OTHER SYSTEMS OF THE BODY

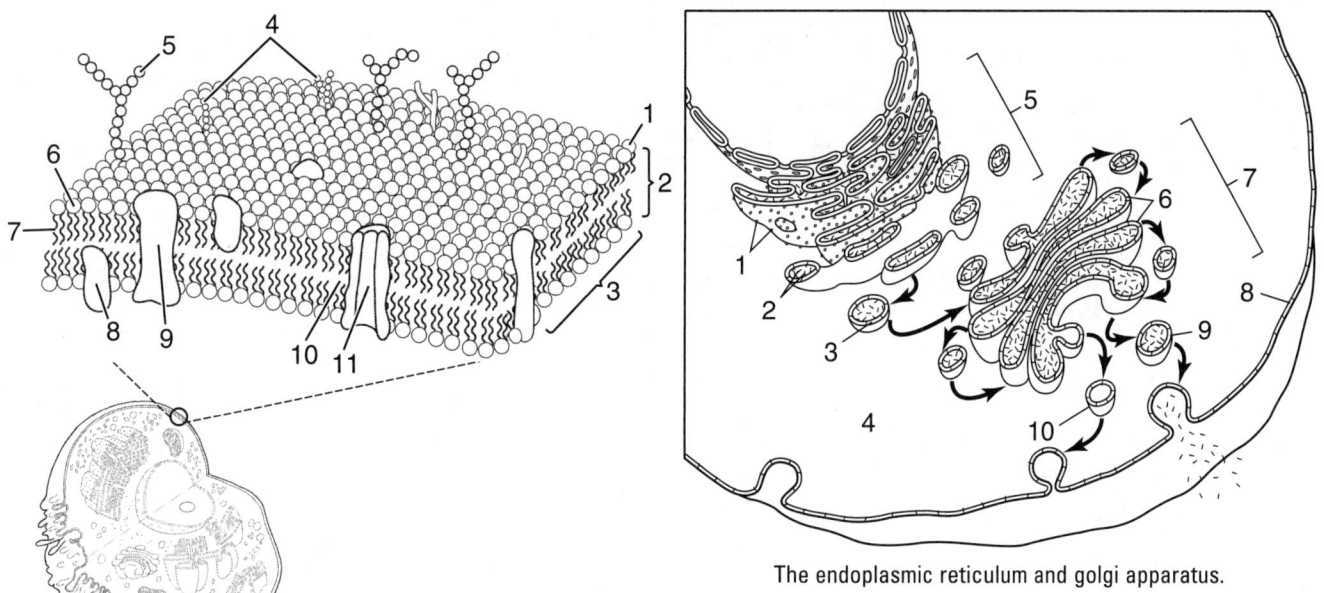

The cell membrane.

The endoplasmic reticulum and golgi apparatus.

Cross section of a mitochondrion.

Cross section of the nucleus.

BONE TISSUE

Longitudinal section of a long bone.

Section of a flat bone.

Magnification of spongy bone tissue.

TISSUE STRUCTURE AND OTHER SYSTEMS OF THE BODY

Longitudinal section of a long bone.

Magnification of compact bone tissue.

MUSCLE TISSUE

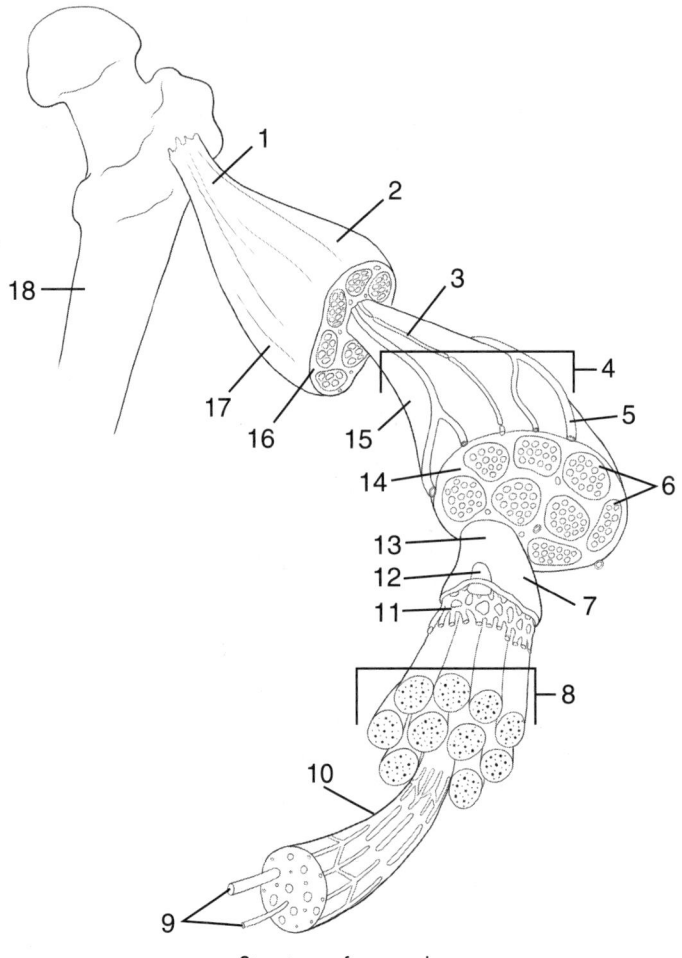

Structure of a muscle.

TISSUE STRUCTURE AND OTHER SYSTEMS OF THE BODY

Structure of a muscle illustrating a sarcomere.

Sarcoplasmic reticulum and T tubules of a muscle fiber.

TISSUE STRUCTURE AND OTHER SYSTEMS OF THE BODY

Myosin and actin filaments.

TISSUE STRUCTURE AND OTHER SYSTEMS OF THE BODY 433

Sliding filament action.

Neuromuscular junction.

TISSUE STRUCTURE AND OTHER SYSTEMS OF THE BODY

NERVE TISSUE

Structure of a neuron.

Types of neuroglial cells.

TISSUE STRUCTURE AND OTHER SYSTEMS OF THE BODY

Myelinated axon of the peripheral nervous system.

Central and peripheral nervous systems.

Convergence of neurons.

Divergence of neurons.

JOINTS

Three types of fibrous joints.

Two types of cartilaginous joints.

TISSUE STRUCTURE AND OTHER SYSTEMS OF THE BODY

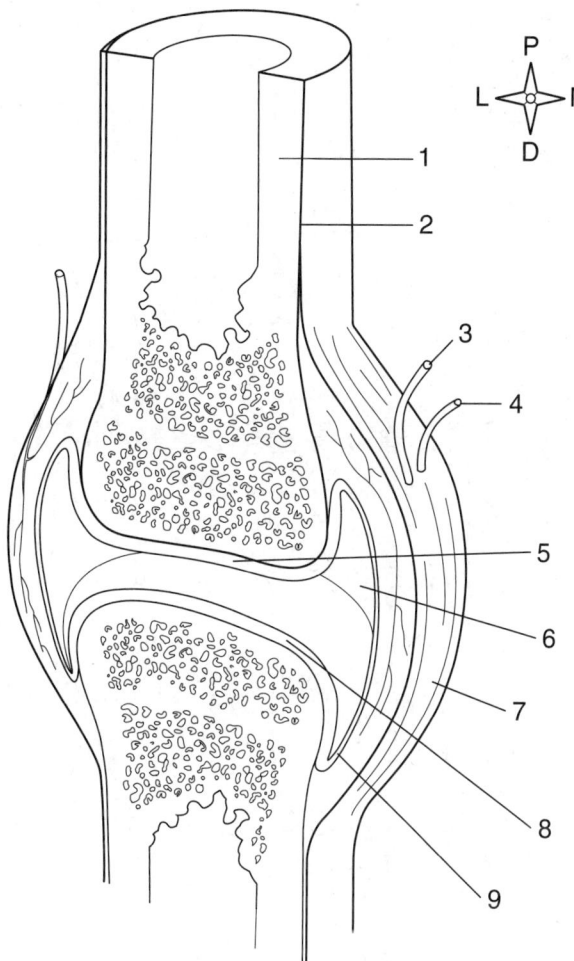

Structure of a typical synovial joint.

Various types of synovial joints.

INTEGUMENTARY SYSTEM

Diagram of the skin.

Glands of the skin.

TISSUE STRUCTURE AND OTHER SYSTEMS OF THE BODY 439

Hair follicle.

Structure of a nail.

CARDIAC SYSTEM
(THE HEART)

Anterior view of the heart.

Posterior view of the heart.

TISSUE STRUCTURE AND OTHER SYSTEMS OF THE BODY

Anterior view of the interior heart.

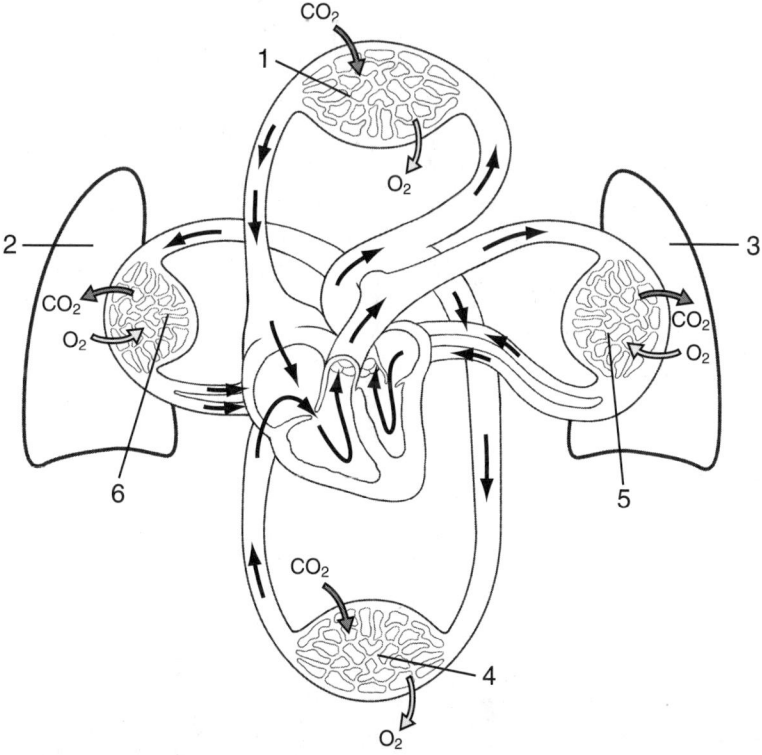

Systemic and pulmonic circulations of the heart.

VENOUS SYSTEM

Major veins of the body.

TISSUE STRUCTURE AND OTHER SYSTEMS OF THE BODY

Venous drainage of the brain.

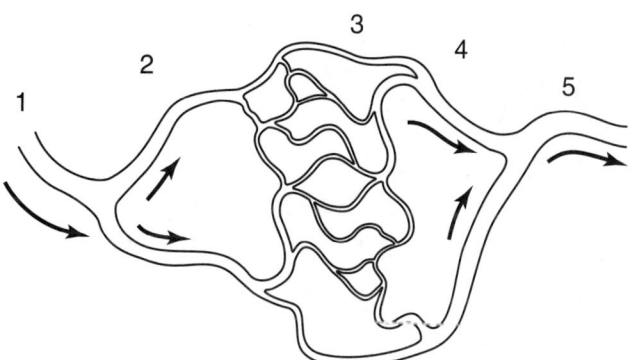

Creation of venous blood flow from capillaries.

Unidirectional venous valves.

TISSUE STRUCTURE AND OTHER SYSTEMS OF THE BODY

LYMPHATIC SYSTEM

Major organs of the lymphatic system.

Lymphatic capillary structure.

Role of lymphatic capillary in draining intercellular fluid.

TISSUE STRUCTURE AND OTHER SYSTEMS OF THE BODY

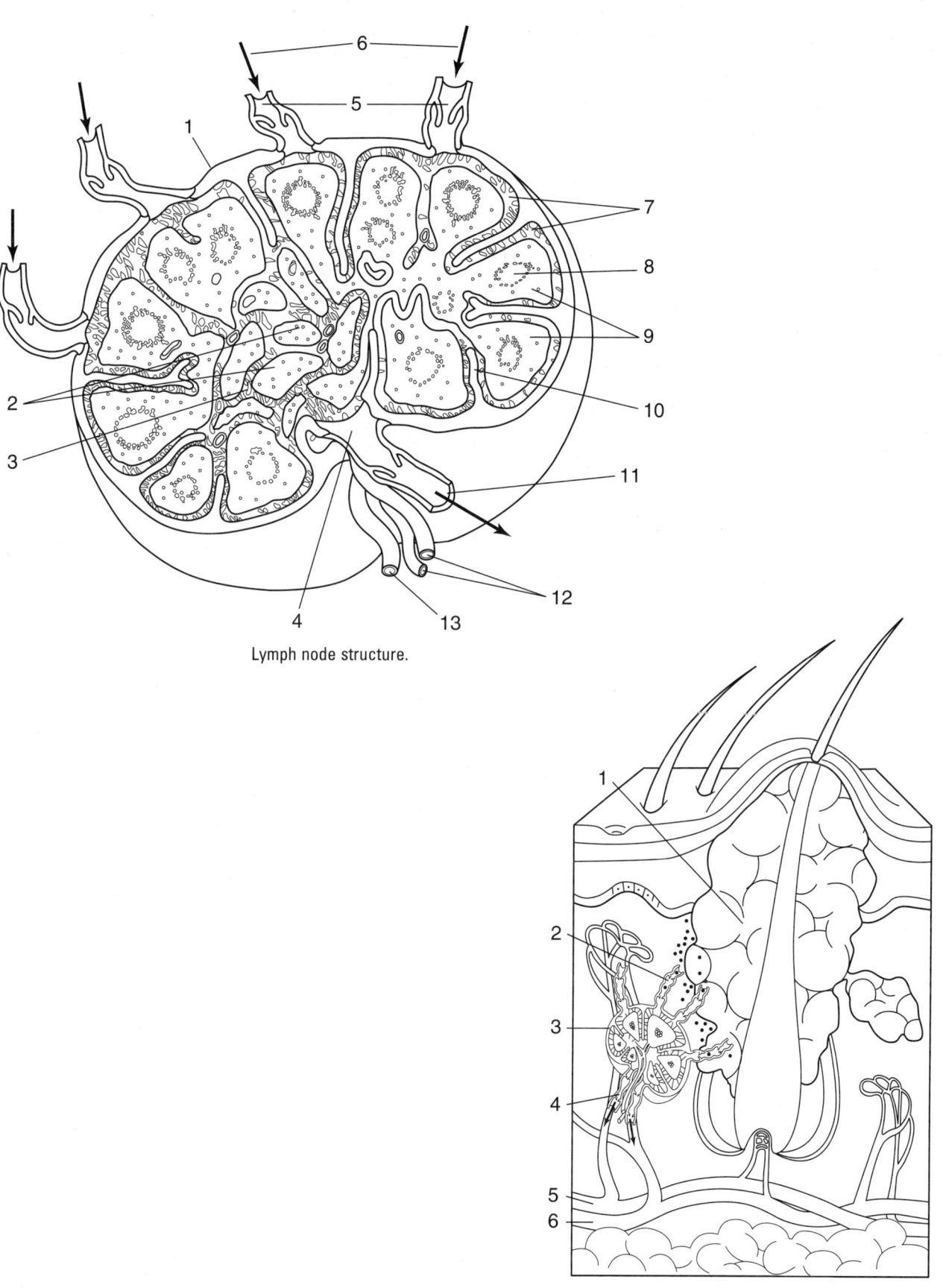

Lymph node structure.

Role of a lymph node in a skin infection.

446 TISSUE STRUCTURE AND OTHER SYSTEMS OF THE BODY

RESPIRATORY SYSTEM

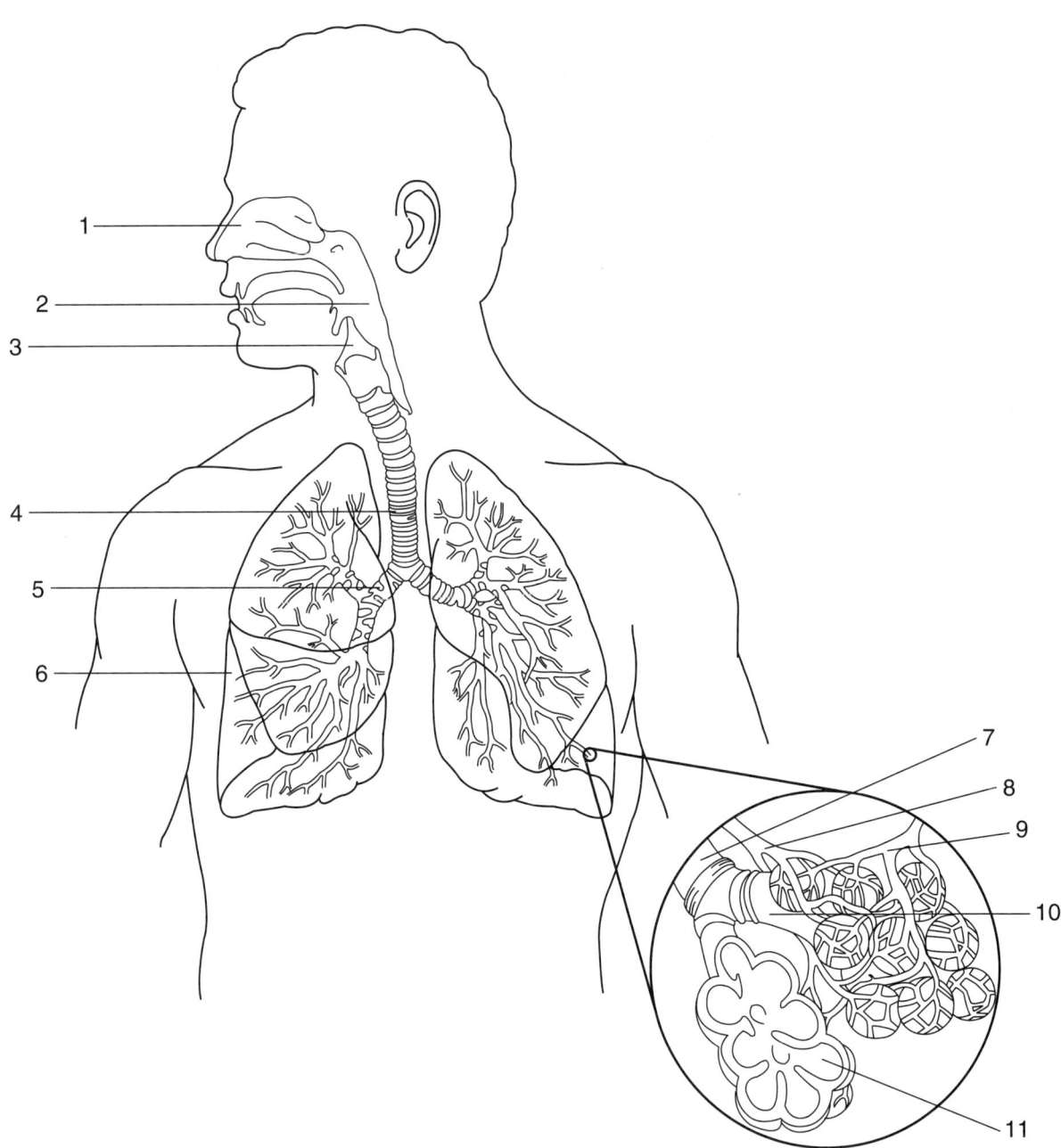

Structures of the respiratory system.

TISSUE STRUCTURE AND OTHER SYSTEMS OF THE BODY

Lobes of the lungs.

Bronchi of the lungs.

Bronchiole and alveoli.

TISSUE STRUCTURE AND OTHER SYSTEMS OF THE BODY

URINARY SYSTEM

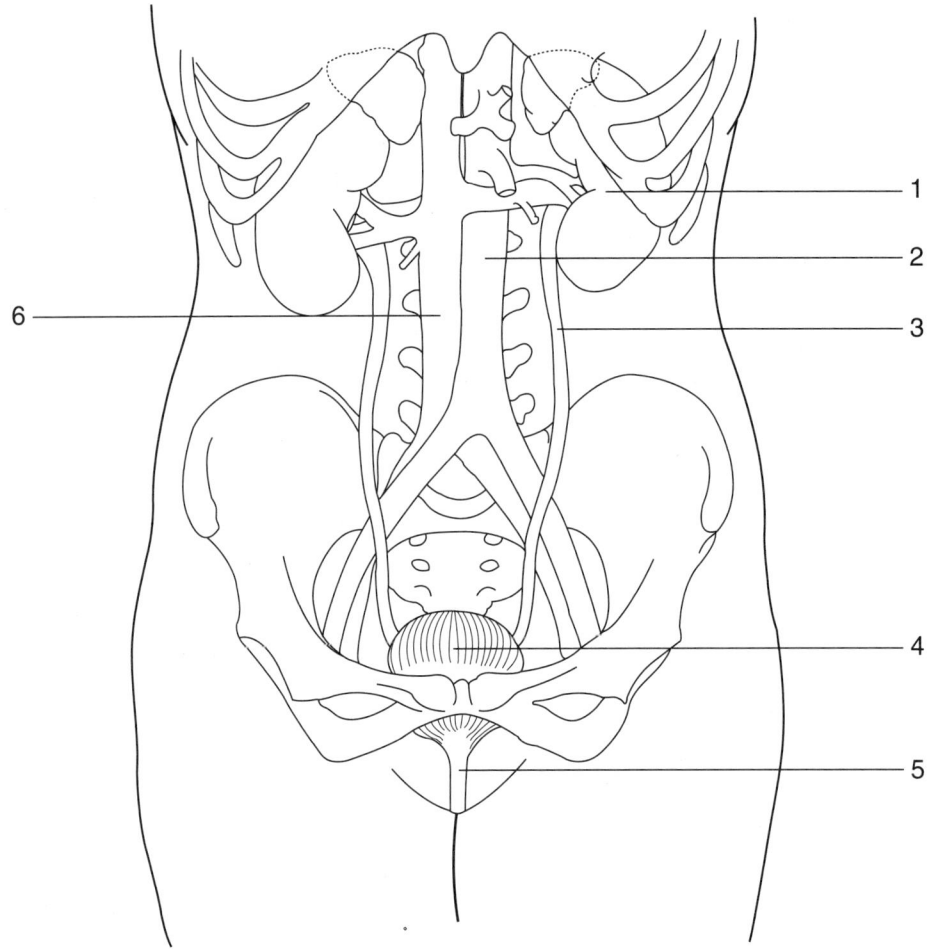

Anterior view of the structures of the urinary system.

TISSUE STRUCTURE AND OTHER SYSTEMS OF THE BODY

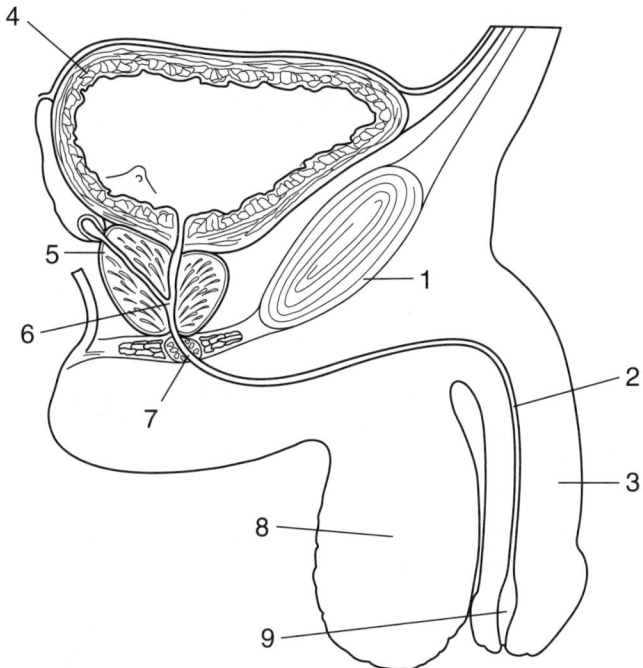

Right lateral view of the bladder and urethra of a male.

Structures of a nephron.

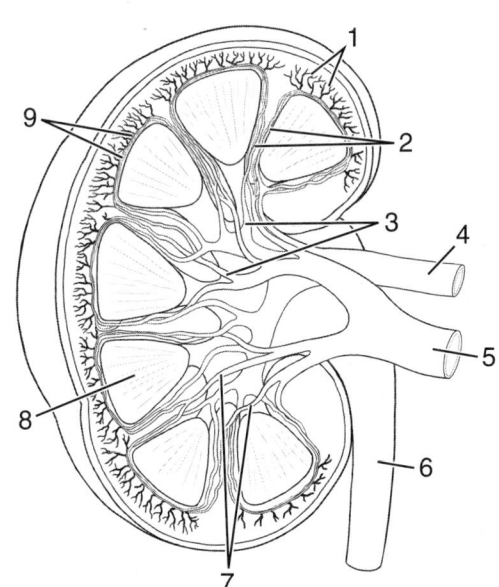

Section through a kidney.

GASTROINTESTINAL SYSTEM

Structures of the gastrointestinal system.

TISSUE STRUCTURE AND OTHER SYSTEMS OF THE BODY

Accessory organs of the gastrointestinal system.

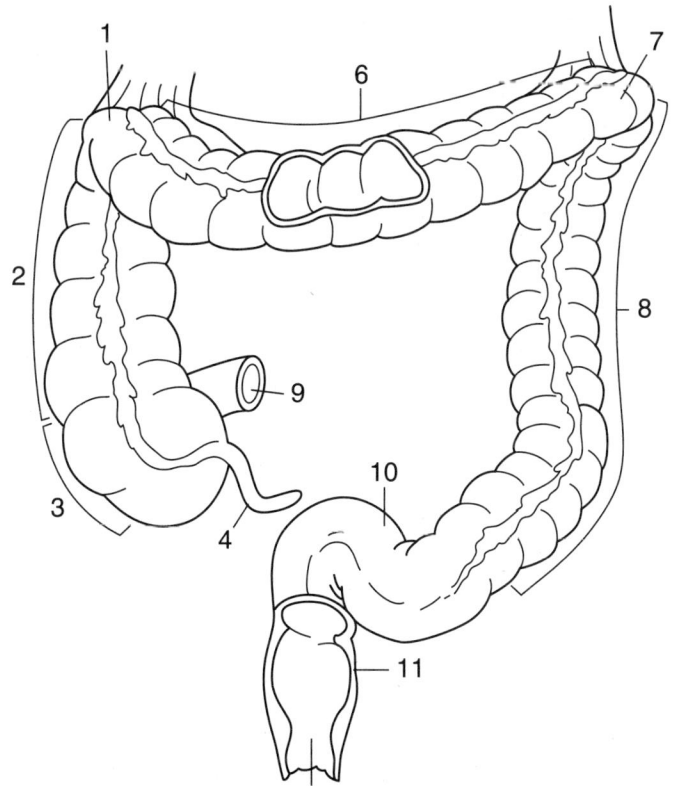

Divisions of the large intestine.

Section through the abdominopelvic cavity.

IMMUNE SYSTEM

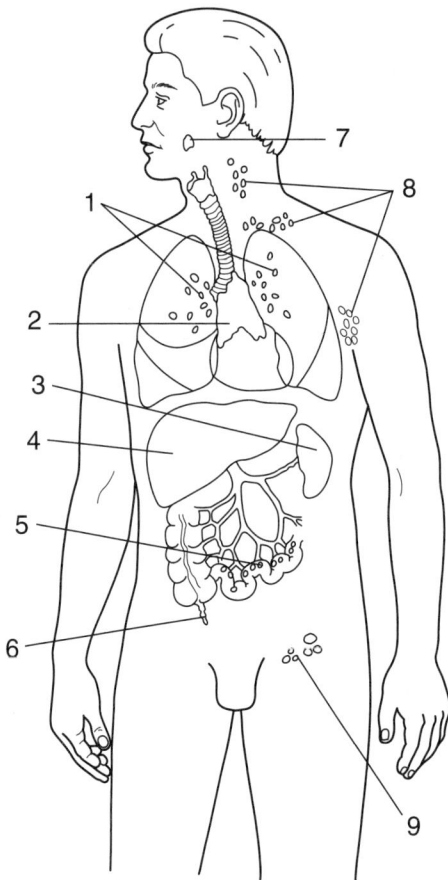

Organization of the immune system.

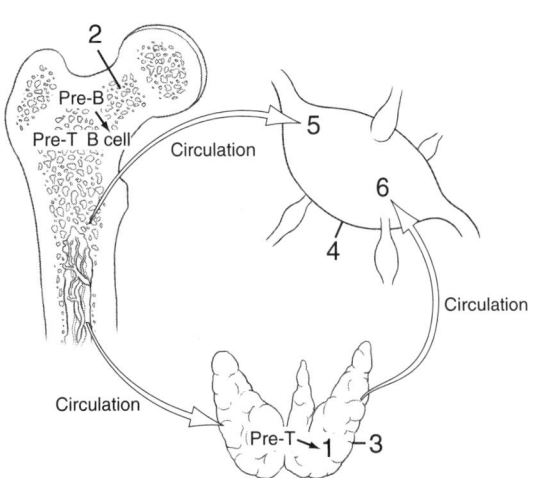

Creation of B cells and T cells by the bone marrow.

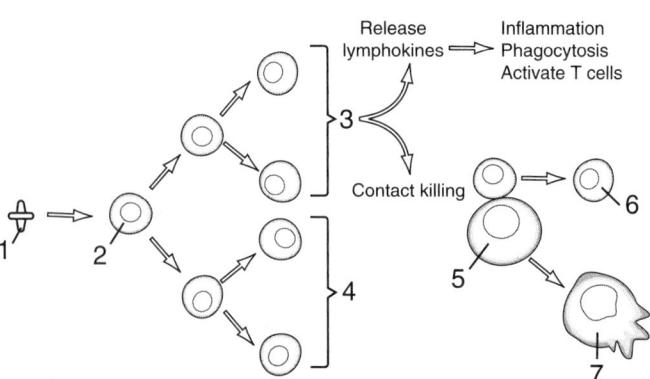

Activation and effects of T cells.

TISSUE STRUCTURE AND OTHER SYSTEMS OF THE BODY

Actions of antibodies.

Action of antibody-activated complement and death of bacterial cell.

Types of antibodies (immunoglobulins).

ENDOCRINE SYSTEM

The major endocrine glands of the body.

The thyroid gland.

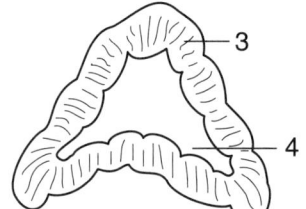

The adrenal gland.

TISSUE STRUCTURE AND OTHER SYSTEMS OF THE BODY

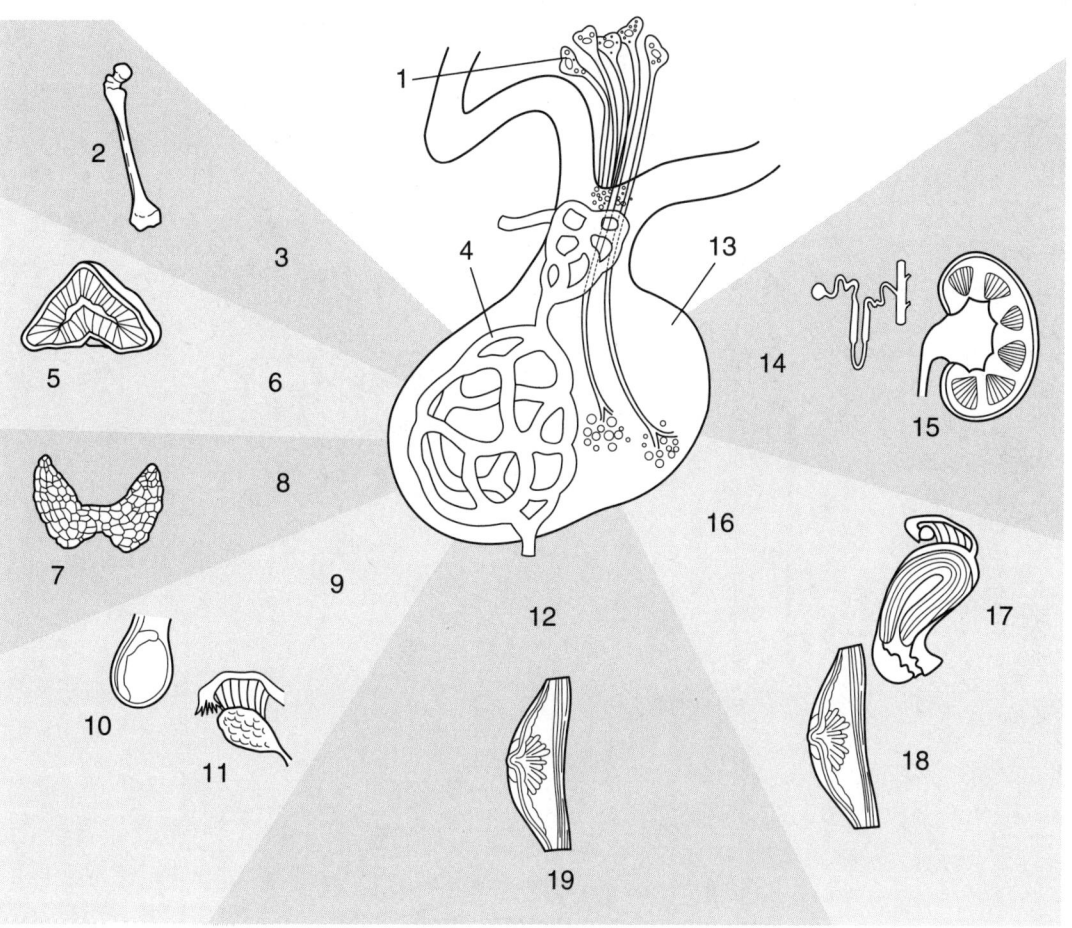

The hypothalamus and pituitary hormones.

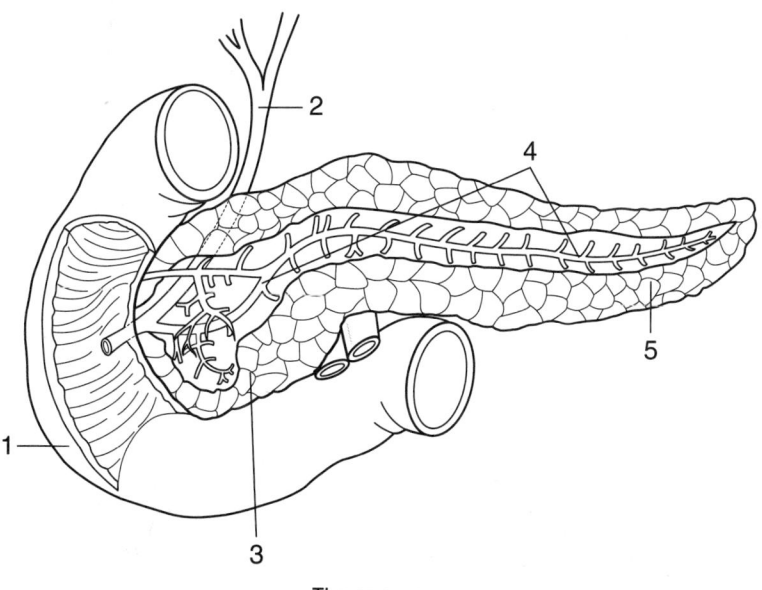

The pancreas.

SENSORY SYSTEM

Somatic and stretch receptors.

Superior view of a horizontal section of the eye.

TISSUE STRUCTURE AND OTHER SYSTEMS OF THE BODY

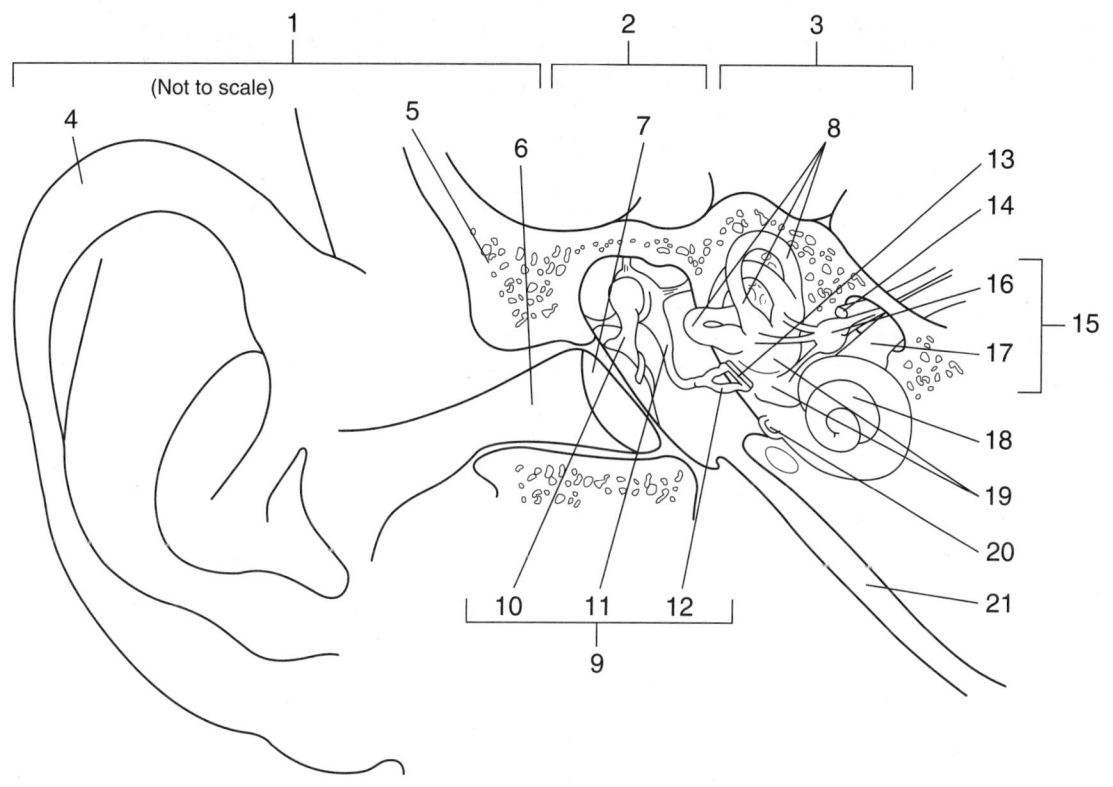

External, middle, and internal ear.

TISSUE STRUCTURE AND OTHER SYSTEMS OF THE BODY

Lateral view of the internal nose.

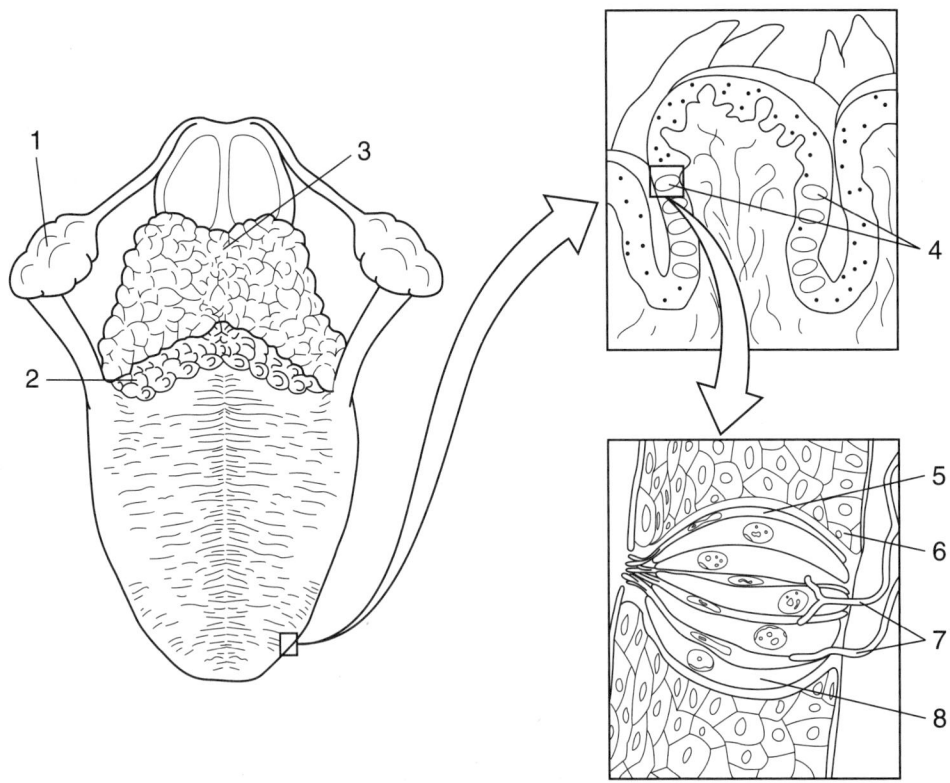

Dorsal surface of a tongue, cross-section through a papilla and a taste bud.

TISSUE STRUCTURE AND OTHER SYSTEMS OF THE BODY

REPRODUCTIVE SYSTEM

Male reproductive organs.

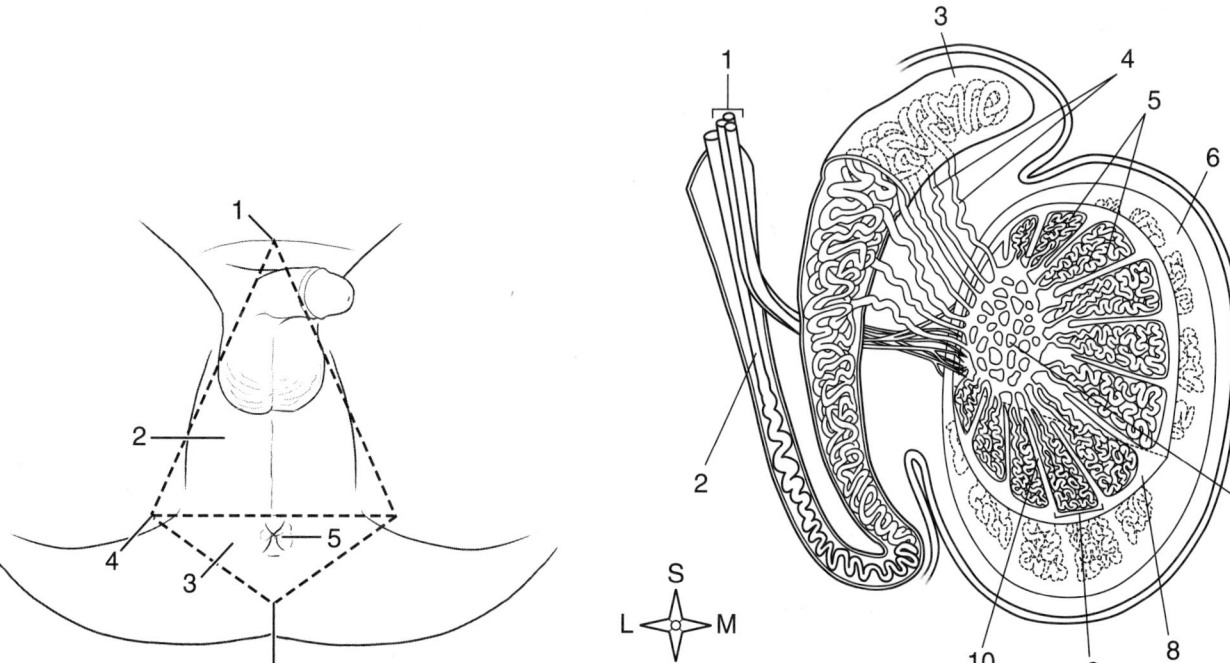

Male perineum.

Tubules of the testis and epididymis.

460 TISSUE STRUCTURE AND OTHER SYSTEMS OF THE BODY

Female reproductive organs.

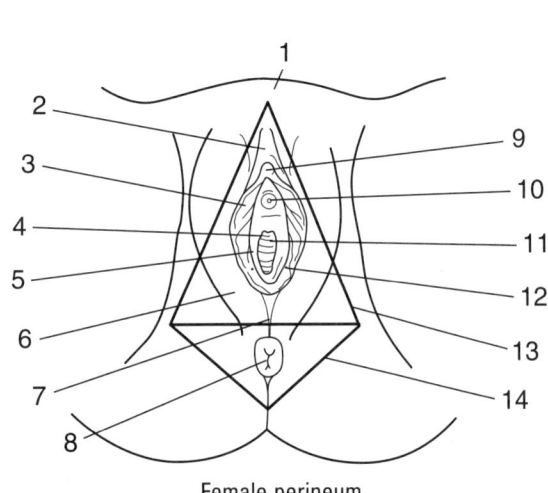

Female perineum.

Anterior view of female reproductive organs.

Answer Key

CHAPTER 1 LABELING ANSWERS: THE SKELETAL SYSTEM

Page 3 Anterior View of the Bones and Bony Landmarks of the Head

1. Frontal bone. 2. Nasal bone. 3. Sphenoid bone. 4. Temporal bone. 5. Lacrimal bone. 6. Ethmoid bone. 7. Zygomatic bone. 8. Zygomaticomaxillary suture. 9. Maxilla. 10. Vomer. 11. Alveolar process of the maxilla. 12. Alveolar process of the mandible. 13. Mandible. 14. Superciliary arch of the frontal bone. 15. Parietal bone. 16. Lesser wing of the sphenoid. 17. Greater wing of the sphenoid. 18. Palatine bone. 19. Frontal process of the maxilla. 20. Infraorbital foramen of the maxilla. 21. Canine fossa of the maxilla. 22. Incisive fossa of the maxilla. 23. Ramus of the mandible. 24. Incisive fossa of the mandible. 25. Angle of the mandible. 26. Mental foramen of the mandible. 27. Oblique line of the mandible. 28. Mental tubercle of the mandible. 29. Symphysis menti of the mandible.

Page 4 Lateral View of the Bones and Bony Landmarks of the Head

1. Temporal fossa (within dotted lines). 2. Temporomandibular joint (TMJ). 3. Highest nuchal line of the occipital bone. 4. Temporal bone. 5. Occipital bone. 6. Mastoid process of the temporal bone. 7. Zygomatic arch of the temporal bone. 8. Neck of the mandible. 9. Zygomaticotemporal suture. 10. Coronoid process of the mandible. 11. Zygomaticomaxillary suture. 12. Ramus of the mandible. 13. Angle of the mandible. 14. Mandible. 15. Oblique line of the mandible. 16. Mental foramen of the mandible. 17. Parietal bone. 18. Frontal bone. 19. Sphenoid bone. 20. Superciliary arch of the frontal bone. 21. Lacrimal bone. 22. Nasal bone. 23. Zygomatic bone. 24. Frontal process of the maxilla. 25. Canine fossa of the maxilla. 26. Maxilla. 27. Incisive fossa of the maxilla. 28. Alveolar process of the maxilla. 29. Alveolar process of the mandible. 30. Incisive fossa of the mandible. 31. Mental tubercle of the mandible.

Page 5 Inferior View of the Bones and Bony Landmarks of the Head

1. Maxilla. 2. Palatine bone. 3. Frontal bone. 4. Zygomatic bone. 5. Zygomatic arch (of the temporal & zygomatic bones). 6. Parietal bone. 7. Sphenoid bone. 8. Temporal bone. 9. Parietal bone. 10. Occipital bone. 11. Incisive fossa of the maxilla. 12. Zygomaticomaxillary suture. 13. Tuberosity of the maxilla. 14. Zygomaticotemporal suture. 15. Greater wing of the sphenoid. 16. Medial pterygoid plate of the pterygoid process of the sphenoid bone. 17. Lateral pterygoid plate of the pterygoid process of the sphenoid bone. 18. Vomer. 19. Styloid process of the temporal bone. 20. Mastoid process of the temporal bone. 21. Mastoid notch of the temporal bone. 22. Jugular process of the occipital bone. 23. Foramen magnum. 24. Highest nuchal line of the occipital bone.

Page 6 Anterior View of the Bones and Bony Landmarks of the Neck

1. Temporal bone. 2. Mastoid process of the temporal bone. 3. Styloid process of the temporal bone. 4. Greater cornu of the hyoid bone. 5. Body of the hyoid bone. 6. Hyoid bone. 7. Lamina of the thyroid cartilage. 8. Thyroid cartilage. 9. Sternoclavicular joint. 10. Acromioclavicular joint. 11. Shoulder joint. 12. Clavicle. 13. Scapula. 14. Costal cartilage of the first rib. 15. Manubrium of the sternum. 16. Basilar part of the occiput. 17. Occiput. 18. Anterior arch of the atlas. 19. Atlas (C1). 20. Axis (C2). 21. Vertebral body. 22. Vertebral transverse process (TP). 23. Posterior tubercle of the transverse process. 24. Anterior tubercle of the transverse process. 25. Humerus. 26. Acromion process of the scapula. 27. Superior border of the scapula. 28. Medial border of the scapula.

Page 7 Posterior View of the Bones and Bony Landmarks of the Neck

1. External occipital protuberance (EOP). 2. Occiput. 3. Superior nuchal line of the occiput. 4. Inferior nuchal line of the occiput. 5. Superior angle of the scapula. 6. Clavicle. 7. Acromioclavicular joint. 8. Acromion process of the scapula. 9. Scapula. 10. Spine of the scapula. 11. Tubercle at the root of the spine of the scapula. 12. Medial border of the scapula. 13. Root of the spine of the scapula. 14. Temporal bone. 15. Mastoid process of the temporal bone. 16. Mandible. 17. Atlas (C1). 18. Axis (C2). 19. Vertebral spinous process (SP). 20. Vertebral transverse process (TP). 21. C7. 22. First rib. 23. T3.

Page 8 Anterior View of the Bones and Bony Landmarks of the Trunk

1. Clavicle. 2. Coracoid process of the scapula. 3. Scapula. 4. Medial border of the scapula. 5. Inferior angle of the scapula. 6. Intercostal space. 7. Costal cartilage. 8. Sacro-iliac joint. 9. Iliac crest. 10. Pelvic bone. 11. Pubic crest. 12. Pubic tubercle. 13. Pubic symphysis. 14. Sacrum. 15. Cervical transverse process. 16. Body of C7. 17. Humerus. 18. Medial lip of the bicipital groove of the humerus. 19. Lateral lip of the bicipital groove of the humerus. 20. Sternum. 21. Xiphoid process of the sternum. 22. Intervertebral disc (L3-L4). 23. Ilium. 24. Ischium. 25. Pubis.

Page 9 Posterior View of the Bones and Bony Landmarks of the Trunk

1. Clavicle. 2. Spine of the scapula. 3. Root of the spine of the scapula. 4. Medial border of the scapula. 5. Scapula. 6. Inferior angle of the scapula. 7. Vertebral transverse process (TP). 8. Vertebral lamina. 9. Vertebral spinous process (SP). 10. Iliac crest. 11. Posterior superior iliac spine (PSIS). 12. Pelvic bone. 13. Sacrum. 14. Ischium. 15. Pubis. 16. Pubic symphysis. 17. C7. 18. Tubercle (of the 5th rib). 19. Angle (of the 5th rib). 20. Intercostal space. 21. Inferior articular process (of L1). 22. Superior articular process (of L2). 23. Mamillary process (of L3). 24. Ilium. 25. Sacro-iliac joint. 26. Medial sacral crest. 27. Lateral sacral crest.

Page 10 Anterior View of the Bones and Bony Landmarks of the Right Thigh and Pelvis

1. Vertebral transverse process (TP). 2. Sacral ala. 3. Iliac crest. 4. Iliac fossa. 5. Internal ilium. 6. Ilium. 7. Anterior superior iliac spine (ASIS). 8. Anterior inferior iliac spine (AIIS). 9. Hip joint. 10. Greater trochanter of the femur. 11. Lesser trochanter of the femur. 12. Femur. 13. Fibula. 14. Intervertebral disc. 15. Vertebral body (L3). 16. Sacrum. 17. Iliopectineal eminence (of the ilium and the pubis). 18. Apex of the sacrum. 19. Coccyx. 20. Pectineal line of the pubis on the superior ramus of the pubis. 21. Pubis. 22. Obturator foramen. 23. Inferior ramus of the pubis. 24. Ramus of the ischium. 25. Ischial tuberosity. 26. Ischium. 27. Patella. 28. Knee (tibiofemoral) joint. 29. Medial tibial condyle. 30. Tibial tuberosity. 31. Tibia.

Page 11 Posterior View of the Bones and Bony Landmarks of the Right Thigh and Pelvis
1. Vertebral transverse process (TP) (of L5). 2. Sacrum. 3. Sacrotuberous ligament. 4. Apex of the sacrum. 5. Coccyx. 6. Pectineal line on the superior ramus of the pubis. 7. Pubis. 8. Obturator foramen. 9. Inferior ramus of the pubis. 10. Ramus of the ischium. 11. Ischium. 12. Ischial tuberosity. 13. Trochanteric fossa. 14. Pectineal line of the femur. 15. Medial lip of the linea aspera. 16. Femur. 17. Medial supracondylar line. 18. Adductor tubercle. 19. Medial tibial condyle. 20. Tibia. 21. Iliac crest. 22. Posterior gluteal line of the ilium. 23. Anterior gluteal line of the ilium. 24. Pelvic bone (Ilium). 25. Anterior superior iliac spine (ASIS). 26. Inferior gluteal line of the ilium. 27. Anterior inferior iliac spine (AIIS). 28. Ischial spine. 29. Head of the femur. 30. Hip (femoroacetabular) joint. 31. Greater trochanter. 32. Intertrochanteric crest. 33. Lesser trochanter. 34. Gluteal tuberosity. 35. Lateral lip of the linea aspera. 36. Linea aspera. 37. Lateral supracondylar line. 38. Knee (tibiofemoral) joint. 39. Lateral tibial condyle. 40. Head of the fibula. 41. Fibula.

Page 12 Anterior View of the Bones and Bony Landmarks of the Right Leg
1. Lateral supracondylar line of the femur. 2. Lateral condyle of the femur. 3. Knee joint. 4. Lateral condyle of the tibia. 5. Head of the fibula. 6. Fibula. 7. Lateral malleolus of the fibula. 8. Calcaneus. 9. Cuboid. 10. Base of (5th) metatarsal. 11. Proximal phalanx of (5th) toe. 12. Middle phalanx of (5th) toe. 13. Distal phalanx of (5th) toe. 14. Femur. 15. Medial condyle of the femur. 16. Tibia. 17. Interosseus membrane. 18. Ankle joint. 19. Medial malleolus of the tibia. 20. Talus. 21. Navicular. 22. 1st cuneiform. 23. 2nd cuneiform. 24. 3rd cuneiform. 25. Metatarsals #1-5. 26. Proximal phalanx of the big toe. 27. Distal phalanx of the big toe.

Page 13 Posterior View of the Bones and Bony Landmarks of the Right Leg
1. Femur. 2. Medial condyle of the femur. 3. Knee joint. 4. Soleal line of the tibia. 5. Tibia. 6. Calcaneus. 7. Medial malleolus of the tibia. 8. Tuberosity of the calcaneus. 9. Talus. 10. Navicular. 11. 3rd cuneiform. 12. 2nd cuneiform. 13. 1st cuneiform. 14. Metatarsals #1-5. 15. Proximal phalanx of the big toe. 16. Distal phalanx of the big toe. 17. Lateral supracondylar line of the femur. 18. Lateral condyle of the femur. 19. Lateral condyle of the tibia. 20. Head of the fibula. 21. Fibula. 22. Interosseus membrane. 23. Lateral malleolus of the fibula. 24. Cuboid. 25. Base of (5th) metatarsal. 26. Proximal phalanx of (5th) toe. 27. Middle phalanx of (5th) toe. 28. Distal phalanx of (5th) toe.

Page 14 Dorsal View of the Bones and Bony Landmarks of the Right Foot
1. Cuboid. 2. Metatarsals #1-5 (Numbering begins with the big toe as toe #1 and ends with the little toe as toe #5.). 3. Metatarsophalangeal joint (MTP joint). 4. Proximal phalanx of a toe. 5. Proximal interphalangeal joint (PIP joint). 6. Middle phalanx of a toe. 7. Distal interphalangeal joint (DIP joint). 8. Distal phalanx of a toe. 9. Calcaneus. 10. Talus. 11. Navicular. 12. 1st cuneiform. 13. 2nd cuneiform. 14. 3rd cuneiform. 15. Base of a metatarsal. 16. Head of a metatarsal. 17. Base of a phalanx. 18. Proximal phalanx of the big toe. 19. Head of a phalanx. 20. Interphalangeal joint (IP joint). 21. Distal phalanx of the big toe.

Page 15 Plantar View of the Bones and Bony Landmarks of the Right Foot
1. Talus. 2. Navicular. 3. 3rd cuneiform. 4. 2nd cuneiform. 5. 1st cuneiform. 6. Base of a metatarsal. 7. Sesamoid bones. 8. Base of a phalanx. 9. Proximal phalanx of the big toe. 10. Interphalangeal joint (IP joint). 11. Distal phalanx of the big toe. 12. Calcaneal tuberosity. 13. Calcaneus. 14. Cuboid. 15. Metatarsals #1-5 (Numbering begins with the big toe as toe #1 and ends with the little toe as toe #5.). 16. Metatarsophalangeal joint (MTP joint). 17. Proximal phalanx of a toe. 18. Proximal interphalangeal joint (PIP joint). 19. Middle phalanx of a toe. 20. Distal interphalangeal joint (DIP joint). 21. Distal phalanx of a toe. 22. Base of a phalanx. 23. Head of a phalanx.

Page 16 Anterior View of the Bones and Bony Landmarks of the Right Scapula/Arm
1. Acromion process of the scapula. 2. Supraglenoid tubercle of the scapula. 3. Superior facet of the greater tubercle of the humerus. 4. Greater tubercle of the humerus. 5. Bicipital groove of the humerus. 6. Lesser tubercle of the humerus. 7. Deltoid tuberosity of the humerus. 8. Humerus. 9. Shaft of the humerus. 10. Elbow joint. 11. Radius. 12. Radial tuberosity. 13. Clavicle. 14. Coracoid process of the scapula. 15. Shoulder joint. 16. Scapula. 17. Subscapular fossa of the scapula. 18. Infraglenoid tubercle of the scapula. 19. Lateral border of the scapula. 20. Coronoid process of the ulna. 21. Ulna. 22. Ulnar tuberosity.

Page 17 Posterior View of the Bones and Bony Landmarks of the Right Scapula/Arm
1. Clavicle. 2. Supraspinous fossa of the scapula. 3. Shoulder joint. 4. Spine of the scapula. 5. Scapula. 6. Infraspinous fossa of the scapula. 7. Lateral border of the scapula. 8. Infraglenoid tubercle of the scapula. 9. Olecranon process of the ulna. 10. Ulna. 11. Acromion process of the scapula. 12. Supraglenoid tubercle of the scapula. 13. Superior facet of the greater tubercle of the humerus. 14. Middle facet of the greater tubercle of the humerus. 15. Greater tubercle of the humerus. 16. Inferior facet of the greater tubercle of the humerus. 17. Deltoid tuberosity of the humerus. 18. Humerus. 19. Shaft of the humerus. 20. Head of the radius. 21. Radius. 22. Radial tuberosity.

Page 18 Anterior View of the Bones and Bony Landmarks of the Right Forearm
1. Lateral supracondylar ridge of the humerus. 2. Lateral epicondyle of the humerus. 3. Head of the radius. 4. Radial tuberosity. 5. Radial shaft. 6. Radius. 7. Interosseus membrane. 8. Wrist joint. 9. Styloid process of the radius. 10. Metacarpals #1-5. 11. Proximal phalanx of the thumb. 12. Distal phalanx of the thumb. 13. Humerus. 14. Medial supracondylar ridge of the humerus. 15. Medial epicondyle of the humerus. 16. Elbow joint. 17. Coronoid process of the ulna. 18. Supinator crest of the ulna. 19. Ulna. 20. Pisiform. 21. Hook of hamate. 22. Base of a metacarpal. 23. Base of a phalanx. 24. Proximal phalanx of a finger (the little finger). 25. Middle phalanx of a finger (the little finger). 26. Distal phalanx of a finger (the little finger).

Page 19 Posterior View of the Bones and Bony Landmarks of the Right Forearm
1. Medial supracondylar ridge of the humerus. 2. Medial epicondyle of the humerus. 3. Coronoid process of the ulna. 4. Supinator crest of the ulna. 5. Ulna. 6. Interosseus membrane. 7. Styloid process of the ulna. 8. Pisiform. 9. Base of a metacarpal. 10. Base of a phalanx. 11. Proximal phalanx of a finger (the little finger). 12. Middle phalanx of a finger (the little finger). 13. Distal phalanx of a finger (the little finger). 14. Humerus. 15. Lateral supracondylar ridge of the humerus. 16. Lateral epicondyle of the humerus. 17. Olecranon process of the ulna. 18. Head of the radius. 19. Radial tuberosity. 20. Radial shaft. 21. Radius. 22. Styloid process of the radius. 23. Metacarpals #1-5. 24. Proximal phalanx of the thumb. 25. Distal phalanx of the thumb.

ANSWER KEY 463

Page 20 Palmar View of the Bones and Bony Landmarks of the Right Hand
1. Scaphoid. 2. Scaphoid tubercle. 3. Trapezium. 4. Tubercle of trapezium. 5. Trapezoid. 6. Interphalangeal joint (IP joint). 7. Sesamoid bones. 8. Proximal phalanx of the thumb. 9. Distal phalanx of the thumb. 10. Proximal phalanx of a finger (index finger). 11. Middle phalanx of a finger (index finger). 12. Distal phalanx of a finger (index finger). 13. Capitate. 14. Lunate. 15. Triquetrum. 16. Pisiform. 17. Hamate. 18. Hook of hamate. 19. Base of a metacarpal. 20. Metacarpals #1-5 (Numbering begins with the thumb as finger #1 and ends with the little finger as finger #5.). 21. Head of a metacarpal. 22. Base of a phalanx. 23. Head of a phalanx. 24. Proximal interphalangeal joint (PIP joint). 25. Distal interphalangeal joint (DIP joint). 26. Metacarpophalangeal joint (MCP joint).

Page 21 Dorsal View of the Bones and Bony Landmarks of the Right Hand
1. Lunate. 2. Pisiform. 3. Triquetrum. 4. Hamate. 5. Base of a metacarpal. 6. Metacarpals #1-5 (Numbering begins with the thumb as finger #1 and ends with the little finger as finger #5.). 7. Head of a metacarpal. 8. Metacarpophalangeal joint (MCP joint). 9. Base of a phalanx. 10. Head of a phalanx. 11. Proximal interphalangeal joint (PIP joint). 12. Distal interphalangeal joint (DIP joint). 13. Capitate. 14. Scaphoid. 15. Trapezium. 16. Trapezoid. 17. Proximal phalanx of the thumb. 18. Interphalangeal joint (IP joint). 19. Sesamoid bone. 20. Distal phalanx of the thumb. 21. Proximal phalanx of a finger. 22. Middle phalanx of a finger. 23. Distal phalanx of a finger.

CHAPTER 2 LABELING ANSWERS: MUSCLES OF THE HEAD

Page 60 Anterior View of the Head
1. Occipitofrontalis. 2. Temporoparietalis. 3. Orbicularis oculi. 4. Procerus. 5. Levator labii superioris alaeque nasi. 6. Nasalis. 7. Zygomaticus minor. 8. Levator labii superioris. 9. Zygomaticus major. 10. Levator anguli oris. 11. Masseter. 12. Risorius. 13. Depressor anguli oris. 14. Depressor labii inferioris. 15. Mentalis. 16. Platysma. 17. Occipitofrontalis (frontalis belly, cut). 18. Corrugator supercillii. 19. Orbicularis oculi (partially cut away). 20. Levator palpebrae superioris. 21. Levator labii superioris alaeque nasi (cut). 22. Levator labii superioris (cut). 23. Zygomaticus minor (cut). 24. Zygomaticus major (cut). 25. Levator anguli oris (cut). 26. Depressor septi nasi. 27. Buccinator. 28. Orbicularis oris. 29. Depressor anguli oris (cut). 30. Depressor labii inferioris (cut).

Page 61 Lateral View of the Head
1. Temporoparietalis. 2. Occipitofrontalis (occipitalis belly). 3. Auricularis muscles. 4. Splenius capitis. 5. Sternocleidomastoid. 6. Levator scapulae. 7. Trapezius. 8. Occipitofrontalis (frontalis belly). 9. Temporalis (deep to facia). 10. Corrugator supercilii. 11. Procerus. 12. Orbicularis oculi (partially cut). 13. Levator labii superioris alaeque nasi. 14. Nasalis. 15. Levator labii superioris. 16. Lateral pterygoid. 17. Depressor septi nasi. 18. Zygomaticus minor. 19. Levator anguli oris. 20. Zygomaticus major. 21. Orbicularis oris. 22. Mentalis. 23. Depressor labii inferioris. 24. Depressor anguli oris. 25. Risorius. 26. Buccinator. 27. Platysma.

Muscles of the Head: Answers to Review Questions (pp 63–65)
1. Lateral pterygoid. 2. Deep. 3. Mentalis. 4. Occipitofrontalis and temporoparietalis. 5. 2. 6. Depressor labii inferioris. 7. Levator labii superioris alaeque nasi. 8. The depressor labii inferioris depresses the lower lip; the mentalis elevates it. 9. Levator labii superioris alaeque nasi. 10. Depressor labii inferioris and mentalis. 11. 3. 12. Occipitofrontalis. 13. It shortens. 14. Depressor labii inferioris. 15. Temporalis, masseter, medial pterygoid. 16. They both elevate the angle of the mouth. 17. Levator labii superioris alaeque nasi. 18. Masseter. 19. Orbicularis oris. 20. Occipitalis and frontalis. 21. They both contralaterally deviate and protract the mandible at the temporomandibular joints. 22. Trapezius. 23. The temporalis elevates the mandible at the temporomandibular joints; the digastric depresses it. 24. Depressor septi nasi and nasalis. 25. Procerus. 26. They both draw laterally the angle of the mouth. 27. Levator labii superioris alaeque nasi and zygomaticus minor. 28. Nasalis. 29. Galea aponeurotica. 30. Auricularis posterior. 31. Corrugator supercilii frontalis (occipitofrontalis). 32. Frontalis (occipitofrontalis). 33. Zygomaticus minor. 34. Levator anguli oris. 35. Levator anguli oris. 36. Masseter. 37. Depressor anguli oris. 38. They both evert the lower lip. 39. Risorius and buccinator. 40. Mandible. 41. Procerus. 42. Levator labii superioris alaeque nasi. 43. Levator labii superioris, levator labii superioris alaeque nasi, zygomaticus minor. 44. Temporalis. 45. Orbicularis oculi. 46. Mentalis. 47. Zygomaticus minor. 48. Orbicularis oris. 49. It shortens. 50. Transverse and alar parts. 51. Risorius and zygomaticus major. 52. Orbicularis oculi. 53. Auricularis, superior, temporoparietalis. 54. Levator labii superioris. 55. Temporalis, masseter, lateral pterygoid, medial pterygoid. 56. Their fibers run in the same direction, but the masseter is superficial to the mandible and the medial pterygoid is deep to it. 57. Levator labii superioris alaeque nasi. 58. Frontalis. 59. Procerus. 60. Anterior, superior, posterior auriculares. 61. Depressor labii inferioris. 62. Depressor septi nasi. 63. Orbicularis oculi. 64. Buccinator. 65. Orbicularis oris. 66. Auricularis superior. 67. Levator labii superioris. 68. Medial pterygoid. 69. Laughing. 70. Orbicularis oculi. 71. It raises it. 72. The temporalis is deep. 73. Depressor anguli oris, depressor labii inferioris, mentalis, buccinator, platysma. 74. It lengthens. 75. Procerus. 76. It lengthens. 77. Levator labii superioris alaeque nasi. 78. 3.

CHAPTER 2 LABELING ANSWERS: MUSCLES OF THE NECK

Page 102 Anterior View of the Neck (Superficial)
1. Omohyoid. 2. Platysma. 3. Sternothyroid. 4. Digastric (anterior belly). 5. Mylohyoid. 6. Stylohyoid. 7. Digastric (posterior belly). 8. Thyrohyoid. 9. Sternocleidomastoid (sternal head). 10. Sternocleidomastoid (clavicular head). 11. Levator scapulae. 12. Sternohyoid. 13. Middle scalene. 14. Posterior scalene. 15. Omohyoid (inferior belly). 16. Trapezius. 17. Anterior scalene. 18. Deltoid. 19. Pectoralis major.

Page 103 Anterior View of the Neck (Intermediate)
1. Mylohyoid. 2. Sternocleidomastoid (cut). 3. Omohyoid (superior belly). 4. Omohyoid (inferior belly). 5. Sternocleidomastoid (cut). 6. Sternohyoid. 7. Digastric (anterior belly). 8. Stylohyoid. 9. Digastric (posterior belly). 10. Sternocleidomastoid (cut). 11. Thyrohyoid. 12. Levator scapulae. 13. Omohyoid (cut and reflected). 14. Sternothyroid. 15. Middle scalene. 16. Posterior scalene. 17. Trapezius. 18. Anterior scalene. 19. Deltoid. 20. Pectoralis major. 21. Sternohyoid (cut and reflected).

Page 104 Anterior View of the Neck (Deep)
1. Rectus capitis lateralis. 2. Rectus capitis anterior. 3. Longus capitis. 4. Longus colli. 5. Middle scalene. 6. Anterior scalene. 7. Posterior scalene. 8. Longus capitis (cut). 9. Rectus capitis anterior. 10. Rectus capitis lateralis. 11. Longus colli. 12. Middle scalene. 13. Anterior scalene (cut). 14. Posterior scalene.

ANSWER KEY

Page 105 Lateral View of the Neck
1. Stylohyoid. 2. Digastric (posterior belly). 3. Splenius capitis. 4. Longus capitis. 5. Sternocleidomastoid. 6. Levator scapulae. 7. Anterior scalene. 8. Middle scalene. 9. Posterior scalene. 10. Trapezius. 11. Omohyoid (inferior belly). 12. Deltoid. 13. Masseter (cut). 14. Mylohyoid. 15. Digastric (anterior belly). 16. Thyrohyoid. 17. Omohyoid (superior belly). 18. Sternohyoid. 19. Sternothyroid. 20. Sternocleidomastoid (sternal head). 21. Sternocleidomastoid (clavicular head). 22. Pectoralis major.

Page 106 Posterior View of the Neck (Superficial and Intermediate)
1. Sternocleidomastoid. 2. Splenius capitis. 3. Levator scapulae. 4. Trapezius. 5. Deltoid. 6. Triceps brachii. 7. Latissimus dorsi. 8. Semispinalis capitis (of transversospinalis group). 9. Splenius capitis. 10. Splenius cervicis. 11. Levator scapulae. 12. Rhomboid minor. 13. Supraspinatus. 14. Infraspinatus. 15. Teres minor. 16. Rhomboid major. 17. Teres major. 18. Erector spinae. 19. Latissimus dorsi.

Page 107 Posterior View of the Neck (Intermediate and Deep)
1. Semispinalis capitis (of transversospinalis group). 2. Longissimus capitis (of erector spinae group). 3. Splenius capitis. 4. Splenius cervicis. 5. Iliocostalis cervicis (of erector spinae group). 6. Serratus posterior superior. 7. Iliocostalis and longissimus (of erector spinae group). 8. Splenius cervicis. 9. Rectus capitis posterior minor. 10. Rectus capitis posterior major. 11. Obliquus capitis superior. 12. Obliquus capitis inferior. 13. Interspinales. 14. Rotatores (of transversospinalis group). 15. Levatores costarum. 16. External intercostals.

Muscles of the Neck: Answers to Review Questions (pp 108–111)
1. Left rotation. 2. Semispinalis capitis. 3. Trapezius. 4. Depression of the mandible at the temporomandibular joints. 5. Two bellies. 6. Digastric. 7. Elevation of the hyoid bone. 8. Thyrohyoid. 9. The right one does right rotation and the left one does left rotation of the atlas at the atlantoaxial joint. 10. Inferior and superior bellies. 11. Right lateral flexion of the neck at the spinal joints. 12. Rhomboids. 13. Platysma. 14. The sternohyoid depresses the hyoid; the stylohyoid elevates the hyoid. 15. It would lengthen and stretch it. 16. Rectus capitis posterior major and minor. 17. Sternothyroid. 18. Digastric [anterior belly]. 19. Elevation of the hyoid bone. 20. Extension, right lateral flexion, and right rotation of the head and neck at the spinal joints. 21. Obliquus capitis inferior. 22. Levator scapulae, serratus anterior and rhomboids major and minor. 23. Geniohyoid. 24. Serratus anterior and the upper and lower trapezius. 25. Digastric, stylohyoid, mylohyoid, geniohyoid. 26. It lengthens. 27. They both left laterally flex the neck at the spinal joints. 28. Anterior, middle, and posterior scalenes. 29. Levator scapulae. 30. Middle scalene. 31. They lengthen. 32. Flexion of the neck at the spinal joint. 33. They both flex the neck at the spinal joints. 34. Longus capitis. 35. The scalenes. 36. C1-C5. 37. Left lateral flexion of the head at the atlanto-occipital joint. 38. Longus colli and capitis and rectus capitis anterior and lateralis. 39. Flexion of the neck at the spinal joints. 40. The transverse process of the atlas (C1). 41. Longus capitis. 42. The occiput. 43. Thyroid cartilage. 44. They both do left lateral flexion and right rotation of the head and neck at the spinal joints. 45. The digastric depresses the mandible at the temporomandibular joints; the masseter elevates the mandible. 46. Flexion, left lateral flexion, and left rotation of the neck at the spinal joints. 47. Rectus capitis posterior major and minor, obliquus capitis inferior and superior. 48. It would shorten and slacken it. 49. Right lateral flexion. 50. Lateral flexion of the neck at the spinal joints. 51. Flexion of the head at the atlanto-occipital joint. 52. Sternohyoid, sternothyroid, thyrohyoid, omohyoid. 53. Middle scalene. 54. Trapezius and deltoid. 55. Flexion of the neck at the spinal joints [the lateral flexion and rotation components would cancel each other out]. 56. Obliquus capitis inferior and superior. 57. Stylohyoid, mylohyoid, geniohyoid. 58. Trapezius. 59. It would lengthen and stretch it. 60. Depression of the hyoid bone. 61. Levator scapulae. 62. They both do left rotation and right lateral flexion of the head and neck at the spinal joints. 63. It lengthens. 64. Anterior scalene and omohyoid. 65. Elevation and protraction of the mandible at the temporomandibular joints and depression of the hyoid bone. 66. Depression of the hyoid bone. 67. Sternocleidomastoid, longissimus capitis. 68. Omohyoid. 69. Upper trapezius. 70. Posterior scalene. 71. It lengthens. 72. Right lateral flexion. 73. Left rotation. 74. 3.75. Obliquus capitis inferior and rectus capitis posterior major. 76. Obliquus capitis inferior. 77. Omohyoid. 78. Elevation and protraction [abduction] of the left scapula at the scapulocostal joint. 79. Retraction [adduction] of the scapula at the scapulocostal joint. 80. The *golf tee* muscles. 81. They both depress the hyoid bone. 82. Right rotation of the head at the atlantooccipital joint. 83. Sternocleidomastoid. 84. Between the anterior and middle scalenes.

CHAPTER 2 LABELING ANSWERS: MUSCLES OF THE TRUNK

Page 160 Posterior View of the Trunk (Superficial and Intermediate)
1. Splenius capitis. 2. Sternocleidomastoid. 3. Rhomboid minor (cut). 4. Rhomboid major (cut). 5. Deltoid. 6. Trapezius. 7. Teres major. 8. Triceps brachii. 9. Latissimus dorsi. 10. External abdominal oblique. 11. Gluteus medius. 12. Gluteus maximus. 13. Semispinalis capitis (of transversospinalis group). 14. Splenius capitis. 15. Splenius cervicis. 16. Levator scapulae. 17. Supraspinatus. 18. Serratus posterior superior. 19. Infraspinatus. 20. Teres minor. 21. Teres major. 22. Longissimus (of erector spinae group). 23. Latissimus dorsi (cut). 24. Spinalis (of erector spinae group). 25. Triceps brachii. 26. Iliocostalis (of erector spinae group). 27. Serratus anterior. 28. Serratus posterior inferior. 29. External abdominal oblique. 30. Latissimus dorsi (cut and reflected). 31. Internal abdominal oblique. 32. Gluteus medius. 33. Gluteus maximus.

Page 161 Posterior View of the Trunk (Deep Layers)
1. Semispinalis capitis (of transversospinalis group). 2. Longissimus (of erector spinae group). 3. Splenius capitis. 4. Splenius cervicis. 5. Iliocostalis (of erector spinae group). 6. Spinalis (of erector spinae group). 7. Longissimus (of erector spinae group). 8. Transversus abdominis. 9. Internal abdominal oblique. 10. External abdominal oblique (cut). 11. Iliocostalis (of erector spinae group). 12. Rectus capitis posterior minor. 13. Rectus capitis posterior major. 14. Obliquus capitis superior. 15. Obliquus capitis inferior. 16. Interspinales. 17. Rotatores (of transversospinalis group). 18. Semispinalis (of transversospinalis group). 19. External intercostals. 20. Levatores costarum. 21. Quadratus lumborum. 22. Multifidus (of transversospinalis group). 23. Intertransversarii. 24. Sacrum.

Page 162 Anterior View of the Trunk (Superficial and Intermediate)
1. Platysma. 2. Deltoid. 3. Pectoralis major. 4. Triceps brachii. 5. Biceps brachii. 6. Latissimus dorsi. 7. Serratus anterior. 8. External abdominal oblique. 9. Iliopsoas. 10. Sartorius. 11. Rectus femoris (of quadriceps femoris group). 12. Pectineus. 13. Adductor longus.

14. Sternocleidomastoid. 15. Trapezius. 16. Subclavius. 17. External intercostals. 18. Pectoralis minor. 19. Coracobrachialis. 20. Internal intercostals. 21. Biceps brachii. 22. External intercostals. 23. Rectus abdominis. 24. External abdominal oblique (cut). 25. Internal abdominal oblique. 26. Gluteus medius. 27. Tensor fasciae latae. 28. Gracilis.

Page 163 Anterior View of the Trunk (Intermediate and Deep)
1. Sternocleidomastoid. 2. Trapezius. 3. Subclavius. 4. External intercostals. 5. Pectoralis minor. 6. Coracobrachialis. 7. Internal intercostals. 8. Biceps brachii. 9. External intercostals. 10. Rectus abdominis. 11. External abdominal oblique (cut). 12. Internal abdominal oblique. 13. Gracilis. 14. Internal intercostals. 15. Rectus abdominis. 16. External abdominal oblique (cut). 17. Transversus abdominis. 18. Internal abdominal oblique (cut). 19. Gluteus medius. 20. Iliopsoas. 21. Tensor fasciae latae. 22. Sartorius. 23. Rectus femoris (of quadriceps femoris group). 24. Pectineus. 25. Adductor longus.

Page 164 Lateral View of the Trunk
1. Trapezius. 2. Supraspinatus (cut). 3. Biceps brachii (cut). 4. Subscapularis (cut). 5. Infraspinatus (cut). 6. Teres minor (cut). 7. Triceps brachii (cut). 8. Teres major (cut). 9. Serratus anterior. 10. Erector spinae. 11. External intercostals. 12. Serratus posterior inferior. 13. Internal abdominal oblique. 14. Gluteus medius. 15. Gluteus maximus. 16. Vastus lateralis (of quadriceps femoris group). 17. Sternocleidomastoid. 18. Subclavius. 19. External intercostals. 20. Internal intercostals. 21. Pectoralis minor. 22. External abdominal oblique. 23. Tensor fasciae latae. 24. Sartorius. 25. Rectus femoris (of quadriceps femoris group). 26. Vastus lateralis (of quadriceps femoris group).

Page 165 Cross Section Views of the Trunk (Thoracic)
1. Transversus thoracis. 2. Internal intercostals. 3. Erector spinae and transversospinalis groups. 4. Rhomboid major. 5. Trapezius. 6. Infraspinatus. 7. Teres major. 8. Subscapularis. 9. Latissimus dorsi. 10. Serratus anterior. 11. External intercostals.

Page 165 Cross Section Views of the Trunk (Lumbar)
1. Diaphragm. 2. Psoas major. 3. Quadratus lumborum. 4. Transversus abdominis. 5. Erector spinae and transversospinalis groups. 6. Serratus posterior inferior. 7. Latissimus dorsi. 8. Internal abdominal oblique. 9. External abdominal oblique.

Muscles of the Trunk: Answers to Review Questions (pp 166–169)
1. Multifidus. 2. Pectoralis major. 3. Rotatores. 4. Clavicular and sternocostal heads. 5. External and internal abdominal obliques. 6. Left lateral flexion of the neck and trunk at the spinal joints. 7. Protraction and depression of the scapula at the scapulocostal joint. 8. Pectoralis major. 9. True. 10. Opposite, i.e., perpendicular. 11. Latissimus dorsi and teres major. 12. Brachial plexus of nerves, subclavian artery and vein. 13. Flexion of the neck and trunk at the spinal joints. 14. It is shortening. 15. Psoas major and quadratus lumborum. 16. Subclavius. 17. Lengthen. 18. Spinalis. 19. External abdominal oblique. 20. Erector spinae group. 21. Pectoralis major and minor. 22. The lower rib will elevate at the sternocostal and costospinal joints. 23. External abdominal obliques. 24. It is lengthening. 25. Internal abdominal oblique and transversus abdominis. 26. They lengthen. 27. The rhomboids. 28. Transversus thoracis. 29. The upper rib will depress at the sternocostal and costospinal joints. 30. Serratus anterior and trapezius (upper and lower fibers). 31. They both depress the twelfth rib at the costospinal and sternocostal joints. 32. Trapezius. 33. It lengthens. 34. Latissimus dorsi. 35. Left rotation. 36. Between costal cartilages. 37. Retracting. 38. Iliocostalis. 39. Multifidus. 40. External abdominal oblique on that side of the body. 41. They are synergistic because they both do flexion and right lateral flexion of the trunk at the spinal joints; they are antagonistic because the right external abdominal oblique does left rotation and the right internal abdominal oblique does right rotation of the trunk. 42. Longissimus. 43. It shortens. 44. Posterior tilt and/or depression of the pelvis at the lumbosacral joint. 45. External and internal abdominal obliques and the transversus abdominis. 46. It shortens. 47. They lengthen. 48. Quadratus lumborum. 49. Rotatores. 50. Right rotation. 51. Spinalis. 52. Iliocostalis. 53. Semispinalis. 54. It is shortening. 55. Trapezius. 56. Transverse processes inferiorly to spinous processes superiorly. 57. Internal abdominal oblique. 58. They both elevate upper ribs (ribs #1-2) at the costospinal and sternocostal joints. 59. Transversus abdominis. 60. It lengthens. 61. It drops. 62. The low back. 63. Serratus posterior superior. 64. Quadratus lumborum. 65. Rectus sheath (abdominal aponeurosis). 66. Spinalis. 67. Serratus anterior, pectoralis major. 68. It lengthens. 69. Internal abdominal oblique. 70. Erector spine group. 71. Costoclavicular syndrome, a type of thoracic outlet syndrome. 72. Rotatores, because they are oriented most horizontally. 73. Lamina of the vertebrae (spinous processes of the vertebrae). 74. Subcostales. 75. Internal intercostals. 76. They both retract (adduct) the scapula at the scapulocostal joint. 77. Upper trapezius. 78. Elevation of ribs #9-12 at the costospinal and sternocostal joints. 79. Left rotation. 80. The neck. 81. It is lengthening. 82. Erector spinae group. 83. Its central tendon/dome. 84. Clavicular head. 85. Antagonistic; they laterally flex the spine to opposite sides. 86. Teres major. 87. Transversospinalis group. 88. Transversus abdominis. 89. Biceps brachii (long head proximal attachment). 90. It lengthens. 91. Internal abdominal oblique on that side of the body. 92. Thoracic. 93. Extension. 94. External intercostals. 95. The levatores costarum elevate ribs; the subcostales depress ribs.

CHAPTER 2 LABELING ANSWERS: MUSCLES OF THE PELVIS

Page 196 Anterior View of the Right Pelvis
1. Transversus abdominis (cut). 2. Quadratus lumborum. 3. Psoas major. 4. Iliacus. 5. Psoas minor.

Page 197 Lateral View of the Right Pelvis
1. Gluteus medius. 2. Gluteus maximus. 3. Vastus lateralis. 4. Biceps femoris. 5. Semimembranosus. 6. Plantaris. 7. Gastrocnemius (lateral head). 8. Soleus. 9. Fibularis longus. 10. Tensor fasciae latae. 11. Sartorius. 12. Rectus femoris. 13. Vastus lateralis. 14. Tibialis anterior. 15. Extensor digitorum longus.

Page 198 Posterior View of the Right Pelvis (Superficial)
1. Gluteus maximus. 2. Adductor magnus. 3. Semitendinosus. 4. Gracilis. 5. Semimembranosus. 6. Sartorius. 7. Gluteus medius. 8. Tensor fasciae latae. 9. Biceps femoris.

Page 199 Posterior View of the Right Pelvis (Deep)
1. Piriformis. 2. Superior gemellus. 3. Obturator internus. 4. Inferior gemellus. 5. Semitendinosus (cut). 6. Biceps femoris (long head, cut). 7. Gracilis. 8. Adductor magnus. 9. Semimembranosus. 10. Gluteus medius (cut). 11. Gluteus minimus. 12. Tensor fasciae latae. 13. Gluteus medius (cut and reflected). 14. Quadratus femoris. 15. Gluteus maximus (cut and reflected). 16. Pectineus. 17. Adductor magnus.

Muscles of the Pelvis: Answers to Review Questions (pp 200–201)

1. Obturator internus. 2. Piriformis. 3. Medial rotation and/or abduction. 4. Piriformis and quadratus femoris, respectively. 5. Obturator internus and externus. 6. Lengthen and stretch it. 7. Gluteus maximus, medius, minimus. 8. Gluteus maximus. 9. Superior gemellus and inferior gemellus. 10. Tensor fasciae latae, anterior fibers of the gluteus medius and minimus (they are medial rotators). 11. Synergistic. 12. Psoas major. 13. It lengthens. 14. Left rotation of the pelvis. 15. Tensor fasciae latae. 16. Both: the upper and lower fibers both extend and laterally rotate the thigh and posteriorly tilt and contralaterally rotate the pelvis at the hip joint, hence they are synergistic; however, the upper fibers abduct the thigh, but the lower fibers adduct the thigh, hence they are antagonistic. 17. Psoas major and iliacus. 18. Depression of the pelvis at the hip joint. 19. Adduction of the thigh at the hip joint. 20. Deep. 21. Deep lateral rotators of the thigh. 22. Inferior to it. 23. They are synergistic for every action. 24. It shortens. 25. Either lateral rotation or abduction (horizontal abduction or horizontal extension of the thigh). 26. Gluteus maximus. 27. Superior gemellus. 28. They share the same spinal joint actions. 29. The posterior fibers do extension and lateral rotation of the thigh and posterior tilt and contralateral rotation of the pelvis at the hip joint; the anterior fibers do flexion and medial rotation of the thigh and anterior tilt and ipsilateral rotation of the pelvis at the hip joint. 30. The right quadratus femoris does left rotation of the pelvis; the left quadratus femoris does right rotation of the pelvis. 31. Gluteus maximus. 32. Extension of the right thigh at the hip joint. 33. Lateral rotation and adduction of the thigh at the hip joint. 34. Synergistic, they both flex and laterally rotate the thigh and anteriorly tilt the pelvis at the hip joint. 35. Gluteus maximus and tensor fasciae latae. 36. Lengthen. 37. Either medial rotation or adduction (horizontal adduction or horizontal flexion) of the thigh. 38. All three hamstrings and the adductor magnus also attach to the ischial tuberosity. 39. It lengthens. 40. Lengthen and stretch. 41. Flexion or left lateral flexion of the trunk at the spinal joints or posterior tilt of the pelvis at the lumbosacral joint. 42. Quadratus femoris. 43. Psoas major and minor. 44. It shortens. 45. Inferior gemellus. 46. Piriformis, superior and inferior gemelli, obturator internus and externus, quadratus femoris. 47. Inferior gemellus. 48. Psoas minor. 49. Left rotation of the pelvis at the right hip joint. 50. Psoas major. 51. Sartorius. 52. Gluteus minimus. 53. Medial rotation of the thigh at the hip joint. 54. Obturator externus.

CHAPTER 2 LABELING ANSWERS: MUSCLES OF THE THIGH

Page 230 Anterior View of the Right Thigh (Superficial)
1. Iliacus. 2. Gluteus medius. 3. Tensor fasciae latae. 4. Rectus femoris. 5. Vastus lateralis. 6. Tibialis anterior. 7. Gastrocnemius. 8. Fibularis longus. 9. Psoas major. 10. Pectineus. 11. Adductor longus. 12. Gracilis. 13. Adductor magnus. 14. Sartorius. 15. Vastus medialis. 16. Gastrocnemius.

Page 231 Anterior View of the Right Thigh (Deep)
1. Iliopsoas (cut). 2. Quadratus femoris. 3. Pectineus (cut and reflected). 4. Vastus intermedius. 5. Adductor longus (cut and reflected). 6. Vastus lateralis (cut). 7. Rectus femoris (cut). 8. Vastus medialis (cut). 9. Pectineus (cut and reflected). 10. Adductor longus (cut and reflected). 11. Obturator externus. 12. Gracilis (cut). 13. Adductor brevis. 14. Adductor magnus. 15. Gracilis (cut). 16. Sartorius (cut). 17. Semitendinosus.

Page 232 Posterior View of the Right Thigh (Superficial)
1. Gluteus maximus. 2. Adductor magnus. 3. Gracilis. 4. Semitendinosus. 5. Semimembranosus. 6. Sartorius. 7. Gastrocnemius (medial head). 8. Soleus. 9. Gluteus medius. 10. Tensor fasciae latae. 11. Biceps femoris (long head). 12. Biceps femoris (short head). 13. Plantaris. 14. Gastrocnemius (lateral head). 15. Soleus.

Page 233 Posterior View of the Right Thigh (Deep)
1. Semitendinosus (cut and reflected). 2. Biceps femoris (long head, cut and reflected). 3. Semimembranosus. 4. Semitendinosus (cut and reflected). 5. Biceps femoris (short head). 6. Biceps femoris (long head, cut and reflected).

Page 234 Lateral View of the Right Thigh
1. Gluteus medius. 2. Gluteus maximus. 3. Vastus lateralis. 4. Biceps femoris. 5. Semimembranosus. 6. Plantaris. 7. Gastrocnemius (lateral head). 8. Soleus. 9. Fibularis longus. 10. Tensor fasciae latae. 11. Sartorius. 12. Rectus femoris. 13. Vastus lateralis. 14. Tibialis anterior. 15. Extensor digitorum longus.

Page 235 Medial View of the Right Thigh
1. Iliacus. 2. Adductor longus. 3. Gracilis. 4. Adductor magnus. 5. Rectus femoris. 6. Sartorius. 7. Vastus medialis. 8. Sartorius. 9. Gracilis. 10. Semitendinosus. 11. Tibialis anterior. 12. Piriformis. 13. Obturator internus. 14. Gluteus maximus. 15. Semitendinosus. 16. Semimembranosus. 17. Gastrocnemius (medial head). 18. Soleus.

Muscles of the Thigh: Answers to Review Questions (pp 236–237)

1. Tensor fasciae latae and sartorius. 2. Gluteus maximus. 3. 3. 4. Semitendinosus. 5. Flexion of the leg at the knee joint. 6. Gluteus maximus, posterior fibers of the gluteus medius and minimus. 7. Adductor magnus. 8. It lengthens. 9. Short head of the biceps femoris. 10. Sartorius. 11. Articularis genu. 12. Posterior tilt of the pelvis at the hip joint. 13. Vastus lateralis, medialis, and intermedius; and the tensor fasciae latae and gluteus maximus. 14. 4. 15. The biceps femoris laterally rotates the thigh and leg; the semitendinosus medially rotates the thigh and leg. 16. They all extend the leg at the knee joint. 17. The TFL flexes the thigh and anteriorly tilts the pelvis at the hip joint; the hamstrings extend the thigh and posteriorly tilts the pelvis at the hip joint. 18. Short head of the biceps femoris. 19. Tibial tuberosity. 20. Tensor fasciae latae and gluteus maximus. 21. Sartorius, gracilis, semitendinosus. 22. It lengthens. 23. Iliopsoas. 24. They both flex the thigh and anteriorly tilt the pelvis at the hip joint. 25. Posterior tilt and depression of the same-side pelvis at the hip joint. 26. Extension. 27. Posterior tilt and depression of the pelvis same-side at the hip joint. 28. Semitendinosus, gracilis, and sartorius. 29. Adductor magnus. 30. Articularis genu. 31. Adductor magnus. 32. Biceps femoris, semitendinosus, semimembranosus. 33. It shortens. 34. Flexion of the thigh at the hip joint. 35. Vastus lateralis. 36. It shortens. 37. Gracilis. 38. Biceps femoris. 39. It shortens. 40. The sartorius flexes the thigh and anteriorly tilts the pelvis at the hip joint; the semitendinosus extends the thigh and posteriorly tilts the pelvis at the hip joint. 41. Gluteus medius, anterior fibers. 42. It is extending. 43. Adductor longus. 44. Vastus lateralis. 45. Iliopsoas. 46. Adductor brevis. 47. They both posteriorly tilt the pelvis. 48. 3. 49. Sartorius. 50. Adductor longus. 51. Vastus intermedius. 52. It lengthens. 53. All three vastus muscles of the quadriceps femoris group, all three 'adductor' muscles of the adductor group, and the biceps femoris of the hamstring group. 54. It shortens. 55. Pectineus, gracilis, adductors longus, brevis, and magnus. 56. It lengthens. 57. Rectus femoris. 58. Rectus femoris,

vastus lateralis, medialis, and intermedius. 59. Vastus lateralis or medialis, rectus femoris, tensor fasciae latae and gluteus maximus.

CHAPTER 2 LABELING ANSWERS: MUSCLES OF THE LEG

Page 262 Anterior View of the Right Leg
1. Vastus lateralis. 2. Rectus femoris. 3. Biceps femoris. 4. Fibularis longus. 5. Tibialis anterior. 6. Extensor digitorum longus. 7. Fibularis brevis. 8. Fibularis tertius. 9. Fibularis tertius tendon. 10. Extensor digitorum brevis. 11. Vastus medialis. 12. Sartorius. 13. Gracilis. 14. Semitendinosus. 15. Gastrocnemius. 16. Soleus. 17. Extensor hallucis longus. 18. Extensor hallucis brevis.

Page 263 Posterior View of the Right Leg (Superficial)
1. Semimembranosus. 2. Gracilis. 3. Sartorius. 4. Semitendinosus. 5. Gastrocnemius (medial head). 6. Soleus. 7. Plantaris (tendon). 8. Tibialis posterior. 9. Flexor digitorum longus. 10. Flexor hallucis longus. 11. Biceps femoris. 12. Plantaris. 13. Gastrocnemius (lateral head). 14. Soleus. 15. Fibularis longus. 16. Fibularis brevis.

Page 264 Posterior View of the Right Leg (Intermediate)
1. Gastrocnemius (medial head, cut). 2. Semimembranosus (cut). 3. Popliteus. 4. Soleus. 5. Gastrocnemius (medial head, cut). 6. Tibialis posterior. 7. Flexor digitorum longus. 8. Flexor hallucis longus. 9. Plantaris. 10. Gastrocnemius (lateral head, cut). 11. Biceps femoris (cut). 12. Fibularis longus. 13. Gastrocnemius (lateral head, cut). 14. Fibularis brevis.

Page 265 Posterior View of the Right Leg (Deep)
1. Gastrocnemius (cut). 2. Semimembranosus. 3. Popliteus. 4. Tibialis posterior. 5. Flexor digitorum longus. 6. Biceps femoris. 7. Gastrocnemius (lateral head, cut). 8. Plantaris (cut and reflected). 9. Soleus (cut and reflected). 10. Fibularis longus. 11. Flexor hallucis longus. 12. Fibularis brevis.

Page 266 Lateral View of the Right Leg
1. Biceps femoris. 2. Plantaris. 3. Fibularis longus. 4. Gastrocnemius. 5. Soleus. 6. Fibularis brevis. 7. Fibularis tertius. 8. Extensor digitorum brevis & extensor hallucis brevis. 9. Vastus lateralis. 10. Rectus femoris. 11. Tibialis anterior. 12. Extensor digitorum longus. 13. Extensor hallucis longus.

Page 267 Medial View of the Right Leg
1. Gracilis. 2. Rectus femoris. 3. Sartorius. 4. Vastus medialis. 5. Sartorius (pes anserine tendon). 6. Gracilis (pes anserine tendon). 7. Semitendinosus (pes anserine tendon). 8. Tibialis anterior. 9. Extensor hallucis longus. 10. Extensor digitorum longus. 11. Adductor magnus. 12. Semitendinosus. 13. Semimembranosus. 14. Gastrocnemius. 15. Soleus. 16. Plantaris. 17. Flexor digitorum longus. 18. Tibialis posterior. 19. Flexor hallucis longus.

Muscles of the Leg: Answers to Review Questions (pp 268–269)
1. They both evert the foot at the subtalar joint. 2. In the distal medial leg. 3. Popliteus. 4. The fibula. 5. The fibularis tertius dorsiflexes the foot at the ankle joint; the fibularis brevis plantarflexes it. 6. Extensor digitorum longus. 7. Dorsiflexion and inversion of the foot at the ankle and subtalar joints, respectively. 8. Fibularis longus. 9. They both dorsiflex the foot at the ankle joint. 10. Gastrocnemius, soleus, plantaris. 11. Fibularis brevis and tertius. 12. Nothing; the flexor digitorum longus does not cross the knee joint. 13. Medial and lateral gastrocnemius and the soleus. 14. Distal. 15. Gastrocnemius and soleus. 16. Tom is tibialis posterior; Dick is the flexor digitorum longus, Harry is the flexor hallucis longus. 17. Extensor hallucis longus. 18. Gastrocnemius. 19. Soleus. 20. Tibialis anterior, extensors digitorum and hallucis longus, fibularis tertius. 21. Dorsiflexion and/or inversion of the foot at the ankle and subtalar joints, respectively. 22. Plantaris and lateral head of the gastrocnemius. 23. It lengthens. 24. Tibialis posterior. 25. Flexor digitorum longus. 26. Soleus. 27. Tibialis anterior and fibularis longus. 28. Both synergistic and antagonistic. 29. Fibularis brevis. 30. The popliteus. 31. It medially rotates the leg at the knee joint; it laterally rotates the thigh at the knee joint. 32. Plantarflexion and inversion of the foot at the ankle and subtalar joints, respectively. 33. Tibialis anterior and fibularis longus. 34. Fibularis longus and brevis. 35. Soleus. 36. Extensor digitorum longus and fibularis tertius. 37. Talus. 38. Flexor digitorum longus. 39. Inversion and/or dorsiflexion of the foot at the subtalar and ankle joints, respectively. 40. Soleus. 41. It shortens. 42. Popliteus, flexors digitorum and hallucis longus, tibialis posterior.

CHAPTER 2 LABELING ANSWERS: INTRINSIC MUSCLES OF THE FOOT

Page 288 Dorsal View of the Right Foot
1. Fibularis longus tendon. 2. Fibularis brevis. 3. Extensor digitorum longus. 4. Fibularis brevis tendon. 5. Fibularis tertius tendon. 6. Extensor digitorum brevis. 7. Abductor digiti minimi pedis. 8. Dorsal interossei pedis. 9. Extensor hallucis longus. 10. Tibialis anterior. 11. Soleus. 12. Extensor hallucis brevis. 13. Abductor hallucis. 14. Dorsal interossei pedis.

Page 289 Plantar View of the Right Foot (Superficial Muscular Layer)
1. Flexor digitorum longus tendons. 2. Flexor digitorum brevis tendons. 3. Adductor hallucis (transverse head). 4. Lumbricals pedis. 5. Flexor digiti minimi pedis. 6. Abductor digiti minimi pedis. 7. Flexor hallucis longus tendon. 8. Flexor hallucis brevis. 9. Flexor digitorum brevis. 10. Abductor hallucis.

Page 290 Plantar View of the Right Foot (Intermediate Muscular Layer)
1. Flexor digitorum longus tendons. 2. Flexor digitorum brevis tendons (cut). 3. Adductor hallucis (transverse head). 4. Lumbricals pedis. 5. Flexor digiti minimi pedis. 6. Plantar interossei. 7. Abductor digiti minimi pedis (partially cut). 8. Quadratus plantae. 9. Flexor digitorum brevis (cut). 10. Flexor hallucis longus tendon. 11. Flexor hallucis brevis. 12. Abductor hallucis (cut). 13. Tibialis posterior tendon. 14. Flexor digitorum longus tendon. 15. Flexor hallucis longus tendon. 16. Abductor hallucis (cut).

Page 291 Plantar View of the Right Foot (Deep Muscular Layer)
1. Flexor digitorum longus tendons (cut). 2. Flexor digitorum brevis tendons (cut). 3. Lumbricals pedis (cut). 4. Adductor hallucis (transverse head). 5. Flexor digiti minimi pedis. 6. Abductor digiti minimi pedis (cut). 7. Plantar interossei. 8. Fibularis brevis tendon. 9. Fibularis longus tendon. 10. Quadratus plantae (cut). 11. Flexor digitorum brevis (cut). 12. Abductor digiti minimi pedis (cut). 13. Flexor hallucis longus tendon (cut). 14. Flexor hallucis brevis. 15. Adductor hallucis (oblique head). 16. Abductor hallucis (cut). 17. Tibialis posterior tendon. 18. Flexor digitorum longus tendon (cut and reflected). 19. Flexor hallucis longus tendon (cut). 20. Abductor hallucis (cut).

Intrinsic Muscles of the Foot: Answers to Review Questions (pp 292–293)

1. Flexor digitorum accessorius. 2. Extensor digitorum longus. 3. Flexion of toes #2–5 at the metatarsophalangeal and proximal interphalangeal joints. 4. Extensors hallucis brevis and longus. 5. Adduction or flexion of the big toe at the metatarsophalangeal joint. 6. Abductor hallucis. 7. It shortens. 8. The 2nd dorsal interosseus pedis muscle. 9. Flexor hallucis brevis, flexor digiti minimi pedis, adductor hallucis. 10. Flexor hallucis brevis. 11. Flexor hallucis brevis. 12. 2; the extensors hallucis and digitorum brevis; the dorsal interossei pedis are technically plantar muscles. 13. Plantar interossei. 14. Abductor hallucis, abductor digiti minimi pedis, flexor digitorum brevis. 15. The lumbricals pedis are superficial. 16. DAB and PAD; Dorsals Abduct. Plantars ADDuct. 17. Quadratus plantae. 18. Calcaneus. 19. 3rd plantar interosseus. 20. Extensor digitorum longus and fibularis tertius. 21. Quadratus plantae and lumbricals pedis. 22. Dorsal interossei pedis. 23. Flexor digitorum longus. 24. Tuberosity of the calcaneus. 25. Oblique and transverse heads. 26. The 1st and 2nd DIP; the 1st DIP tibially abducts the 2nd toe; the 2nd DIP fibularly abducts the 2nd toe. 27. Flexor digitorum brevis. 28. Abductor digiti minimi pedis. 29. Abductor hallucis, abductor digiti minimi pedis, flexor digitorum brevis. 30. Fibularis longus. 31. Extensor hallucis longus. 32. Flexor digitorum brevis. 33. Extension of toes #2–5 at the metatarsophalangeal and/or proximal interphalangeal joints. 34. Abductor digiti minimi pedis. 35. Adductor hallucis. 36. Adduction of the big toe at the metatarsophalangeal joint. 37. Flexor digitorum longus. 38. The distal tendons of the flexor digitorum longus. 39. Plantar interossei and dorsal interossei pedis. 40. The flexor hallucis brevis. 41. It lengthens. 42. Both; they flex the toes at the metatarsophalangeal joints and extend the toes at the interphalangeal joints.

CHAPTER 2 LABELING ANSWERS: MUSCLES OF THE SCAPULA/ARM

Page 316 Anterior View of the Right Shoulder
1. Anterior scalene. 2. Middle scalene. 3. Levator scapulae. 4. Omohyoid. 5. Posterior scalene. 6. Trapezius. 7. Deltoid. 8. Biceps brachii. 9. Triceps brachii. 10. Latissimus dorsi. 11. Serratus anterior. 12. External abdominal oblique. 13. Sternocleidomastoid. 14. Pectoralis major.

Page 317 Posterior View of the Shoulders (Superficial and Intermediate)
1. Sternocleidomastoid. 2. Splenius capitis. 3. Levator scapulae. 4. Trapezius. 5. Deltoid. 6. Triceps brachii. 7. Latissimus dorsi. 8. Semispinalis capitis (of transversospinalis group). 9. Splenius capitis. 10. Splenius cervicis. 11. Levator scapulae. 12. Rhomboid minor. 13. Supraspinatus. 14. Infraspinatus. 15. Rhomboid major. 16. Teres minor. 17. Teres major. 18. Triceps brachii. 19. Erector spinae.

Page 318 Anterior View of the Right Arm (Superficial)
1. Deltoid. 2. Pectoralis major (cut and reflected). 3. Biceps brachii (long head). 4. Biceps brachii (short head). 5. Biceps brachii. 6. Brachialis. 7. Brachioradialis. 8. Pectoralis minor (cut). 9. Coracobrachialis. 10. Subscapularis. 11. Teres major. 12. Latissimus dorsi. 13. Triceps brachii. 14. Pronator teres. 15. Flexor carpi radialis. 16. Palmaris longus. 17. Flexor carpi ulnaris.

Page 319 Anterior View of the Right Arm (Deep)
1. Supraspinatus. 2. Biceps brachii (cut). 3. Deltoid (cut). 4. Biceps brachii (cut). 5. Pectoralis minor (cut). 6. Subscapularis. 7. Teres major. 8. Latissimus dorsi. 9. Coracobrachialis. 10. Brachialis.

Page 320 Medial View of the Right Arm
1. Biceps brachii (long head, cut). 2. Subscapularis (cut). 3. Pectoralis major (cut). 4. Biceps brachii (short head, cut). 5. Coracobrachialis (cut). 6. Biceps brachii. 7. Bicipital aponeurosis of the biceps brachii. 8. Brachioradialis. 9. Flexor carpi radialis. 10. Supraspinatus (cut). 11. Infraspinatus (cut). 12. Teres minor (cut). 13. Deltoid (cut). 14. Teres major (cut). 15. Latissimus dorsi (cut). 16. Triceps brachii (long head). 17. Triceps brachii (medial head). 18. Brachialis. 19. Pronator teres. 20. Palmaris longus. 21. Flexor carpi ulnaris.

Page 321 Lateral View of the Right Arm
1. Deltoid. 2. Triceps brachii. 3. Anconeus. 4. Extensor carpi ulnaris. 5. Extensor digitorum. 6. Extensor digiti minimi. 7. Biceps brachii. 8. Brachialis. 9. Brachioradialis. 10. Extensor carpi radialis longus. 11. Extensor carpi radialis brevis.

Page 322 Posterior View of the Right Arm
1. Supraspinatus. 2. Infraspinatus. 3. Teres minor. 4. Teres major. 5. Triceps brachii (medial head). 6. Flexor carpi ulnaris. 7. Deltoid (cut and reflected). 8. Triceps brachii (lateral head). 9. Triceps brachii (long head). 10. Brachioradialis. 11. Extensor carpi radialis longus. 12. Anconeus. 13. Extensor carpi radialis brevis. 14. Extensor digitorum. 15. Extensor digiti minimi. 16. Extensor carpi ulnaris.

Page 323 Anterior View of the Right Glenohumeral Joint
1. Supraspinatus. 2. Coracobrachialis (cut). 3. Biceps brachii (short head, cut). 4. Biceps brachii (long head, cut). 5. Triceps brachii. 6. Coracobrachialis (cut). 7. Biceps brachii (cut). 8. Supraspinatus. 9. Pectoralis minor (cut). 10. Subscapularis. 11. Teres major. 12. Latissimus dorsi.

Page 323 Posterior View of the Right Glenohumeral Joint
1. Supraspinatus (cut). 2. Infraspinatus (cut and reflected). 3. Teres major. 4. Teres minor. 5. Supraspinatus (cut). 6. Infraspinatus (cut and reflected). 7. Deltoid (cut and reflected). 8. Triceps brachii (medial head). 9. Triceps brachii (long head). 10. Triceps brachii (lateral head).

Muscles of the Scapula/Arm: Answers to Review Questions (pp 324–325)

1. Triceps brachii, anconeus, extensor carpi ulnaris. 2. Synergistic; they both flex and adduct the arm at the shoulder joint. 3. Superficial. 4. Medial rotation of the arm at the shoulder joint. 5. They both do abduction of the arm at the shoulder joint. 6. Teres major and teres minor. 7. Deep; anterior. 8. Medial head. 9. Anterior fibers flex while the posterior fibers extend; anterior fibers medially rotate while the posterior fibers laterally rotate. 10. Anterior. 11. Deltoid. 12. Coracobrachialis, pectoralis minor, and biceps brachii, short head. 13. Subscapularis; they both do medial rotation of the arm at the shoulder joint. 14. Long head. 15. Inferior. 16. Antagonistic; the pronator teres flexes the elbow joint; the triceps brachii extends it. 17. Brachialis. 18. Shorten. 19. Neither; pronation and supination have no effect upon the length of the brachialis. 20. Shortened. 21. Deep. 22. Brachialis. 23. Synergistic; they both flex the elbow joint. 24. Lateral rotation, abduction, and flexion of the arm at the shoulder joint. 25. Latissimus dorsi. 26. Supraspinatus. 27. Lateral. 28. 3; The elbow, radioulnar, and shoulder joints. 29. Supraspinatus and teres minor. 30. Shortened. 31. Supraspinatus, infraspinatus, teres minor, subscapularis. 32. Antagonistic; minor does lateral rotation; major does medial rotation. 33. Infraspinatus. 34. They both do abduction of the arm at the shoulder joint. 35. Supraspinatus, infraspinatus, teres minor. 36. Clavicular head. 37. Extension and abduction. 38. Inferior. 39. Superior. 40. Latissimus dorsi. 41. Trapezius and deltoid. 42. Deltoid.

ANSWER KEY

CHAPTER 2 LABELING ANSWERS: MUSCLES OF THE FOREARM

Page 360 Anterior View of the Right Forearm (Superficial)
1. Biceps brachii. 2. Brachialis. 3. Brachioradialis. 4. Extensor carpi radialis longus. 5. Extensor carpi radialis brevis. 6. Flexor pollicis longus. 7. Pronator quadratus. 8. Abductor pollicis longus. 9. Triceps brachii (medial head). 10. Brachialis (deep to median nerve and brachial artery from this view). 11. Bicipital aponeurosis of the biceps brachii. 12. Pronator teres. 13. Flexor carpi radialis. 14. Palmaris longus. 15. Flexor carpi ulnaris. 16. Flexor digitorum superficialis. 17. Flexor digitorum profundus.

Page 361 Anterior View of the Right Forearm (Intermediate)
1. Biceps brachii. 2. Brachialis. 3. Brachialis (tendon). 4. Biceps brachii (tendon). 5. Supinator. 6. Brachioradialis. 7. Pronator teres (cut). 8. Flexor pollicis longus. 9. Abductor pollicis longus. 10. Pronator quadratus. 11. Flexor carpi radialis (cut). 12. Triceps brachii (medial head). 13. Pronator teres (humeral head, cut and reflected). 14. Brachialis. 15. Flexor carpi radialis (cut). 16. Palmaris longus (cut). 17. Pronator teres (ulnar head, cut and reflected). 18. Flexor digitorum profundus. 19. Flexor carpi ulnaris. 20. Flexor digitorum superficialis. 21. Flexor digitorum profundus.

Page 362 Anterior View of the Right Forearm (Deep)
1. Brachialis. 2. Biceps brachii (tendon). 3. Supinator. 4. Flexor digitorum superficialis (cut). 5. Pronator teres (cut and reflected). 6. Flexor pollicis longus (cut). 7. Pronator quadratus. 8. Brachioradialis (cut). 9. Flexor carpi radialis (cut). 10. Flexor pollicis longus (cut). 11. Triceps brachii (medial head). 12. Pronator teres (humeral head, cut and reflected). 13. Flexor carpi radialis (cut). 14. Palmaris longus (cut). 15. Flexor carpi ulnaris (cut and reflected). 16. Flexor digitorum superficialis (cut). 17. Pronator teres (ulnar head, cut). 18. Flexor digitorum profundus (cut). 19. Flexor carpi ulnaris (cut).

Page 363 Anterior Views of the Pronators and Supinator of the Right Radius
1. Supinator: ulnar head. 1. Supinator: humeral head. 2. Pronator quadratus. 3. Pronator teres: humeral head. 3. Pronator teres: ulnar head.

Page 364 Posterior View of the Right Forearm (Superficial)
1. Triceps brachii. 2. Flexor carpi ulnaris. 3. Extensor carpi ulnaris. 4. Extensor digiti minimi. 5. Abductor digiti minimi manus. 6. Dorsal interossei manus. 7. Brachioradialis. 8. Anconeus. 9. Extensor carpi radialis longus. 10. Extensor carpi radialis brevis. 11. Extensor digitorum. 12. Abductor pollicis longus. 13. Extensor pollicis brevis. 14. Extensor pollicis longus. 15. Dorsal interossei manus. 16. Extensor indicis tendon.

Page 365 Posterior View of the Right Forearm (Deep)
1. Flexor carpi ulnaris. 2. Extensor digitorum tendons (cut). 3. Extensor indicis. 4. Extensor digiti minimi (cut). 5. Extensor carpi ulnaris (cut). 6. Abductor digiti minimi manus. 7. Dorsal interossei manus. 8. Triceps brachii tendon (cut). 9. Brachioradialis. 10. Anconeus. 11. Extensor carpi radialis longus. 12. Extensor carpi radialis brevis. 13. Supinator. 14. Pronator teres. 15. Abductor pollicis longus. 16. Extensor pollicis longus. 17. Extensor pollicis brevis. 18. Dorsal interossei manus. 19. Extensor indicis tendon.

Page 366 Posterior View of the Right Forearm and Hand (Superficial)
1. Extensor digiti minimi. 2. Extensor carpi ulnaris. 3. Extensor carpi radialis longus. 4. Extensor carpi radialis brevis. 5. Extensor digitorum. 6. Abductor pollicis longus. 7. Extensor pollicis brevis. 8. Extensor pollicis longus. 9. Extensor indicis (tendon).

Page 367 Posterior View of the Right Forearm and Hand (Deep)
1. Extensor digiti minimi (cut). 2. Extensor carpi ulnaris (cut). 3. Extensor pollicis longus. 4. Extensor indicis. 5. Extensor carpi ulnaris tendon (cut). 6. Extensor carpi radialis longus. 7. Extensor carpi radialis brevis. 8. Extensor digitorum (cut). 9. Abductor pollicis longus. 10. Extensor pollicis brevis.

Muscles of the Forearm: Answers to Review Questions (pp 368–371)
1. Flexor digitorum superficialis. 2. Deep. 3. Extensor carpi ulnaris. 4. Palmaris longus and flexor carpi radialis. 5. Brachioradialis. 6. Extension and/or ulnar deviation of the hand at the wrist joint. 7. Anconeus, extensor carpi radialis brevis, extensors digitorum and digiti minimi, extensor carpi ulnaris, and supinator. 8. Metacarpals 2, 3, and 5, respectively. 9. Extension and ulnar deviation of the hand at the wrist joint. 10. Extensor digitorum. 11. The anconeus extends the forearm at the elbow joint; the flexor carpi radialis flexes it. 12. Both muscles can supinate the forearm at the radioulnar joints. 13. Extensor carpi ulnaris. 14. Flexor pollicis longus. 15. Brachioradialis and extensor carpi radialis longus. 16. Extension of the elbow joint. 17. Flexor digitorum profundus. 18. Median nerve. 19. The common flexor tendon. 20. Flexor pollicis longus. 21. Extensor carpi radialis longus. 22. Both do flexion of the hand at the wrist joint and flexion of the forearm at the elbow joint. 23. Extensors carpi radialis longus and brevis, extensor carpi ulnaris. 24. Extensor digiti minimi. 25. Supinator and anconeus. 26. Abductor pollicis longus. 27. Extensor digiti minimi and extensor indicis. 28. Abductor pollicis longus and extensor pollicis brevis laterally; extensor pollicis longus medially. 29. Extensor carpi radialis brevis and extensor digitorum. 30. The extensor pollicis brevis radially deviates the hand at the wrist joint; the extensor carpi ulnaris ulnar deviates it. 31. Extensors carpi radialis brevis and longus and the brachioradialis. 32. Radial deviation. 33. Anconeus. 34. Extensor pollicis brevis. 35. Abductor pollicis longus, extensors pollicis brevis and longus, extensor indicis. 36. Flexor digitorum profundus. 37. Extensors carpi radialis longus and brevis. 38. It lengthens. 39. Extensor pollicis brevis. 40. Flexor digitorum profundus. 41. Brachioradialis, extensors carpi radialis longus and brevis. 42. Triceps brachii. 43. Flexor carpi ulnaris. 44. The FCR radially deviates the hand at the wrist joint; the FCU ulnar deviates the hand at the wrist joint. 45. Pronator teres. 46. Pronators teres and quadratus. 47. The radius. 48. They shorten. 49. It shortens. 50. Flexor pollicis longus and brevis, opponens and adductor pollicis. 51. Common flexor tendon at the medial epicondyle of the humerus. 52. Triceps brachii. 53. Flexors carpi radialis and ulnaris, palmaris longus. 54. Pronator teres. 55. They both flex the hand at the wrist joint and flex the forearm at the elbow joint. 56. Supinator, abductor pollicis longus, extensors pollicis longus and brevis, extensor indicis. 57. Extensor carpi ulnaris. 58. Flexor digitorum profundus. 59. Extensor digitorum. 60. Brachioradialis, abductor or extensor pollicis longus, extensor indicis. 61. Brachialis, biceps brachii, pronator teres. 62. Flexor carpi radialis. 63. Pronator quadratus. 64. Flexors digitorum superficialis and profundus. 65. Pronation of the forearm at the radioulnar joints. 66. Extensors digitorum, digiti minimi, carpi ulnaris and carpi radialis brevis. 67. Flexor digitorum superficialis. 68. It shortens. 69. Extensor carpi radialis longus. 70. Extension and/or radial deviation of the hand at the wrist joint. 71. It lengthens. 72. Extensor digitorum. 73. They lengthen. 74. It lengthens. 75. Extension of the elbow joint. 76. It shortens. 77. Extension of the fingers at the metacarpophalangeal and/or

proximal interphalangeal joints, and/or extension of the hand at the wrist joint and the forearm at the elbow joint. 78. Flexor digitorum profundus.

CHAPTER 2 LABELING ANSWERS: MUSCLES OF THE HAND

Page 388 Palmar View of the Right Hand (Superficial)
1. Palmaris longus. 2. Flexor pollicis brevis (deep to fascia). 3. Abductor pollicis brevis (deep to fascia). 4. Adductor pollicis (deep to fascia). 5. Lumbricals manus (partially deep to fascia). 6. Flexor pollicis longus. 7. Dorsal interossei manus. 8. Flexor digitorum profundus. 9. Flexor digitorum superficialis. 10. Palmar interossei. 11. Dorsal interossei manus. 12. Lumbricals manus. 13. Palmaris brevis. 14. Hypothenar muscle group (deep to fascia). 15. Palmar interossei. 16. Flexor digitorum profundus. 17. Flexor digitorum superficialis. 18. Lumbricals manus. 19. Dorsal interossei manus. 20. Lumbricals manus. 21. Dorsal interossei manus.

Page 389 Palmar View of the Right Hand (Superficial Muscular Layer)
1. Flexor pollicis brevis. 2. Abductor pollicis brevis. 3. Adductor pollicis (deep to fascia). 4. Dorsal interossei manus. 5. Lumbricals manus. 6. Lumbricals manus. 7. Flexor digitorum profundus. 8. Flexor digitorum superficialis. 9. Palmar interossei. 10. Dorsal interossei manus. 11. Opponens digiti minimi. 12. Abductor digiti minimi manus. 13. Flexor digiti minimi manus. 14. Lumbricals manus. 15. Lumbricals manus. 16. Palmar interossei. 17. Flexor digitorum profundus. 18. Flexor digitorum superficialis. 19. Dorsal interossei manus. 20. Dorsal interossei manus.

Page 390 Palmar View of the Right Hand (Deep Muscular Layer)
1. Pronator quadratus. 2. Abductor pollicis brevis (cut). 3. Opponens pollicis. 4. Flexor pollicis brevis. 5. Abductor pollicis brevis (cut). 6. Adductor pollicis. 7. Dorsal interossei manus. 8. Lumbricals manus (cut and reflected). 9. Lumbricals manus (cut and reflected). 10. Palmar interossei. 11. Dorsal interossei manus. 12. Flexor carpi ulnaris. 13. Abductor digiti minimi manus (cut). 14. Flexor digiti minimi manus (cut). 15. Opponens digiti minimi. 16. Palmar interossei. 17. Dorsal interossei manus. 18. Abductor digiti minimi manus (cut). 19. Flexor digiti minimi manus (cut). 20. Dorsal interossei manus. 21. Lumbricals manus (cut and reflected). 22. Palmar interossei. 23. Lumbricals manus (cut and reflected).

Page 391 Dorsal View of the Right Hand
1. Extensor digitorum. 2. Extensor digiti minimi. 3. Extensor carpi ulnaris. 4. Abductor digiti minimi manus. 5. Dorsal interossei manus. 6. Dorsal interossei manus. 7. Palmar interossei. 8. Lumbricals manus. 9. Lumbricals manus. 10. Extensor carpi radialis brevis. 11. Extensor carpi radialis longus. 12. Extensor pollicis brevis. 13. Abductor pollicis longus. 14. Extensor indicis. 15. Extensor pollicis longus. 16. Dorsal interossei manus. 17. Dorsal interossei manus. 18. Adductor pollicis. 19. Palmar interossei.

Muscles of the Hand: Answers to Review Questions (pp 392–393)
1. Thenar, hypothenar, central compartment. 2. Abductor and flexor pollicis brevis. 3. Lumbricals manus, palmar interossei, dorsal interossei manus, adductor pollicis. 4. They both flex fingers at the metacarpophalangeal joints and extend fingers at the interphalangeal joints. 5. Hypothenar group. 6. Palmaris longus. 7. 3rd palmar interosseus. 8. Flexion of the thumb at the carpometacarpal and/or metacarpophalangeal joints and/or abduction of the thumb at the carpometacarpal joint. 9. Trapezium. 10. Adductor pollicis. 11. Deep. 12. Adductor pollicis, lumbricals manus, palmar interossei, dorsal interossei manus. 13. Abductor and flexor pollicis brevis, opponens pollicis. 14. Abductor and flexor pollicis brevis, opponens pollicis. 15. Palmar interossei. 16. It has no bony attachments; it attaches only into soft tissues. 17. Abductor and flexor pollicis brevis; adductor pollicis. 18. The abductor digiti minimi manus abducts the little finger at the metacarpophalangeal joint; the opponens digiti minimi adducts it. 19. When objects are being gripped in the hand. 20. No joint action occurs when any muscle isometrically contracts. 21. Flexor pollicis brevis. 22. Deep. 23. Abductor pollicis brevis. 24. Lumbricals manus, palmar interossei, dorsal interossei manus, adductor pollicis. 25. It lengthens. 26. Pisiform and hamate. 27. Extension of the little finger at the metacarpophalangeal joint. 28. Abductor and flexor digiti minimi manus and opponens digiti minimi. 29. Lateral rotation of the little finger. 30. It lengthens. 31. Palmar interossei. 32. Abductor and flexor digiti minimi manus, opponens digiti minimi. 33. Their distal attachments are onto metacarpals. 34. Both; the metacarpophalangeal joints are flexed; the interphalangeal joints are extended. 35. Flexor digiti minimi manus. 36. The palmar interossei adduct fingers at the metacarpophalangeal joints; the dorsal interossei manus abduct fingers at the metacarpophalangeal joints.

CHAPTER 3 LABELING ANSWERS: OTHER SKELETAL MUSCLES

Page 396 Anterior Views of the Other Muscles of the Abdomen
1. External abdominal oblique. 2. Rectus abdominis. 3. Pyramidalis. 4. External abdominal oblique. 5. Internal abdominal oblique. 6. Cremaster.

Page 397 Views of the Muscles of the Perineum
1. Ischiocavernosus. 2. Bulbospongiosus. 3. Deep transverse perineal. 4. Superficial transverse perineal. 5. Gluteus maximus. 6. External anal sphincter. 7. Compressor urethrae. 8. Sphincter urethrae. 9. Sphincter urethrovaginalis. 10. Levator ani. 11. Coccygeus. 12. Sphincter urethrae. 13. Deep transverse perineal. 14. Superficial transverse perineal. 15. External anal sphincter. 16. Gluteus maximus. 17. Ischiocavernosus. 18. Bulbospongiosus. 19. Deep transverse perineal. 20. Superficial transverse perineal. 21. Levator ani. 22. Coccygeus.

Page 398 Views of the Muscles of the Tongue
1. Superior longitudinal muscle. 2. Vertical muscle. 3. Transverse muscle. 4. Inferior longitudinal muscle. 5. Genioglossus. 6. Stylohyoid. 7. Styloglossus. 8. Buccinator. 9. Platysma. 10. Hyoglossus. 11. Digastric. 12. Inferior longitudinal muscle. 13. Genioglossus. 14. Mylohyoid. 15. Geniohyoid. 16. Hyoglossus. 17. Palatoglossus. 18. Palatopharyngeus. 19. Superior pharyngeal constrictor (partially cut). 20. Digastric (cut). 21. Styloglossus. 22. Stylopharyngeus. 23. Stylohyoid. 24. Middle pharyngeal constrictor. 25. Digastric (cut).

Page 399 Views of the Muscles of the Palate
1. Tensor veli palatini. 2. Levator veli palatini. 3. Palatoglossus. 4. Mylohyoid. 5. Geniohyoid. 6. Hyoglossus. 7. Middle pharyngeal constrictor. 8. Stylopharyngeus. 9. Salpingopharyngeus. 10. Musculus uvulae. 11. Superior pharyngeal constrictor. 12. Palatopharyngeus.

Page 400 Views of the Muscles of the Pharynx
1. Levator veli palatini. 2. Accessory muscle bundle from temporal bone. 3. Digastric. 4. Stylohyoid. 5. Medial pterygoid.

6. Stylopharyngeus. 7. Circular esophageal muscle. 8. Longitudinal esophageal muscle. 9. Superior pharyngeal constrictor. 10. Salpingopharyngeus. 11. Palatopharyngeus. 12. Middle pharyngeal constrictor. 13. Musculus uvulae. 14. Longitudinal pharyngeal muscle. 15. Transverse and oblique arytenoids. 16. Posterior cricoarytenoid. 17. Inferior pharyngeal constrictor.

Page 401 Views of the Muscles of the Larynx
1. Transverse arytenoid. 2. Oblique arytenoid. 3. Posterior cricoarytenoid. 4. Cricothyroid. 5. Cricothyroid. 6. Transverse arytenoid. 7. Oblique arytenoid. 8. Lateral cricoarytenoid. 9. Posterior cricoarytenoid. 10. Thyroarytenoid. 11. Cricothyroid (cut).

Page 402 Views of the Muscles of the Larynx: Superior/Inferior View
1. Transverse arytenoid. 2. Oblique arytenoid. 3. Posterior cricoarytenoid.

Page 402 Views of the Muscles of the Larynx: Posterior/Anterior View
1. Posterior cricoarytenoid. 2. Transverse arytenoid. 3. Oblique arytenoid. 4. Lateral cricoarytenoid. 5. Thyroarytenoid. 6. Cricothyroid.

Page 403 Views of the Extrinsic Muscles of the Right Eye: Top Illustration
1. Levator palpebrae superioris. 2. Superior oblique. 3. Superior rectus. 4. Medial rectus. 5. Lateral rectus (cut). 6. Inferior rectus. 7. Inferior oblique.

Bottom Left Illustration
1. Superior rectus (cut). 2. Lateral rectus (cut). 3. Inferior rectus (cut). 4. Inferior oblique (cut). 5. Superior oblique (cut). 6. Medial rectus (cut).

Bottom Right Illustration
1. Superior oblique. 2. Medial rectus. 3. Inferior rectus. 4. Levator palpebrae superioris. 5. Superior rectus. 6. Lateral rectus. 7. Levator palpebrae superioris.

Page 404 Views of the Muscles of the Tympanic Cavity
1. Tensor tympani. 2. Stapedius.

CHAPTER 4 LABELING ANSWERS: THE NERVOUS SYSTEM

Page 406 Cranial Nerves
1. CN IV (trochlear nerve). 2. CN VI (adbucens nerve). 3. CN VII (facial nerve). 4. CN VIII (acoustic nerve, also known as vestibulocochlear nerve). 5. CN IX (glossopharyngeal nerve). 6. CN X (vagus nerve). 7. CN XI (spinal accessory nerve). 8. CN I (olfactory nerve). 9. CN II (optic nerve). 10. CN III (occulomotor nerve). 11. CN V (trigeminal nerve). 12. CN XII (hypoglossal nerve).

Page 407 Cross Section View of the Spinal Cord through a Cervical Vertebra—Spinal Nerve Diagram
1. Sympathetic ganglion. 2. Vertebral artery. 3. Ventral nerve root. 4. Spinal cord. 5. Dura mater. 6. Vertebral spinous process (SP). 7. Dorsal nerve root. 8. Gray ramus communicans of a spinal nerve. 9. Ventral ramus of a spinal nerve. 10. Dorsal ramus of a spinal nerve. 11. Dorsal root ganglion.

Page 408 View of the Cervical Plexus
1. Lesser occipital nerve. 2. to the vagus nerve. 3. Greater auricular nerve. 4. to sternocleidomastoid. 5. to levator scapulae. 6. Transverse cutaneous nerve of the neck. 7. to trapezius. 8. to levator scapulae. 9. to middle scalene. 10. Supraclavicular nerve. 11. to rectus lateralis. 12. to rectus capitis anterior and longus capitis. 13. to geniohyoid. 14. to longus capitis and longus colli. 15. to longus capitis, longus colli, and middle scalene. 16. to thyrohyoid. 17. Ansa cervicalis. 18. to longus colli. 19. Phrenic nerve.

Page 409 View of the Brachial Plexus
1. Dorsal scapular nerve. 2. to the phrenic nerve. 3. Suprascapular nerve. 4. Lateral pectoral nerve. 5. Axillary nerve. 6. Musculocutaneous nerve. 7. Radial nerve. 8. Median nerve. 9. Ulnar nerve. 10. Medial antebrachial cutaneous nerve. 11. Medial brachial cutaneous nerve. 12. Lower subscapular nerve. 13. Thoracodorsal nerve. 14. Nerve to scalenes. 15. Nerve to scalenes. 16. Nerve to subclavius. 17. Nerve to scalenes. 18. Long thoracic nerve. 19. Nerve to scalenes. 20. First intercostal nerve. 21. Medial pectoral nerve. 22. Upper subscapular nerve.

Page 410 View of the Lumbar Plexus
1. Iliohypogastric nerve. 2. Ilio-inguinal. 3. Genitofemoral. 4. Lateral cutaneous nerve of the thigh. 5. to psoas and iliacus (iliopsoas). 6. Femoral nerve. 7. Accessory obturator nerve. 8. Obturator nerve. 9. Lumbosacral trunk.

Page 411 View of the Sacral and Coccygeal Plexuses
1. Superior gluteal nerve. 2. Inferior gluteal nerve. 3. to piriformis. 4. to superior gemellus and obturator internus. 5. to inferior gemellus and quadratus femoris. 6. Common fibular nerve of the sciatic nerve. 7. Tibial nerve of the sciatic nerve. 8. Posterior femoral cutaneous nerve. 9. Perforating cutaneous nerve. 10. Pelvic splanchnic nerves. 11. Pudendal nerve. 12. to levator ani, coccygeous, and external anal sphincter. 13. Anococcygeal nerves. 14. Visceral branches. 15. Visceral branches.

Page 412 Views of Innervation to the Right Lower Extremity
1. Femoral nerve. 2. Common fibular nerve of the sciatic nerve. 3. Superficial fibular nerve. 4. Obturator nerve. 5. Deep fibular nerve. 6. Sciatic nerve. 7. Tibial nerve of the sciatic nerve. 8. Medial plantar nerve. 9. Common fibular nerve of the sciatic nerve. 10. Superficial fibular nerve. 11. Lateral plantar nerve.

Page 413 Anterior View of Innervation to the Right Upper Extremity
1. Axillary nerve. 2. Musculocutaneous nerve. 3. Radial nerve. 4. Brachial plexus. 5. Median nerve. 6. Ulnar nerve.

CHAPTER 5 LABELING ANSWERS: THE ARTERIAL SYSTEM

Page 416 Lateral View of Arterial Supply to the Head and Neck
1. Posterior auricular artery. 2. Superficial temporal artery. 3. Occipital artery. 4. Ascending pharyngeal artery. 5. Vertebral artery. 6. Internal carotid artery. 7. Deep cervical artery. 8. Dorsal scapular artery. 9. Costocervical trunk. 10. Axillary artery. 11. Transverse facial artery. 12. Supraorbital artery. 13. Supratrochlear artery. 14. Ophthalmic artery. 15. Infraorbital artery. 16. Maxillary artery. 17. Inferior alveolar artery. 18. Facial artery. 19. Lingual artery. 20. Superior thyroid artery. 21. External carotid artery. 22. Ascending cervical artery. 23. Inferior thyroid artery. 24. Transverse cervical artery. 25. Thyrocervical trunk. 26. Common carotid artery. 27. Subclavian artery. 28. Brachiocephalic trunk. 29. Internal thoracic artery.

Page 417 **Anterior View of Arterial Supply to the Trunk and Pelvis**
1. Costocervical trunk. 2. Dorsal scapular artery. 3. Thoracoacromial trunk. 4. Internal thoracic artery. 5. Anterior intercostal artery. 6. Posterior intercostal artery. 7. Musculophrenic artery. 8. Superior epigastric artery. 9. Lumbar artery. 10. Subcostal artery. 11. Iliolumbar artery. 12. Inferior epigastric artery. 13. Deep circumflex iliac artery. 14. Common carotid artery. 15. Subclavian artery. 16. Brachiocephalic trunk. 17. Axillary artery. 18. Ascending aorta. 19. Descending aorta. 20. Common iliac artery. 21. Internal iliac artery. 22. External iliac artery. 23. Median sacral artery.

Page 418 **Anterior View of Arterial Supply to the Right Lower Extremity**
1. Common iliac artery. 2. Iliolumbar artery. 3. External iliac artery. 4. Perforating branches of the deep femoral artery. 5. Popliteal artery. 6. Anterior tibial artery. 7. Lateral plantar artery. 8. Plantar arch. 9. Internal iliac artery. 10. Superior gluteal artery. 11. Inferior gluteal artery. 12. Femoral artery. 13. Obturator artery. 14. Deep femoral artery. 15. Posterior tibial artery. 16. Fibular artery. 17. Medial plantar artery. 18. Dorsalis pedis artery.

Page 419 **Anterior View of Arterial Supply to the Right Upper Extremity**
1. Suprascapular artery. 2. Thoracoacromial trunk. 3. Axillary artery. 4. Anterior circumflex humeral artery. 5. Posterior circumflex humeral artery (posterior to the humerus). 6. Brachial artery. 7. Deep brachial artery. 8. Radial artery. 9. Interosseus recurrent artery (posterior to the radius and humerus). 10. Posterior interosseus artery. 11. Deep palmar arterial arch. 12. Thyrocervical trunk. 13. Subclavian artery. 14. Dorsal scapular artery. 15. Superior thoracic artery. 16. Subscapular artery. 17. Lateral thoracic artery. 18. Thoracodorsal artery. 19. Circumflex scapular artery. 20. Ulnar artery. 21. Anterior interosseus artery. 22. Superficial palmar arterial arch.

CHAPTER 6 LABELING ANSWERS: OTHER STRUCTURES AND SYSTEMS OF THE BODY

Page 426 A Typical Cell
1. Centrosome. 2. Centrioles. 3. Smooth endoplasmic reticulum. 4. Mitochondrion. 5. Lysosome. 6. Rough endoplasmic reticulum. 7. Peroxisome. 8. Cytoskeleton. 9. Intermediate filament. 10. Microtubule. 11. Microfilament. 12. Nuclear envelope. 13. Ribosomes. 14. Mitochondrion. 15. Smooth endoplasmic reticulum. 16. Cilia. 17. Free ribosomes. 18. Golgi apparatus. 19. Microvilli. 20. Vesicle. 21. Nucleolus. 22. Nucleus.

Page 426 Major Components of a Cell
1. Cell membrane. 2. Cytoplasm. 3. Nucleus. 4. Organelles.

Page 426 The Cytoskeleton
1. Intermediate filament. 2. Endoplasmic reticulum. 3. Ribosome. 4. Microtubule. 5. Mitochondrion. 6. Microfilament. 7. Plasma membrane.

Page 427 The Cell Membrane
1. External membrane surface. 2. Phospholipid bilayer. 3. Internal membrane surface. 4. Carbohydrate chains. 5. Glycolipid. 6. Polar region of phospholipid. 7. Nonpolar region of phospholipid. 8. Protein. 9. Glycoprotein. 10. Cholesterol. 11. Membrane channel protein.

Page 427 The Endoplasmic Reticulum and Golgi Apparatus
1. Ribosomes. 2. Proteins. 3. Vesicle. 4. Cytoplasm. 5. Endoplasmic reticulum. 6. Cisternae. 7. Golgi apparatus. 8. Plasma membrane. 9. Secretory vesicle. 10. Vesicle containing plasma membrane components.

Page 427 Cross Section of a Mitochondrion
1. Outer membrane. 2. Inner membrane. 3. Matrix. 4. Cristae.

Page 427 Cross Section of the Nucleus
1. Nucleolus. 2. Nuclear pores. 3. Chromatin. 4. Nucleoplasm. 5. Nuclear envelope.

Page 428 Longitudinal Section of a Long Bone
1. Proximal epiphysis. 2. Diaphysis. 3. Distal epiphysis. 4. Articular cartilage. 5. Spongy bone. 6. Epiphyseal plate. 7. Red marrow cavities. 8. Compact bone. 9. Medullary cavity. 10. Endosteum. 11. Yellow marrow. 12. Periosteum.

Page 428 A. Section of a Flat Bone
1. Compact bone. 2. Spongy bone.

Page 428 B. Magnification of Spongy Bone Tissue
1. Trabeculae.

Page 429 Longitudinal Section of a Long Bone and Magnification of Compact Bone Tissue
1. Osteonic canal. 2. Osteon. 3. Periosteum. 4. Blood vessels and nerve in osteonic canal. 5. Volkmann's canal. 6. Compact bone. 7. Spongy bone. 8. Nerve. 9. Blood vessel. 10. Canaliculus. 11. Osteocyte. 12. Nerve. 13. Blood vessel. 14. Endosteum. 15. Compact bone. 16. Osteon.

Page 430 Structure of a Muscle
1. Tendon. 2. Muscle (fibrous fascia). 3. Axon of motor neuron. 4. Fascicle. 5. Blood vessel. 6. Muscle fibers. 7. Muscle fiber. 8. Myofibrils. 9. Filaments. 10. Myofibril. 11. Sarcoplasmic reticulum. 12. Nucleus. 13. Sarcolemma. 14. Endomysium. 15. Perimysium. 16. Perimysium. 17. Epimysium. 18. Bone.

Page 431 Structure of a Muscle Illustrating a Sarcomere
1. Actin filaments. 2. Myosin filament. 3. Myosin head. 4. Z-line. 5. M-line. 6. H-band. 7. A-band. 8. I-band. 9. Striations of skeletal muscle tissue. 10. Nuclei. 11. Muscle fiber. 12. Z-line. 13. Sarcomere. 14. Myofibril. 15. M-line.

Page 431 Sarcoplasmic Reticulum and T Tubules of a Muscle Fiber
1. Motor neuron fiber. 2. T tubule. 3. Synapse. 4. T tubule. 5. Sarcoplasmic reticulum. 6. Neurotransmitters in synapse. 7. Motor endplate. 8. Myofibrils. 9. Nucleus. 10. Sarcolemma.

Page 432 Myosin and Actin Filaments – Top
1. Actin subunits. 2. Actin filament. 3. Actin molecules. 4. Troponin. 5. Tropomyosin.

Page 432 Myosin and Actin Filaments – Bottom Left
1. Titin. 2. Actin filament. 3. Myosin filament.

Page 432 Myosin and Actin Filaments – Bottom Right
1. Titin. 2. Actin filament. 3. Myosin filament.

ANSWER KEY

Page 433 Sliding Filament Action – Top
1. Actin filaments. 2. Troponin. 3. Tropomyosin. 4. Myosin heads. 5. Myosin filament.

Page 433 Neuromuscular Junction
1. Motor neuron fiber. 2. Muscle fiber nucleus. 3. Myofibril of muscle fiber. 4. Mitochondria. 5. Synaptic vesicles. 6. Synapse (synaptic cleft). 7. Neurotransmitters. 8. Motor end plate.

Page 434 Structure of a Neuron
1. Dendrites. 2. Cell body. 3. Nucleus. 4. Axon hillock. 5. Node of Ranvier. 6. Myelin sheath. 7. Axon. 8. Synapses with another neuron. 9. Collateral branch. 10. Synapses with muscle fibers. 11. Nucleus of Schwann cell.

Page 434 Types of Neuroglial Cells
1. Capillary. 2. Astrocytes. 3. Microglial cell. 4. Cilia. 5. Ependymal cells. 6. Oligodendrocyte. 7. Nerve fiber. 8. Myelin sheath. 9. Schwann cell.

Page 435 Central and Peripheral Nervous Systems
1. Cerebrum. 2. Brainstem. 3. Cerebellum. 4. Medulla oblongata. 5. Spinal cord. 6. Nerve. 7. Dorsal root ganglion. 8. Afferent nerve. 9. Efferent nerve to muscle. 10. Action potential (impulse propagation). 11. Muscle fibers. 12. Muscle fiber. 13. Neurotransmitters.

Page 435 Myelinated Axon of the Peripheral Nervous System
1. Node of Ranvier. 2. Neurolemma (sheath of Schwann cell). 3. Nucleus of Schwann cell. 4. Myelin sheath. 5. Plasma membrane of axon. 6. Neurofibrils.

Page 435 Convergence of Neurons
1. Cell body of postsynaptic neuron. 2. Axon of postsynaptic neuron. 3. Axon of presynaptic neuron.

Page 435 Divergence of Neurons
1. Axon of presynaptic neuron. 2. Cell body of postsynaptic neuron. 3. Axon of postsynaptic neuron.

Page 436 Three Types of Fibrous Joints
1. Bone. 2. Fibrous tissue. 3. Radius. 4. Ulna. 5. Interosseus membrane. 6. Parietal bone. 7. Frontal bone. 8. Coronal suture. 9. Coronal suture. 10. Periodontal ligament. 11. Root (of tooth).

Page 436 Two Types of Cartilaginous Joints
1. Ribs. 2. Costal cartilages. 3. Sternum. 4. Sternocostal joint. 5. Growth plate. 6. Bone. 7. Symphysis pubis. 8. Intervertebral disc.

Page 437 Structure of a Typical Synovial Joint
1. Bone. 2. Periosteum. 3. Blood vessel. 4. Nerve. 5. Articular cartilage. 6. Joint cavity. 7. Fibrous joint capsule. 8. Articular cartilage. 9. Synovial membrane.

Page 437 Various Types of Synovial Joints
1. Pivot joint (uniaxial). 2. Hinge joint (uniaxial). 3. Condyloid joint (biaxial). 4. Saddle joint (biaxial). 5. Ball and socket joint (triaxial). 6. Gliding joint (nonaxial).

Page 438 Diagram of the Skin
1. Hair shaft. 2. Stratum corneum. 3. Stratum granulosum. 4. Stratum germinativum. 4a. Stratum spinosum. 4b. Stratum basale. 5. Dermal papilla. 6. Tactile (Meissner) corpuscle. 7. Sebaceous (oil) gland. 8. Hair follicle. 9. Papilla of hair. 10. Cutaneous nerve. 11. Openings of sweat ducts. 12. Epidermis. 13. Dermis. 14. Subcutaneous layer (hypodermis). 15. Sweat gland. 16. Artery. 17. Vein. 18. Arrector pili muscle. 19. Pacinian corpuscle (joint receptor).

Page 438 Glands of the Skin
1. Epidermis. 2. Dermis. 3. Subcutaneous layer (hypodermis). 4. Hair follicle. 5. Sebaceous (oil) gland. 6. Eccrine sweat gland (in subcutaneous tissue). 7. Apocrine sweat gland (in dermis).

Page 439 Hair Follicle

Left Illustration
1. Dermal root sheath. 2. External epithelial root sheath. 3. Internal epithelial root sheath. 4. Germinal matrix. 5. Papilla. 6. Artery. 7. Vein. 8. Hair shaft. 9. Medulla. 10. Cortex. 11. Cuticle. 12. Hair root. 13. Arrector pili muscle. 14. Sebaceous (oil) gland. 15. Hair bulb. 16. Fat.

Right Illustration
1. Germinal matrix (growth zone). 2. Papilla. 3. Hair follicle. 3a. Medulla. 3b. Cortex. 3c. Cuticle. 4. Hair follicle wall. 4a. Dermal root sheath. 4b. External epithelial root sheath. 4c. Internal epithelial root sheath. 5. Melanocyte. 6. Stratum basale. 7. Basement membrane.

Page 439 Structure of a Nail
1. Free edge. 2. Nail body. 3. Lunula. 4. Cuticle. 5. Nail root. 6. Stratum germinativum. 7. Stratum granulosum. 8. Stratum corneum. 9. Nail body. 10. Cuticle. 11. Nail root. 12. Nail matrix. 13. Nail bed.

Page 440 Anterior View of the Heart
1. Superior vena cava. 2. Pulmonary trunk. 3. Right pulmonary veins. 4. Auricle of right atrium. 5. Right coronary artery. 6. Right cardiac vein. 7. Right ventricle. 8. Aorta. 9. Auricle of left atrium. 10. Left pulmonary veins. 11. Great cardiac vein. 12. Anterior interventricular branch of left coronary artery. 13. Left ventricle. 14. Apex.

Page 440 Posterior View of the Heart
1. Left pulmonary artery. 2. Left pulmonary veins. 3. Auricle of left atrium. 4. Left atrium. 5. Great cardiac vein. 6. Posterior artery of left ventricle. 7. Left ventricle. 8. Apex. 9. Aorta. 10. Superior vena cava. 11. Right pulmonary artery. 12. Right pulmonary veins. 13. Right atrium. 14. Inferior vena cava. 15. Coronary sinus. 16. Posterior interventricular branch of right coronary artery. 17. Middle cardiac vein. 18. Right ventricle.

Page 441 Anterior View of the Interior Heart
1. Superior vena cava. 2. Right pulmonary arteries. 3. Pulmonic valve. 4. Right pulmonary veins. 5. Right atrium. 6. Tricuspid (AV) valve. 7. Right ventricle. 8. Inferior vena cava. 9. Trabeculae carneae. 10. Aorta (thoracic). 11. Aorta (arch). 12. Pulmonary trunk. 13. Left pulmonary arteries. 14. Cut edge of pericardium. 15. Left pulmonary veins. 16. Left atrium. 17. Aortic valve. 18. Mitral (left AV) valve. 19. Chordae tendineae. 20. Papillary muscle. 21. Left ventricle. 22. Interventricular septum.

Page 441 Systemic and Pulmonic Circulations of the Heart
1. Systemic capillaries. 2. Right lung. 3. Left lung. 4. Systemic capillaries. 5. Pulmonary capillaries. 6. Pulmonary capillaries.

Page 442 Major Veins of the Body
1. Right internal jugular. 2. Right external jugular. 3. Right brachiocephalic. 4. Axillary. 5. Cephalic. 6. Basilic. 7. Brachial. 8. Median cubital. 9. Ulnar. 10. Radial. 11. Popliteal. 12. Small saphenous. 13. Anterior tibial. 14. Fibular. 15. Posterior tibial. 16. Left external jugular. 17. Left internal jugular. 18. Vertebral. 19. Subclavian. 20. Left brachiocephalic. 21. Superior vena cava. 22. Inferior vena cava. 23. Hepatic. 24. Splenic. 25. Hepatic portal. 26. Renal. 27. Inferior mesenteric. 28. Superior mesenteric. 29. Gonadal. 30. Common iliac. 31. Internal iliac. 32. External iliac. 33. Femoral. 34. Great saphenous.

Page 443 Venous Drainage of the Brain
1. Straight sinus. 2. Transverse sinus. 3. Occipital sinus. 4. Sigmoid sinus. 5. Superior petrosal sinus. 6. Inferior petrosal sinus. 7. Internal jugular vein. 8. Superior sagittal sinus. 9. Inferior sagittal sinus. 10. Cavernous sinus. 11. Ophthalmic veins. 12. Facial vein.

Page 443 Creation of Venous Blood Flow From Capillaries
1. Artery. 2. Arterioles. 3. Capillaries. 4. Venules. 5. Vein.

Page 443 Unidirectional Venous Valves
1. Normal vein/normal (unidirectional) valve. 2. Varicose vein/incompetent (leaky) valve.

Page 444 Major Organs of the Lymphatic System
1. Right lymphatic duct draining into right subclavian vein. 2. Axillary nodes. 3. Cisterna chyli. 4. Inguinal nodes. 5. Palatine tonsils. 6. Cervical nodes. 7. Thoracic duct draining into left subclavian vein. 8. Thymus. 9. Thoracic duct. 10. Spleen. 11. Area drained by right lymphatic duct. 12. Area drained by thoracic duct.

Page 444 Role of Lymphatic Capillary in Draining Intercellular Fluid
1. Arteriole (from the heart). 2. Intercellular fluid. 3. Blood capillary. 4. Lymphatic capillary. 5. Venule (to the heart). 6. Tissue cells. 7. Lymph fluid (to veins).

Page 444 Lymphatic Capillary Structure
1. Overlapping endothelial cells. 2. Fluid entering lymphatic capillary. 3. Direction of flow. 4. Valve closed. 5. Valve open. 6. Anchoring fibers.

Page 445 Lymph Node Structure
1. Capsule. 2. Medullary cords. 3. Medullary sinus. 4. Hilus. 5. Afferent lymph vessels. 6. Lymph. 7. Sinuses. 8. Germinal center. 9. Cortical nodules. 10. Trabeculae. 11. Efferent lymph vessel. 12. Venules. 13. Arteriole.

Page 445 Role of a Lymph Node in a Skin Infection
1. Site of infection. 2. Afferent lymph vessel. 3. Lymph node. 4. Efferent lymph vessel. 5. Venule. 6. Arteriole.

Page 446 Structures of the Respiratory System
Upper tract
1. Nasal cavity. 2. Pharynx. 3. Larynx.

Lower tract
4. Trachea. 5. Primary bronchus. 6. Lung. 7. Bronchiole. 8. Pulmonary vein. 9. Pulmonary artery. 10. Alveolar duct. 11. Alveolus.

Page 447 Lobes of the Lungs
1. Right upper lobe. 2. Major (oblique) fissure. 3. Horizontal (minor) fissure. 4. Right middle lobe. 5. Right lower lobe. 6. Left upper lobe. 7. Lingula. 8. Oblique fissure. 9. Left lower lobe.

Page 447 Bronchi of the Lungs
1. Trachea. 2. Right primary bronchus. 3. Left primary bronchus. 4. Segmental bronchi. 5. Lobar bronchi.

Page 447 Bronchiole and Alveoli
1. Bronchiole. 2. Pleura. 3. Alveolus.

Page 448 Anterior View of the Structures of the Urinary System
1. Kidney. 2. Aorta. 3. Ureter. 4. Bladder. 5. Urethra. 6. Inferior vena cava.

Page 449 Right Lateral View of the Bladder and Urethra of a Male
1. Pubis. 2. Penile urethra. 3. Penis. 4. Bladder. 5. Prostate. 6. Prostatic urethra. 7. Membranous urethra. 8. Scrotum. 9. Navicular fossa.

Page 449 Section Through a Kidney
1. Cortical arteries and veins. 2. Interlobar arteries and veins. 3. Segmental arteries and veins. 4. Renal artery. 5. Renal vein. 6. Ureter. 7. Lobar arteries and veins. 8. Renal pyramid. 9. Arcuate arteries and veins.

Page 449 Structures of a Nephron
1. Efferent arteriole. 2. Distal convoluted tubule. 3. Collecting tubule. 4. Papilla of pyramid. 5. Afferent arteriole. 6. Proximal convoluted tubule. 7. Glomerulus. 8. Descending limb of loop of Henle. 9. Ascending limb of loop of Henle. 10. Loop of Henle.

Page 450 Structures of the Gastrointestinal System
1. Oral cavity. 2. Salivary glands. 3. Liver. 4. Gall bladder. 5. Duodenum (small intestine). 6. Hepatic flexure (large intestine). 7. Ascending colon (large intestine). 8. Ileum (small intestine). 9. Cecum (large intestine). 10. Appendix. 11. Palate. 12. Uvula. 13. Pharynx. 14. Tongue. 15. Esophagus. 16. Common bile duct. 17. Stomach. 18. Splenic flexure (large intestine). 19. Pancreas. 20. Transverse colon (large intestine). 21. Jejunum (small intestine). 22. Descending colon (large intestine). 23. Sigmoid colon (large intestine). 24. Rectum (large intestine). 25. Anus.

Page 451 Accessory Organs of the Gastrointestinal System
1. Corpus (body) of gall bladder. 2. Neck of gall bladder. 3. Cystic duct. 4. Liver. 5. Lesser duodenal papilla. 6. Greater duodenal papilla. 7. Duodenum. 8. Sphincter muscles. 9. Right and left hepatic ducts. 10. Common hepatic duct. 11. Common bile duct. 12. Pancreas. 13. Pancreatic duct. 14. Superior mesenteric vein. 15. Superior mesenteric artery.

Page 451 Divisions of the Large Intestine
1. Hepatic flexure. 2. Ascending colon. 3. Cecum. 4. Appendix. 5. Anal canal. 6. Transverse colon. 7. Splenic flexure. 8. Descending colon. 9. Terminal ileum. 10. Sigmoid colon. 11. Rectum.

Page 451 Section Through the Abdominopelvic Cavity
1. Diaphragm. 2. Liver. 3. Stomach. 4. Transverse colon. 5. Greater omentum. 6. Mesentery of small intestine. 7. Small intestine. 8. Uterus. 9. Urinary bladder. 10. Symphysis pubis. 11. Lesser omentum. 12. Pancreas. 13. Duodenum. 14. Retroperitoneal space. 15. Sigmoid colon. 16. Rectum.

Page 452 Organization of the Immune System
1. Bronchial-associated lymphoid tissues. 2. Thymus. 3. Spleen. 4. Liver. 5. Gut-associated lymphoid tissues. 6. Appendix. 7. Tonsils. 8. Lymph nodes (cervical, thoracic, and axillary). 9. Lymph nodes (inguinal).

ANSWER KEY

Page 452 Creation of B Cells and T Cells by the Bone Marrow
1. T cell. 2. Red bone marrow. 3. Thymus. 4. Lymph node. 5. B cell. 6. T cell.

Page 452 Activation and Effects of T Cells
1. Antigen. 2. T cell activated. 3. Cytotoxic T cells. 4. T memory cells. 5. Target cell. 6. Cytotoxic T cell. 7. Lysis.

Page 453 Actions of Antibodies
1. Inactivates antigen. 2. Binds antigens together. 3. Facilitates phagocytosis. 4. Antigen. 5. Antibody. 6. Phagocytic body cell. 7. Mast cell. 8. Activates complement cascade. 9. Initiates release of inflammatory chemicals.

Page 453 Action of Antibody-Activated Complement and Death of Bacterial Cell
1. Complement. 2. Bacterial cell.

Page 453 Types of Antibodies (Immunoglobulins)
1. IgM. 2. IgG. 3. IgA. 4. IgE. 5. IgD.

Page 454 The Major Endocrine Glands of the Body
1. Pineal. 2. Parathyroids (on posterior surface of thyroid gland). 3. Testes (male). 4. Hypothalamus. 5. Pituitary. 6. Thyroid. 7. Thymus. 8. Adrenals. 9. Pancreas. 10. Ovaries (female).

Page 454 The Thyroid Gland
1. Thyroid cartilage. 2. Right lobe. 3. Isthmus. 4. Left lobe. 5. Trachea.

Page 454 The Adrenal Gland
1. Adrenal gland. 2. Kidney. 3. Adrenal cortex. 4. Adrenal medulla.

Page 455 The Hypothalamus and Pituitary Hormones
1. Hypothalamic nerve cell. 2. Bone. 3. Growth hormone (GH). 4. Anterior pituitary. 5. Adrenal cortex. 6. Adrenocorticotropic hormone (ACTH). 7. Thyroid gland. 8. Thyroid-stimulating hormone (TSH). 9. Gonadotropic hormones (FSH and LH). 10. Testis. 11. Ovary. 12. Prolactin (PRL). 13. Posterior pituitary. 14. Antidiuretic hormone (ADH). 15. Kidney tubules. 16. Oxytocin (OT). 17. Uterus smooth muscle. 18. Mammary glands. 19. Mammary glands.

Page 455 The Pancreas
1. Duodenum. 2. Common bile duct. 3. Head of pancreas. 4. Pancreatic duct. 5. Tail of pancreas.

Page 456 Somatic and Stretch Receptors
1. Free nerve endings. 2. Krause's end bulb. 3. Pacinian corpuscle. 4. Merkel endings (Merkel's disc). 5. Meissner's corpuscle. 6. Ruffini's corpuscle (Ruffini ending). 7. Tendon. 8. Muscle fibers (extrafusal fibers). 9. Muscle spindle fibers (intrafusal fibers). 9a. Nuclear bag fibers. 9b. Nuclear chain fibers. 10. Neuromuscular spindle. 11. Type Ib sensory fiber. 12. Golgi tendon organ. 13. Capsule. 14. Perimysium of muscle fasciculus. 15. Gamma motor neuron. 16. Connective tissue capsule. 17. Type II sensory ending. 18. Type IA sensory endings. 19. Type II sensory ending. 20. Alpha motor neuron.

Page 456 Superior View of a Horizontal Section of the Eye
1. Fovea centralis. 2. Optic nerve. 3. Optic disc. 4. Retina. 5. Choroid. 6. Sclera. 7. Ciliary body. 8. Suspensory ligament. 9. Cornea. 10. Lens. 11. Pupil. 12. Anterior cavity (filled with aqueous humor). 13. Iris. 14. Posterior cavity (filled with vitreous humor). 15. Conjuctiva. 16. Extraocular muscles.

Page 457 External, Middle, and Internal Ear
1. External ear. 2. Middle ear cavity. 3. Inner ear. 4. Auricle (pinna). 5. Temporal bone. 6. External auditory meatus. 7. Tympanic membrane. 8. Semicircular canals. 9. Auditory ossicles. 10. Malleus. 11. Incus. 12. Stapes. 13. Oval window. 14. Facial nerve (CN VII). 15. Acoustic nerve (vestibulocochlear nerve) (CN VIII). 16. Vestibular nerve (CN VIII). 17. Cochlear nerve (CN VIII). 18. Cochlea. 19. Vestibule. 20. Round window. 21. Auditory (Eustacian) tube.

Page 458 Lateral View of the Internal Nose
1. Olfactory tract. 2. Temporal lobe – Olfactory cortex. 3. Olfactory bulb. 4. Olfactory epithelium. 5. Nasal cavity. 6. Mucous layer. 7. Cilia of receptor cell. 8. Odor molecule. 9. Cell body of olfactory neuron. 10. Supporting cells. 11. Cribiform plate of ethmoid bone.

Page 458 Dorsal Surface of the Tongue, Cross Section Through a Papilla and a Taste Bud
1. Palatine tonsil. 2. Circumvallate papillae. 3. Lingual tonsil. 4. Taste buds. 5. Gustatory cell. 6. Oral epithelium. 7. Nerve fibers. 8. Supporting cell.

Page 459 Male Reproductive Organs
1. Rectum. 2. Seminal vesicle. 3. Levator ani muscle. 4. Ejaculatory duct. 5. Anus. 6. Bulbocavernosus muscle. 7. Urinary bladder. 8. Symphysis pubis. 9. Prostate gland. 10. Corpus cavernosum. 11. Corpus spongiosum. 12. Urethra. 13. Testis. 14. Glans penis.

Page 459 Male Perineum
1. Location of symphysis pubis. 2. Urogenital triangle. 3. Anal triangle. 4. Location of ischial tuberosity. 5. Anus. 6. Location of coccyx.

Page 459 Tubules of the Testis and Epididymis
1. Nerves and blood vessels (vas afferens) in the spermatic cord. 2. Ductus (vas) deferens. 3. Epididymis. 4. Efferent ductules. 5. Seminiferous tubules. 6. Testis. 7. Rete testis. 8. Tunica albuginea. 9. Lobule. 10. Septum.

Page 460 Female Reproductive Organs
1. Sacral promontory. 2. Fallopian (uterine) tube. 3. Ureter. 4. Sacro-uterine ligament. 5. Posterior cul-de-sac (of Douglas). 6. Cervix. 7. Fornix of vagina. 8. Anus. 9. Vagina. 10. Ovarian ligament. 11. Body of uterus. 12. Fundus of uterus. 13. Round ligament. 14. Anterior cul-de-sac. 15. Parietal peritoneum. 16. Urinary bladder. 17. Symphysis pubis. 18. Uretha. 19. Clitoris. 20. Labium minora. 21. Labium majora.

Page 460 Female Perineum
1. Mons pubis (without pubic hair). 2. Prepuce. 3. Labia minora. 4. Hymen. 5. Vestibule. 6. Labia majora (without pubic hair). 7. Perineal body. 8. Anus. 9. Clitoris. 10. Orifice of urethra. 11. Orifice of vagina. 12. Opening of greater vestibular gland. 13. Urogenital triangle. 14. Anal triangle.

Page 460 Anterior View of Female Reproductive Organs
1. Fundus. 2. Corpus. 3. Fimbriae. 4. Ovary. 5. Uterus. 6. Bartholin's gland. 7. Fallopian (uterine) tube. 8. Ovum. 9. Graafian follicle. 10. Perimetrium. 11. Endometrium. 12. Myometrium. 13. Cervix. 14. Vagina.

Illustration Credits

Chapter 6 illustrations are modified from the following titles:

Fehrenbach MJ, editor: *Dental anatomy coloring book*, St. Louis, 2008, Saunders: Pages 434 (top figure), 435 (top left figure), 441 (top figure), 442, 444 (top left figure), 446, 448, 450, 455 (bottom figure), 458 (bottom figure).

LaFleur Brooks M: *Exploring medical language: a student-directed approach*, St. Louis, 2002, Mosby: Pages 426 (bottom left figure), 443 (middle figure), 447 (bottom left figure), 451 (bottom left figure), 454 (right figures), 456 (bottom figure), 460 (bottom right figure).

Mathers LH, Chase RA, John Gosling, et al: *Clinical anatomy principles*, St. Louis, 1995, Mosby: Pages 447 (top and bottom right figures), 449 (top left figure).

Patton KT, Thibodeau GA: *The human body in health and disease,* ed. 6, St. Louis, 2014, Mosby: Pages 427 (top right figure), 428 (left figure), 434 (middle row left and center figures, bottom left figure), 435 (top right figure), 436 (all figures except the top left), 437, 439 (top left figure), 443 (bottom figure), 445, 453 (top and bottom left figures), 455 (top figure), 456 (top left figure), 457, 459 (bottom right figure), 460 (top and bottom left figures).

Thibodeau GA, Patton KT: *Anatomy & physiology*, ed. 5, St. Louis, 2003, Mosby: Pages 438, 439 (top right figure), 440 (top figure), 443 (top figure), 444 (right figure), 451 (top and bottom right figures), 458 (top figures), 459 (top figure).

Thompson JM et al: *Mosby's clinical nursing*, ed. 4, St. Louis, 1997, Mosby: Page 452 (top figure).